P9-APK-029

SLEEP APNEA SYNDROMES

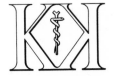

THE KROC FOUNDATION SERIES

Volumes in the Series published by Alan R. Liss, Inc.

Volume 10: Propranolol and Schizophrenia
Eugene Roberts and Peter Amacher, *Editors*

Volume 11: Sleep Apnea Syndromes
Christian Guilleminault and William C Dement, *Editors*

Kroc Foundation Series
Volume 11

SLEEP APNEA SYNDROMES

Editors

Christian Guilleminault, MD
Maître de Recherche
Institut National de la Santé
et Recherche Médicale, and
Sleep Disorders Clinic and Research Center
Stanford University School of Medicine
Stanford, California

William C Dement, MD, PhD
Professor of Psychiatry
Sleep Disorders Clinic and Research Center
Stanford University School of Medicine
Stanford, California

ALAN R. LISS, INC. • NEW YORK • 1978

Address all inquiries to the publisher:

Alan R. Liss, Inc.
150 Fifth Avenue
New York, New York 10011

Printed in the United States of America.

Library of Congress Cataloging in Publication Data

Main Entry Under Title:

Sleep apnea syndromes.

(Kroc Foundation series; v. 11)
Includes the proceedings of a conference sponsored by the Kroc Foundation, held July 1977 in Santa Ynez, Calif.
Includes bibliographical references and index.
1. Sleep apnea syndromes — Congresses. I. Guilleminault, Christian. II. Dement, William Charles, 1928—
III. Kroc Foundation. IV. Series: Kroc Foundation.
Kroc Foundation series; v. 11.
RC737.5.S54   616.2   78-416
ISBN 0-8451-0301-6

This monograph includes the proceedings of a conference
sponsored by the Kroc Foundation, held in July 1977, at
its headquarters in the Santa Ynez Valley, California.

Contents

THE OBSTRUCTION: WHERE IS IT LOCATED?

SPECIFIC SYNDROMES OF SLEEP APNEA

HORMONAL SECRETION IN THE SLEEP APNEA SYNDROME

THERAPEUTIC APPROACHES

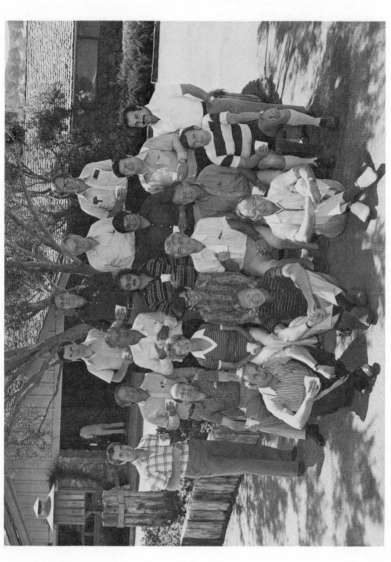

Front L to R: David Read, Peter Amacher, Robert L Kroc
2nd Row: Giorgio Coccagna, Mary Smith, Christian Guilleminault, William C Dement, John Schroeder, David Henderson-Smart
3rd Row: Daniel Kurtz, John V Weil, Elio Lugaresi, Michael Hill, Abbott J Krieger, Ronald Harper, Ara Tilkian
4th Row: Eliot Phillipson, Elliot D Weitzman, William WL Glenn, John W Severinghaus

Participants and Contributors

A Michael Anch, Department of Medicine, University of Texas Medical Branch, Galveston, Texas 77550

Suzanne Austin, Sleep Disorders Clinic and Research Center, Stanford University School of Medicine, Stanford, and Institute for Medical Research, San Jose, California 95128

Bernard Borowiecki, Sleep-Wake Disorders Unit, Department of Neurology, Montefiore Hospital and Medical Center, Bronx, New York, 10467

Jonathan G Briskin, Division of Cardiology, Stanford University School of Medicine, Stanford, California 94305

Bernard Burack, Sleep-Wake Disorders Unit, Department of Neurology, Montefiore Hospital and Medical Center, Bronx, New York 10467

Fabio Cirignotta, Clinica delle Malattie Nervose e Mentali dell'Università di Bologna, Bologna, Italy

Stephen C Coburn, Sleep Disorders Clinic and Research Center, Stanford University School of Medicine, Stanford, California 94305

Giorgio Coccagna, Clinica delle Malattie Nervose e Mentali dell'Università di Bologna, Bologna, Italy

Joseph Cummiskey, Division of Respiratory Medicine, Stanford University School of Medicine, Stanford, California 94305

William J deGroot, Department of Medicine, University of Texas Medical Branch, Galveston, Texas 77550

William C Dement, Sleep Disorders Clinic and Research Center, Stanford University School of Medicine, Stanford, California 94305

Wayne H Flagg, Sleep Disorders Clinic and Research Center, Stanford University School of Medicine, Stanford, California 94305

William WL Glenn, Department of Surgery, Yale University School of Medicine, New Haven, Connecticut 06510

Christian Guilleminault, Institut National de la Santé et Recherche Médicale and Sleep Disorders Clinic and Research Center, Stanford University School of Medicine, Stanford, California 94305

Ronald M Harper, Department of Anatomy, University of California Medical Center, Los Angeles, California 90024

David J Henderson-Smart, Department of Physiology, University of Sydney, and Department of Perinatal Medicine, King George V Memorial Hospital, New South Wales, Australia

Michael W Hill, Division of Otolaryngology, Stanford University School of Medicine, Stanford, California 94305

Abbott J Krieger, Section of Neurological Surgery, New Jersey Medical School, Newark, New Jersey and Veterans Administration Hospital, East Orange, New Jersey 07019

Jean Krieger, Service d'Exploration Fonctionnelle du Système Nerveux, Hôpital Civil, Strasbourg, France

Meir H Kryger, Cardiovascular Pulmonary Research Laboratory and Division of Pulmonary Sciences, Department of Medicine, University of Colorado Medical Center, Denver, Colorado 80220

Daniel Kurtz, Service d'Exploration Fonctionnelle du Système Nerveux, Hôpital Civil, Strasbourg, France

Kenneth L Lehrman, Division of Cardiology, Stanford University School of Medicine, Stanford, California 94305

Elio Lugaresi, Clinica delle Malattie Nervose e Mentali dell'Università di Bologna, Bologna, Italy

Patricia Lynne-Davies, Division of Respiratory Medicine, Veterans Administration Hospital, Palo Alto, California 94304

Laughton E Miles, Sleep Disorders Clinic and Research Center, Stanford University School of Medicine, Stanford, and the Institute for Medical Research, San Jose, California 95128

Merrill M Mitler, Sleep Disorders Clinic and Research Center, Stanford University School of Medicine, Stanford, California 94305

Jorge Motta, Division of Cardiology, Stanford University School of Medicine, Stanford, California 94305

John Orem, Department of Physiology, Texas Tech University School of Medicine, Lubbock, Texas 79409

Eliot A Phillipson, Department of Medicine, University of Toronto, Toronto, Ontario, Canada

Charles P Pollak, Sleep-Wake Disorders Unit, Department of Neurology, Montefiore Hospital and Medical Center, Bronx, New York 10467

Saul Rakoff, Sleep-Wake Disorders Unit, Department of Neurology, Montefiore Hospital and Medical Center, Bronx, New York 10467

David JC Read, Department of Physiology, University of Sydney, New South Wales, Australia

John E Remmers, Department of Medicine, University of Texas Medical Branch, Galveston, Texas 77550

Eberhardt K Sauerland, Department of Anatomy, University of Texas Medical Branch, Galveston, Texas 77550

John S Schroeder, Division of Cardiology, Stanford University School of Medicine, Stanford, California 94305

Charles H Scoggin, Cardiovascular Pulmonary Research Laboratory and Department of Medicine, University of Colorado Medical Center, Denver, Colorado 80220

John W Severinghaus, Department of Anesthesiology, University of California Medical Center, San Francisco, California 94143

Robert Shprintzen, Sleep-Wake Disorders Unit, Department of Neurology, Montefiore Hospital and Medical Center, Bronx, New York 10467

F Blair Simmons, Division of Otolaryngology, Stanford University School of Medicine, Stanford, California 94305

Colin E Sullivan, Department of Medicine, University of Toronto, Toronto, Ontario, Canada

Ara G Tilkian, Division of Cardiology, Stanford University School of Medicine, Stanford, and Division of Cardiology, University of California Medical Center, Los Angeles, California 90024

Johanna van den Hoed, Sleep Disorders Clinic and Research Center, Stanford University School of Medicine, Stanford, California 94305

John V Weil, Cardiovascular Pulmonary Research Laboratory and Division of Pulmonary Science, Department of Medicine, University of Colorado Medical Center, Denver, Colorado 80220

Elliot D Weitzman, Sleep-Wake Disorders Unit, Department of Neurology, Montefiore Hospital and Medical Center, Bronx, New York 10467

Foreword

The chapters in this book were authored in part by participants in a workshop on the sleep apnea syndromes sponsored by the Kroc Foundation and held in July 1977 at the Foundation Headquarters in the Santa Ynez Valley, California, and by other leading researchers in the field. It is our hope that this monograph will provide a multidisciplinary tool for the clinician, gather available information on the physiological and clinical aspects of respiration during sleep, suggest therapeutic possibilities, and pose questions for future research into the puzzling and intriguing sleep apnea syndromes.

The enthusiastic support of the Kroc Foundation, Dr Robert L Kroc, President, and Dr Peter Amacher, Director of Conference Programs, during the preparations for the symposium and the monograph is gratefully acknowledged. We are indebted to Mary W Smith who coordinated preparations at Stanford for the workshop and also played a major role in the organization and edition of this monograph. Technical assistance and manuscript typing were provided by Eileen M Gunther. In addition, a substantial number of the investigations reported here were carried out as part of a research program on the sleep apnea syndromes at the Sleep Disorders Clinic and the Clinical Research Center of the Stanford University Medical Center and were supported by National Institute of Neurological Diseases and Stroke grant NS 10727 and by Public Health Service Research grant RR-70 from the General Clinical Research Centers, Division of Research Resources. Specific acknowledgement of these and other support is made in each chapter.

This research would not have been possible without the cooperation and willing support of the sleep apnea patients. Many participated numerous times in repetitive research protocols not only in the hope of ameliorating their own disabling ailment but also as enlightened participants in the search for further understanding.

Finally, we acknowledge the silent but continuous support and cooperation of the nursing team of the Stanford University Clinical Research Center where a large part of the reported studies have been performed during the past four years.

1

Clinical Overview of the Sleep Apnea Syndromes

Christian Guilleminault, Johanna van den Hoed, and Merrill M Mitler

In the last six years over 150 patients presenting a sleep apnea syndrome have been seen at the Stanford Sleep Disorders Clinic. Although the nature of our clinical work-ups and the variables monitored during sleep have changed over the years as our knowledge of the syndrome has increased, the diagnosis in each case was based on at least one nocturnal polysomnogram. This diagnostic measure also permitted subdivision of patients into three major categories based on the predominant type of apnea seen during an eight-hour nocturnal polygraphic monitoring. The standard protocol included electroencephalogram (C_3/A_2 or C_4/A_1 of the International 10-20 System), chin electromyogram (EMG), and eye movement (electrooculogram) for determination of sleep stages. Respiratory effort was monitored by strain gauges (abdominal and thoracic) and respiratory airflow by thermistors (nasal and buccal). Blood oxygen saturation was measured by an ear oximeter. The electrocardiogram was also monitored systematically on all patients. Depending on the protocol (clinical or research) other variables have been monitored, including hemodynamic (pulmonary and femoral arterial pressures, cardiac output), respiratory (expired CO_2), electromyographic (intercostal, diaphragmatic, laryngeal, pharyngeal muscles), oximetric (arterial oxygen electrode, multiple blood gases), and endoesophageal values. Some patients were monitored for as along as ten successive 24-hour periods or for 24 nearly successive nocturnal periods — four nights a week for six weeks. Results of these studies will be presented in following chapters.

We have tried to obtain a clinical profile of sleep apneic patients by reviewing the charts of our many patients.

Sleep Apnea Syndromes, pages 1—12

TERMINOLOGY AND DEFINITIONS

An apnea has been defined as cessation of airflow at the level of the nostrils and mouth lasting at least ten seconds. A sleep apnea syndrome is diagnosed if, during seven hours of nocturnal sleep, at least 30 apneic episodes are observed in both rapid eye movement (REM) and non-rapid eye movement (NREM) sleep, some of which must appear repetitively in NREM sleep. Apneic episodes at sleep onset or accompanying bursts of rapid eye movement in REM periods are not considered pathological. In one study, we monitored 20 normal control subjects (between 40 and 60 years of age) over four consecutive eight-hour nocturnal sleep periods. This study disclosed a mean number of apneic episodes per night of 7 (range 1–25) in men and 2.1 (range 0–5) in women. All apneic episodes in this group were seen during REM sleep or at sleep onset. In our controls, apneic episodes were never recorded in stages 2, 3, or 4 NREM sleep.

The smallest number of apneas ever recorded in one individual considered "sleep apneic" was 45 during 245 minutes of nocturnal sleep, or 11 apneas per hour of sleep. (We feel that the use of an "Apnea Index," ie, the number of apneas per sleep-hour, frequently gives a better indication of the seriousness of the disorder). This lowest number of apneas in a patient can be compared to a maximum of four apneas per sleep-hour in one of our male controls (mean 0.5 apnea/hour).

With strain gauge and thermistor recording techniques, three types of apnea have been defined. Central apnea is characterized by cessation of both airflow and respiratory movements. In obstructive (or upper airway) apnea, airflow past nasal and buccal thermistors is absent despite persistent respiratory effort recorded by thoracic and abdominal strain gauges. Mixed apnea is defined by cessation of airflow and an absence of respiratory effort early in the episode followed by resumption of respiratory effort in the latter part of the episode that eventually reestablishes airflow.

The number of apneic episodes varied from night to night and from patient to patient. A likely factor in such variability was the amount of externally induced sleep disturbances such as equipment- or protocol-directed arousals. In any case, we have never seen marked changes in percentage of "apnea per sleep-hour" during time intervals free of external disturbance. Patients diagnosed with "sleep apnea syndrome" always presented an abnormally elevated apnea index and a similar predominant type of apnea (central, mixed, or obstructive). We have never observed only one type of apnea during a nocturnal polygraphic recording; however, a predominant type usually could be easily identified.

PATIENT POPULATIONS

Sleep apnea may be seen in patients with damaged respiratory centers in the brain, as in bulbar poliomeylitis, brain stem infarct, bilateral cordotomy, Ondine's curse syndrome, and Shy-Drager syndrome. It may also occur with drug intoxication (barbiturates and tranquilizers) and with abnormalities of the breathing apparatus, as in muscular dystrophy, kyphoscoliosis, Pierre-Robin syndrome, obstructive lung diseases, etc. Some of these entities are considered in other chapters. The 150 patients reported here did not fit into the above diagnostic categories. Forty patients presented a combination of sleep apnea syndrome and narcolepsy. We will not deal here with the relationship between these two disease entities other than to note that both of them are associated with marked disturbances of sleep. Patients with this combination will be separated from the "pure" sleep apnea syndrome patients.

Two major subcategories are distinguished, based on the predominant type of sleep-induced apnea: obstructive and central sleep apnea.

Predominantly Obstructive Sleep Apnea Patients

Fifty patients in this category have been reviewed. All of them are adults, with ages ranging between 28 and 62 years (mean age 45.5 years). Forty-eight patients are male; the two female patients were 58 and 61 years of age, respectively, at the time of referral.

Causes for referral. Thirty-nine patients, including both women, were referred for a chief complaint of excessive daytime sleepiness. One patient sought consultation because at night during sleep he gasped for breath and felt nauseated. One patient was referred because of an abnormal electrocardiographic Holter monitoring during sleep and loud snoring. One patient was referred for essential hypertension and loud snoring. In another patient, referral was instigated because of morning headaches and confusion, and loud snoring at night. In seven patients, the referral complaint came from the spouse: Patients were referred by their wives after the latter had read articles in the lay press relating abnormal behavior during sleep, observation of apnea, and loud snoring at night.

Race. Four patients were black, four were Mexican-Indian, and 42 were white.

Weight. Ten patients were of normal weight (as computed in Metropolitan Life Statistical Bulletin [1] corrected for age and height); ten patients (20%) were 5 to 15% overweight; 15 patients (30%) were 16 to 30% overweight; and 20 patients (40%) were 31 to 400% overweight. Five patients in this last group had been labeled Pickwickian (Burwell type).

Clinical symptomatology. *Loud snoring.* During sleep, all patients had noisy, pharyngeal snoring associated with snorting and interrupted by silences (apneic episodes) of 15 seconds or longer. This symptom was reported as a source of embarrassment and annoyance. Snoring was first noted during childhood in 52% of the cases and before 21 years of age in 94%.

Excessive daytime sleepiness. Thirty-nine patients (78%) complained of excessive daytime somnolence and sleep attacks. Nine patients (23%) had complained of this symptom for longer than ten years, ten patients (26%) for five to ten years, and 20 (51%) for one to five years. Specifically, the patients complained of sudden excessive drowsiness occurring at inappropriate times and producing an irresistible urge to sleep. Twenty-seven patients (54%) had had automobile accidents, and one was nearly struck by a train at a railroad crossing because of his inappropriate sleepiness. Sixteen patients (32%) had difficulties at work or were on the verge of losing their jobs because of daytime sleepiness; seven (14%) were totally unable to work and received disability assistance. Of the 11 patients who denied daytime somnolence, interviews with the families revealed that four of them frequently took naps at work, fell asleep on the couch almost daily while watching television, and often fell asleep while reading the newspaper or when riding in a car.

Excessive daytime sleepiness was accompanied by hypnagogic hallucinations in 22 patients (44%), and automatic behavior was reported by 29 patients (58%).

Intellectual deterioration. This complaint was closely related to automatic behavior. All 39 patients with daytime somnolence reported difficulty in focusing their attention and an inability to concentrate, particularly during the early afternoon hours when somnolence was at its peak. For 12 patients (24%) these problems were more troublesome in the morning hours. Two patients who did not complain of daytime somnolence experienced similar clouding of intellect and deterioration of memory and judgment in the morning. Two patients seemed so confused in the early morning that a brain tumor was suspected.

Personality changes. The families of 24 patients (48%) reported disturbing changes in the patient's personalities; eight patients (16%) had seen psychiatrists for anxiety and/or depression. The personality changes were responsible for three broken marriages in this series. Analysis of Minnesota Multiphasic Personality Inventory (MMPI) profiles in patients revealed abnormal (t scores greater than 70) elevations on at least one clinical scale in 17 patients (34%). Elevations occurred on the depression scale in 12 patients (24%) and on the anxiety scale in 13 (26%). Noticeable confusion, hostility, marked irritability, and aggressiveness were observed in nine patients.

Fourteen spouses (28%) reported dismay at outbursts of completely irrelevant behavior in patients. They reported sudden episodes of jealousy, suspicion, and irrational behavior toward their children. At times the behavior resembled a persecution reaction. These behaviors, in all cases, were totally unlike the patient's normal behavior pattern.

Sexual functioning. Twenty-one patients (42%) reported impotence. These patients noted a diminished libido and difficulty in obtaining erection and ejaculation. Nine of the 21 patients were under 46 years of age.

Nocturnal enuresis. Fifteen patients (30%) complained of intermittent enuretic episodes; four of them had sought urologic evaluations for this complaint.

Morning headaches. Eighteen patients (36%) had recurrent morning headaches that were described as frontal and occasionally diffuse. The headaches, like the nocturnal enuresis, had appeared gradually and intermittently over the years, but had usually become more noticeable during the 18 months before evaluation. Both headaches and enuresis were reported primarily by the overweight patients (88% of the patients were moderately to heavily obese).

Morning nausea. Four patients (8%) reported this symptom. It was the major complaint and cause of referral in one patient.

Abnormal motor activity during sleep. These reports were obtained from spouses and bed partners. All of these patients (100%) moved abnormally during sleep, and some had done so for as long as 34 years. This behavior was observed in every patient during the polygraphic recordings. A patient's sleep is extremely agitated during periods of repetitive apneas; there are frequent abnormal movements, either simple movements of the extremities or gross movements of the whole body. The sleeping patients often unwittingly kicked or slapped their bed partners during large movements of the arms and legs, and this, along with the heavy snoring, led to separate beds for 15 couples. Patients would also sit up abruptly during sleep, as if struggling for breath. Falling out of bed and sleepwalking episodes occurred with varying frequency (weekly to once every six months) in 27 cases (54%). Patients often bruised themselves, and in one case, a humeral fracture was sustained. During these episodes patients might talk or mumble unintelligibly. Patients could not be awakened during these episodes and often spent part of the night sleeping on the floor where they had fallen.

Neck and face. None of our patients could be considered as presenting Pierre-Robin syndrome. However, the two women (4%) fit the "bird-like face" description (see Chapter 17), and 19 men (38%) had a short neck although no obvious cervical abnormalities were detected by standard X ray.

Hypertension. Twenty-six patients (52%) were hypertensive, usually moderately (systolic range 210–150, diastolic range 120–95); ten patients were under treatment for high blood pressure. Seven patients also had pretibial and ankle edema, and five patients had enlarged livers with hepatojuglar reflux.

Neurological evaluation. None of the patients had any neurological defect during wakefulness, and EEGs performed during the daytime were within normal limits.

Nocturnal polygraphic recordings. All patients under consideration here presented a predominance of obstructive (upper airway) apnea. Thirty-seven patients had continuous apnea throughout sleep. Their mean Apnea Index (number of apneas per sleep-hour) was 78 (range 48–160). The apnea durations ranged from ten seconds (by definition) to 92 seconds; the mean was 22 seconds duration. An average of 48% of total sleep time was spent without air exchange.

These patients always presented their longest apneic episodes during REM sleep.

Three patients had repetitive apneas during NREM sleep but had normal respiration during REM sleep. Their mean Apnea Index was 65 (range 48–79).

Ten patients had intermittent apnea during both REM and NREM sleep. Their mean apnea index was 42 (range 17–90). The longest apneas in this group were seen during REM sleep in eight cases out of ten. Stages 3–4 NREM sleep, not recorded in the first two groups, were observed in nine of these ten cases and represented a mean of 3% of total sleep time (range 0–6%). Very few apneic episodes were observed during stages 3–4 NREM sleep.

Relationship between weight and polygraphic findings. Patients of normal weight had as many total apneic episodes or as high an Apnea Index as overweight patients. A comparison was made between five normal-weight patients (mean 70.5 kg) and five obese patients (mean 112 kg) who had continuous apnea during sleep. The mean apnea duration was 22 and 21.5 seconds, respectively.

The ten patients who presented intermittent apnea during both NREM and REM sleep were placed on a drastic diet. Weight loss ranged from 20 to 45 kg in five patients. After weight loss, the Apnea Index improved: The mean Apnea Index was 32 before and 14 after the diet regimen. In these patients, obstructive apnea remained the predominant type. The patient's subjective complaint of daytime sleepiness greatly lessened after weight loss and was no longer considered a problem. However, two patients stated that they still felt "overly tired" at the end of the day and still napped regularly on weekends. No objective measurements of daytime sleepiness were obtained (see Chapter 3). Spouses reported that snoring was reduced and intermittent after weight loss. One reported that the symptoms were "less disturbing and more tolerable." Runs of cyclic sinus arrhythmia were still observed in conjunction with obstructive apneas (see Chapter 12). Apneas were observed during polygraphic recording of stage 2 NREM sleep and REM sleep. The longest durations of apnea occurred during REM sleep.

Two of the three patients with apnea occurring only during NREM sleep were placed on a diet for three months (mean weight before dieting was 76 kg). Their mean weight loss was 7 kg; there were no changes in symptomatology or polygraphic variables.

All patients with continuous apnea throughout sleep were placed on a diet. Some of these patients had been dieting for as long as five years. Three patients were hospitalized and maintained on a controlled diet of 800 calories per day for at least 45 days. Each lost over 30 kg without symptomatic improvement. Our most obese patients, despite rigorous diet supervised by the spouse and reportedly followed accurately, were unable to lose more than a mean of 3.5 kg in over four months. It should be emphasized that despite progressive weight increase with age, most of the obstructive sleep apneic patients and their families stated that overeating was the exception. In fact, most of our overweight obstructive sleep apnea patients reported a continuous and increasingly difficult battle against weight gain since their late teens and had noted that their food consumption was considerably less than that of their peers.

Five grossly overweight obstructive sleep apneic patients (mean weight 115 kg) were compared to a group of five obese patients (three women and two men, mean weight 135.5 kg) who presented alveolar hypoventilation without obstructive apnea during sleep and who also complained of excessive daytime sleepiness. Polygraphic recordings revealed no statistical difference between total sleep time in the two groups. No stages 3–4 NREM sleep occurred; the mean total stage 1 NREM sleep, an index of sleep disruption, was 12% in the first group (obstructive sleep apnea) and 13.25% in the latter. Patients with alveolar hypoventilation had more notable respiratory acidosis during the daytime than sleep apneic patients. The pCO_2 in the five sleep apneic patients was always below 55 mm Hg during sleep (mean 42 mm Hg during wakefulness) in constrast to a mean pCO_2 of 58 mm Hg during sleep in the second group (with a range of 51 to 62 mm Hg during wakefulness). During sleep, oxygen saturation varied much more in sleep apneic patients than in those with alveolar hypoventilation. In the former group, arterial oxygen pressure dropped to 25 mm Hg during REM sleep in association with the longest apneas. There were also fluctuations in the partial pressure of oxygen despite the fact that the mean PaO_2 was usually under 65 mm Hg during the entire sleep period. Hypoxemia varied less in the five obese alveolar hypoventilation patients, usually oscillating between 60 and 40 mm Hg, with low values also seen during REM sleep.

In summary, obese patients with alveolar hypoventilation presented less PaO_2 variation but more severe hypercapnia. Obese sleep apneic patients had marked blood gases variation related to sleep stages and apnea, as well as greater hypoxia and less hypercapnia.

Long-term follow-up of obstructive sleep apnea patients. Twenty-three of the patients reported above have had tracheostomies with positioning of a valve. All subjective symptoms have cleared after surgery. The longest patient follow-up in this group is four years, the shortest one month (see also Chapters 12 and 24). Four other patients are now awaiting surgery. Two patients have had tonsillectomy and adenoidectomy, or submucous resection with marked improvement of symptoms. Two other patients first had similar treatment, did not experience significant subjective or objective improvement, and secondarily had a tracheostomy. Ten tracheostomized patients had previously had, or first requested, nasal repair surgery for deviated septum without improvement.

Three patients who declined surgery died during sleep within six months after diagnosis. Autopsy in two cases revealed no obvious cause of death; a cardiac factor was suspected.

Seven patients who declined surgery have had progressive worsening of their symptoms; one had myocardial infarction during sleep, and two are virtually bedridden because of cardiac failure. Three patients receive disability payments, unable to lead normal lives because of their illness. The remaining patient of these seven, after three years of hesitation, has asked for a new evaluation and is reconsidering surgery.

The ten patients who had intermittent apnea during sleep have been placed under strict diet, medroxy progesterone, and/or aminophylline, and have been regularly followed. Under such a regimen, improvement has been observed as noted above.

We have lost contact with one patient.

Predominantly Central Sleep Apnea Patients

Ten patients with predominantly central sleep apnea were reviewed. All of these patients were male; one was black and nine were white. Their ages ranged from 27 to 79 years (mean 57). They seemed to be a more heterogeneous group than the predominantly obstructive one. In fact, this group could be divided into two subcategories: group A in which over 80% of recorded apneas were central type, and group B in which 50 to 60% of apneas were central with the rest mixed and/or obstructive. Seven patients (mean age 57) were classified group A; three patients (mean age 60) were included in group B.

Six of the seven patients in group A were referred to the Sleep Disorders Clinic for the complaint of insomnia, and one for sudden awakenings at night with a choking feeling and severe shortness of breath. The three patients in group B were seen for the complaint of excessive daytime somnolence combined with awakenings at night, shortness of breath, and gasping for air. Two of these three patients had a past medical history of head trauma, with loss of consciousness, 20 to 25 years before referral.

Clinical symptomatology. *Sleep complaint.* All patients had short sleep latencies, usually falling asleep in less than three minutes, but the majority of them woke up several times during the course of the night, sometimes gasping for air or with a feeling of choking. This feeling was frequently associated with anxiety which sometimes persisted for several minutes after awakening. None of the group A patients took naps during the daytime, and, although they reported feelings of tiredness and fatigue in the morning, none related this lethargy to their sleep complaint. Group B patients, who reported awakening during sleep — an event not perceived by predominantly obstructive patients — took naps during the daytime and also complained of daytime somnolence.

Snoring. All patients presented some degree of snoring when they started to breathe again, but snoring was frequently light and intermittent.

Depression. All patients showed an elevated depression scale (t score over 70) on the MMPI. Four patients recognized suicidal ideas related to their sleep problems which may have existed as long as 25 years before referral.

Sexual functioning. Four patients reported loss of libido and difficulty having an erection; this symptom may possibly be related to the patients' depressive reaction.

Physical aspects. All group A patients were of normal weight or were underweight for age and height. Faces and necks were normal. In group B, two patients were in the 5 to 15% overweight category. One patient had a relatively short neck.

Neurological evaluation. These examinations were within normal limits in all cases despite the reported head trauma in two patients.

Polygraphic monitoring. Nine of the ten patients had intermittent apneas. The mean Apnea Index was 49 with a mean duration of 30 seconds (range 10 to 180 seconds). The longest apneic episodes were seen in association with bursts of rapid eye movements during sleep. It is unclear why some apneic episodes led to a complete behavioral awakening several times during the night, but this did not seem to be related to hypoxia or hypercapnia; similar levels may occur at other times without leading to complete arousal.

Follow-up. One group B patient who had 52% central apnea and a short neck was recorded after intubation and demonstrated considerable improvement. Central apneas decreased, and he reported a decrease in daytime sleepiness the following morning. A tracheostomy was done after this trial. Central apnea was reduced only slightly at first, but three months later a greater reduction in the number of central apneas was observed, as if some central apneas had been induced by the respiratory problem, ie, some degree of obstruction. This patient's condition was suggestive of a vicious circle characterized by obstruction of the airway inducing slight hypoxia, hypercapnia, and acidosis, further depressing the central nervous system control of breathing and inducing central apnea. This progressive decrease of central apnea with time after tracheostomy was also observed in predominantly obstructive sleep apneic patients. None of the other patients, who presented larger percentages of central apnea, was improved by intubation.

Chemotherapy was instituted which included trials with aminophylline, theophylline, and naloxone intravenously during monitoring, and medroxyprogesterone and clomipramine orally. None of these drugs had a dramatic impact. The only drug which produced some positive results in two cases was clomipramine. It was given at doses between 75 and 125 mg at bedtime for three and five years, respectively, and reduced the mean Apnea Index from 42 to 7. However, the sexual side effects (impotence) of this drug limit its usefulness.

Some Special Cases

Narcolepsy and sleep apnea. The combination of the narcolepsy-cataplexy syndrome with sleep apnea is not uncommon; the most common association is with central apnea. Narcoleptics frequently present respiratory pauses during REM sleep, more so than the control population. This is particularly obvious in women, where controls have a very low Apnea Index. But about 10% of our total narcoleptic group (20 patients) have an Apnea Index between 6 and 9, which is clearly above the normal range. These apneas are predominantly central (over 90% of recorded apnea), and the impact of these events on the sleep complaint is difficult to evaluate. The possible hemodynamics and cardiac impacts are reviewed in other chapters (see Chapters 11 and 12).

Five patients with narcolepsy had a combination of predominantly mixed and obstructive apnea. Loud snoring and abnormal nocturnal movements were noted during sleep in these patients, and moderate hypertension was present in three cases. Three patients were in the 5 to 15% overweight category (moderate obesity is frequent in narcoleptics without sleep apnea); the two remaining patients were of normal weight. One patient in this group had a tracheostomy which improved the excessive daytime sleepiness and the cardiovascular anomalies seen with repetitive apnea.

Acromegaly and sleep apnea. Two patients (one male and one female) presenting with typical acromegalic syndromes were referred for excessive daytime sleepiness. In one case the daytime somnolence was the symptom which led the patient to seek medical attention; in the other, acromegaly had previously been diagnosed. All symptoms reported above in the obstructive sleep apnea section were observed. The prognathism, macroglossia, and possible growth of hypopharynx soft tissue easily explain the development of obstructive components. As in some other cases of enlarged tonsils and adenoids and obstructive sleep apnea, we cannot yet explain the precipitating role of sleep in producing a complete obstruction ordinarily nonexistent during wakefulness.

Hodgkin disease, lymphoma, and obstructive sleep apnea. One patient with Hodgkin infiltration of the hypopharynx was also referred for excessive daytime sleepiness, loud snoring, and morning confusion. His obstructive Apnea Index was 65. This case should be related to the recent report by Zorick et al [2] of a typical obstructive sleep apneic symptomatology with lymphoma. Radiotherapy in this patient was helpful in relieving most of the symptoms.

CONCLUSION

The sleep apnea syndromes may induce life-threatening pathology (see Chapters 11 and 12) regardless of their diverse causes. Some cases of sleep apnea syndrome are related to micrognathia, acromegaly, and abnormally enlarged tonsils and adenoids, but frequently none of these is observed in our patients. Why are sleep apnea syndromes not seen in all patients with acromegaly or other reported anatomical causes? Is the syndrome in these cases overlooked by clinicians unaware of its existence and is it, in fact, more frequent than reported, or are some persons particularly susceptible to airway closure during sleep, the anatomical factors then playing only a precipitating role or enhancing a mild defect existent during sleep? When no peripheral causes of obstruction can be found, why does predominantly obstructive sleep apnea still occur? Where is the defect located? What are its causes? These are some of the questions that are considered in the following chapters.

ACKNOWLEDGMENTS

This research was supported by National Institute of Neurological Diseases and Stroke grant NS 10727, Public Health Service Research grant RR-70 from the General Clinical Research Centers, Division of Research Resources, and by INSERM to Dr. Guilleminault.

REFERENCES

1. Metropolitan Life Insurance Company: Statistical Bulletin 40: November–December, 1959.
2. Zorick R, Roth T, Kramer M, Flessa H: Intensification of excessive daytime sleepiness by lymphoma. Sleep Res 6:199, 1977.

DISCUSSION

Dr Lugaresi expressed concern about the division of sleep apnea patients into two groups (central and obstructive). He suggested that there may be a continuum during life wherein patients who are heavy snorers develop a mixed syndrome with obstructive and central apneas. Drs Guilleminault and Weitzman, however, strongly defended this division. In New York and at Stanford, a group of patients with the primary complaint of insomnia surprisingly demonstrated a major degree of recurring diaphragmatic apnea. Dr Weitzman also emphasized that in patients with clear-cut, dramatic obstructive apnea, there were no past histories or present complaints of insomnia, but there were histories of increasing sleepiness.

Dr Phillipson commented that the sleep apneic population, judging from Dr Guilleminault's presentation, appeared a heterogeneous group as far as the state of sleep in which apnea occurred, the type of problem, and more importantly, the patients' symptoms. He observed that they really seem quite different, and that the critical question then is whether the fundamental mechanisms are basically different. For example, if the drive to the neurons in the tractus solitarius is reduced, the diaphragm stops. By a movement of a few microns, the same stimuli also stimulate the upper motor neurons of the upper airway and, if they stop firing, an obstructive apnea occurs. The same withdrawal of stimuli acting less than a millimeter apart can result in diaphragmatic versus obstructive symptomatology. Whether the underlying mechanisms are fundamentally different is yet to be determined.

2
Snoring and Its Clinical Implications

Elio Lugaresi, Giorgio Coccagna, and Fabio Cirignotta

FROM SNORING TO HPA: NATURAL HISTORY OF UPPER AIRWAY OBSTRUCTION SYNDROMES

The study of a phenomenon as apparently trivial as snoring shows that patients who have what is termed "hypersomnia with periodic apneas" (HPA) have in fact been heavy snorers for years, even decades, before becoming hypersomniac. This important relationship between snoring and HPA is supported by two observations: 1) Snoring is due to an hypnogenic stenosis of the upper airway; 2) heavy snorers have been shown to have apneas and series of apneas which are identical to those which characterize HPA.

In heavy snorers slight alveolar hypoventilation may develop during sleep. Pulmonary pressure rises more than in normal subjects, and systemic arterial pressure increases, in contrast to what normally occurs [1]. The hypothesis that snoring represents the first step towards HPA is further strengthened by the fact that, after weight loss, some Pickwickian patients present only snoring without apneas.

These and other data, which cannot be presented here due to space limitations, have led us to conclude that snoring and HPA are the extremes in a series of pathophysiological events which originate with a hypnogenic stenosis of the upper airway [2]. Mechanical narrowing of the upper airways due to obesity, mandibular malformations, adenoidal and tonsillar hypertrophy, or laryngeal stenosis, and possible dynamic factors such as a particular hypotonia of the oropharyngeal muscles, favor the occurrence of snoring. If snoring is light and intermittent, there are no abnormal effects on alveolar ventilation or pulmonary and systemic circulation. However, if snoring is loud and continuous, a certain degree of alveolar hypoventilation may occur, as well as increases in pulmonary

Sleep Apnea Syndromes, pages 13–21

and systemic arterial pressures. In other words, alveolar ventilation and pulmonary and systemic arterial pressures in heavy snorers undergo variations intermediate between those occurring in normal subjects and in HPA patients (Fig 1).
With the aggravation of the respiratory disturbance the first clinical symptoms
appear: diurnal somnolence and alveolar hypoventilation during sleep. This is the
transition from simple snoring to a mild form of HPA.

If the respiratory disturbance worsens, obstructive apneas become particularly numerous and prolonged; they persist for the duration of sleep. The
pathological impact of apneas on alveolar ventilation and pulmonary and systemic arterial pressures is greatly increased. Diurnal somnolence becomes a continuous complaint. Thus, there is a transition from mild to full-blown HPA.

The disease further worsens, and, when the central depression of respiration
exceeds a certain critical level provoking alveolar hypoventilation even during
wakefulness, it leads to the appearance of cor pulmonale and polycythemia. If
the respiratory situation is not corrected at this point (through weight loss or
tracheostomy), death may occur due to respiratory or cardiac failure.

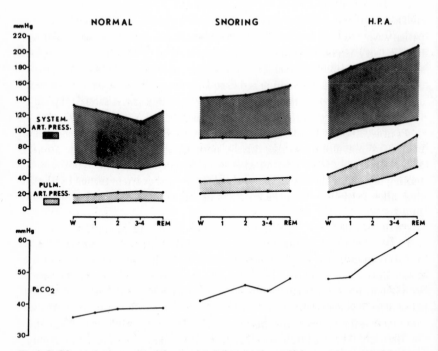

Fig 1. PaCO$_2$, pulmonary arterial pressure, and systemic arterial pressure recorded during
wakefulness and sleep in normal subjects, in heavy snorers, and in patients with HPA.

SUGGESTIONS FOR FURTHER INVESTIGATIONS INTO SNORING

Preliminary Findings Which May Contribute to the Clinical and Pathophysiological Definition of Snoring

1. We have demonstrated that snoring is linked to a hypnogenic stenosis of the upper airway. It is now important to establish whether this phenomenon is favored by particular anatomical situations. Obesity, tonsillar and adenoidal hypertrophy, and mandibular malformation certainly favor the appearance of snoring. Some authors (cf Kleitman [3]) have suggested that other anatomical situations, for example, nasal obstruction and certain conformations of the pharyngeal pillars, may lead to the development of hypnogenic stenosis of the upper airway. In some of our heavy snorers the large size of the pharyngeal pillars and the uvula visibly reduce the air space at the oropharyngeal level. Might this condition be the anatomical cause of snoring? A definitive answer can only be obtained by the study of a large group of heavy snorers.

2. In heavy snorers, incomplete obstruction of the upper airway may be present even during wakefulness (Fig 2). Figure 2 shows a polygraphic recording of an extremely obese 28-year-old subject who has been a heavy snorer since adolescence. Even during wakefulness, endoesophageal pressure oscillations reach $20-25$ cm H_2O (normally, this is no higher than 10 cm H_2O). During snoring, negative endothoracic pressure may reach $50-60$ cm H_2O. We measured inspiratory endothoracic pressure during nocturnal sleep in the same subject and, even without snoring, elevated negative endothoracic pressures were recorded.

3. In heavy snorers, obstructive apneas are facilitated by a relative drop in central input (Fig 3). Figure 3 shows typical obstructive apnea in an habitual snorer. The cessation of snoring and simultaneous apnea onset are accompanied by a marked diminution of intercostal electromyogram (EMG) activity. This is commonly found in heavy snorers. Obstructive apneas occur most often during stages $1-2$ non-rapid eye movement (NREM) and rapid eye movement (REM) sleep when periodic and irregular breathing favors the appearance of apneas. During stages $3-4$ NREM sleep, when respiration is very regular, apneas are absent or extremely rare, despite a greater obstruction of the upper airway.

4. The severity of snoring varies from one night to the next, and the reasons for this variability are, for the most part, unknown. We can state with almost absolute certainty, however, even from personal experience, that fatigue, sleep deprivation, and some hypnotics favor snoring. We do not have information as yet on psychophysiological states or drugs which lessen the tendency to snore.

Two consecutive sleep recordings in a heavy snorer are shown in Figure 4, the first night without drugs and the second after taking 30 mg of flurazepam. The "snoring index" is noted below each histogram. This is the relationship between breaths accompanied by snoring and the total number of breaths per

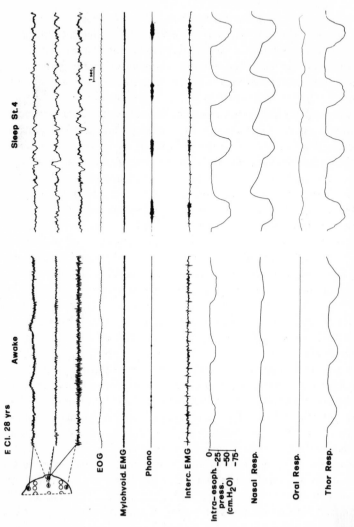

Fig 2. Polygraphic recording of a heavy snorer showing intraesophageal pressure during wakefulness and sleep (stage 4). See text for explanation.

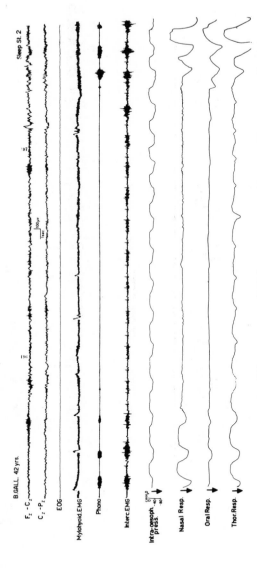

Fig 3. Polygraphic recording of an obstructive apnea in a heavy snorer.

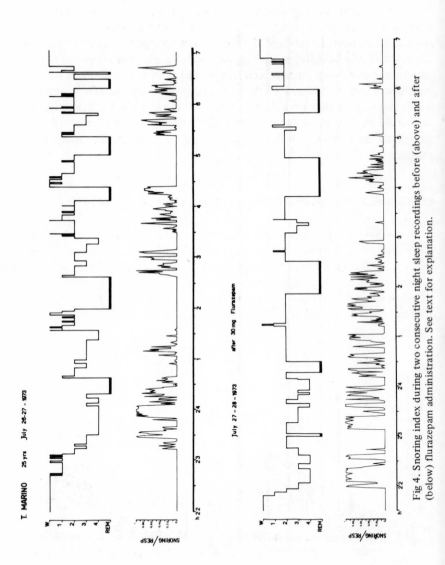

Fig 4. Snoring index during two consecutive night sleep recordings before (above) and after (below) flurazepam administration. See text for explanation.

minute. The "snoring index" is equal to 1 when all breaths are noisy, and to 0 when breathing is silent. Note that the snoring index is lower during the first night than during the second night.

We have also begun to investigate the effect of weight loss on snoring in obese subjects. For example, a young, moderately obese subject was seen for habitual snoring, which started years ago. More recently, he complained of slight daytime somnolence. After weight loss the "snoring index" actually increased but the number and duration of apneas decreased markedly. In this case obesity apparently had a greater influence on the development of apneas than on snoring.

We cannot generalize from the last two observations, especially in consideration of the extreme variability of snoring. These observations are presented only to indicate the methods which we intend to pursue in our further study of snoring.

SOME PRELIMINARY EPIDEMIOLOGICAL FINDINGS ON SNORING

The following is excerpted from epidemiological data collected for an as yet incomplete research project regarding sleep disturbances. Our study will include data on 2,000 people, but at the present time statistics are available for only 1,000 subjects. Of these, 45% state that they snore occasionally, while 25% admit to being habitual snorers. Figure 5 shows the frequency percentage of snoring in 500 males (left) and 500 females (right). Fifty-three percent of males

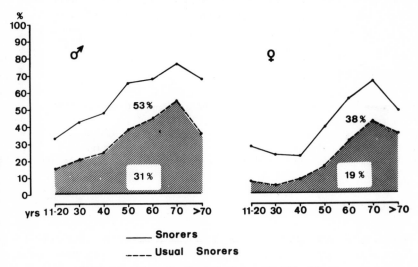

Fig 5. Age and sex distribution of snorers (1,000 subjects).

and 38% of females snore. Habitual snorers represent 31% of males and 19% of females. The frequency of snoring progressively increases in males after 20 years of age; in females, the increase occurs only after 40 years of age. After age 70, the percentage of snorers seems to decrease. We have noted that 6% of the habitual snorers complain of sudden awakenings accompanied by sensations of suffocation.

In our preliminary data obesity, hypertension, and heart disease are more common in heavy snorers than in normal subjects. Due to the relatively small number of cases examined, we cannot yet state that these data are truly significant. With regard to obesity, however, these data do seem indisputable: In our study, 7% of nonsnorers and 21% of habitual snorers are obese. Furthermore, of 122 obese subjects, 70% state that they snore.

Seven percent of nonsnorers and 14% of habitual snorers are affected with hypertension, and 90% of the latter have been heavy snorers for over ten years. This suggests that heavy and continuous snoring may favor the appearance of a hypertensive state.

CONCLUSIONS

Habitual and heavy snoring can no longer be considered merely an annoying noise. It is a definite respiratory disturbance which may have important effects on alveolar ventilation and blood circulation. Future research should be oriented towards a further understanding of the etiology and pathophysiology of snoring. Therapeutic possibilities must be investigated. It is also important to establish whether heavy snoring represents a risk factor for cardiovascular disease.

REFERENCES

1. Lugaresi E, Coccagna G, Farneti P, Mantovani M, Cirignotta F: Snoring. Electroencephalogr Clin Neurophysiol 39:59–64, 1975.
2. Lugaresi E, Coccagna G, Mantovani M: Hypersomnia with periodic apneas. In Weitzman E (ed): "Advances in Sleep Research," vol 4. New York: Spectrum (in press).
3. Kleitman N: "Sleep and Wakefulness." Chicago: University of Chicago Press, 1963, pp 1–552.

DISCUSSION

Dr Guilleminault emphasized that, with male/female ratios reported by different experimenters between 10 and 60 to 1, the data presented here confirm that the sleep apnea syndrome is a *male* disease. Dr Weil added that chronic mountain sickness is also overwhelmingly a male disease. Drs Weitzman and Lugaresi agreed that affected women in their populations either had micrognathia or were older women. Dr Lugaresi also recalled a presentation from the 1977 international physiology meeting in Paris which indicated that the CO_2 response curve during sleep differs in men and women. Dr Guilleminault questioned the possible role of progesterone (which has been used as a theapeutic agent in some Pickwickians). However, other than the data collected by Miles and co-workers (see Chapter 22), we have little information on hormonal levels during sleep, particularly in these female patients.

Dr Phillipson commented on the controversial question of weight loss: Some patients appear to improve following weight loss and others do not. Dr Lugaresi felt there was no absolute value, but he suggested a critical weight for each patient; under it he is a heavy snorer and over it he becomes a "Pickwickian." Dr Weil questioned the concept of a correlation between weight loss and improvement, particularly in "Pickwickians." Dr Guilleminault noted the questions raised earlier as to whether different sleep apnea patients were representative of a continuum or of different problems. He commented also that if a "central" defect exists, external factors such as enlarged adenoids and tonsils, malformations, and obesity may compound the defect. Otherwise, it is difficult to explain why some patients with the same anatomic defect develop sleep apnea and others do not. In addition, the question of how slender patients develop sleep apnea remains.

Dr Severinghaus reported a patient who had always been sleepy, even as a baby, long before he gained excessive weight. His personality progressively changed and by the time he was first seen, he had been charged with felony numerous times and weighed 169 kg. Tracheostomy resolved his sleepiness and psychological difficulties, and was followed also by weight loss. This post-tracheostomy weight loss had also been observed by Dr Guilleminault and Dr Lugaresi in patients who, before surgery, had never been successful in weight reduction.

Dr Hill remarked that only a slight fat infiltration of the muscles of the airway may have a tremendous impact. The airway in tracheostomized patients may become reduced by only 1 to 2 mm and cause the patient to become suddenly symptomatic — leading to dramatic change in the patient's clinical status and performance. This should be remembered in any consideration of the role of fat as well as in the evaluation of patients who still complain of sleepiness after tracheostomy.

3
Excessive Daytime Sleepiness in the Sleep Apnea Syndrome

William C Dement, Mary A Carskadon, and Gary Richardson

The sleep apnea syndrome, specifically upper airway sleep apnea, while it has a number of other serious medical complications, usually presents as a disorder of excessive daytime sleepiness and is a major cause of this symptom. We have found, for example, that 37% of male patients complaining of excessive daytime sleepiness have upper airway sleep apnea [1], and nearly 80% of upper airway sleep apnea patients have excessive daytime sleepiness as their chief complaint (see Chapter 1). Sleepiness, although the term sounds benign and is usually thought to be of minor consequence, represents the single most obvious difficulty for most sleep apnea patients and is responsible for the unremitting misery they experience daily.

The prevalence of upper airway sleep apnea has not been established, but the ultimate figures will probably bear some relation to previous estimates of the prevalence of the symptom of excessive daytime sleepiness [2–4] and to the overall occurrence of notable snoring. The former complaint appears to include several hundred thousand individuals in the United States. The latter symptom is, of course, very difficult to define and has rarely been systematically studied. Nonetheless, a number of surveys have shown that 10 to 50% of all adult males snore in a manner that is noteworthy (see also Chapter 2). To the extent to which snoring represents some impairment of upper airway function during sleep, however small, millions of people have this problem. And to the extent that excessive daytime sleepiness is a major consequence of compromised respiration during sleep, clinical scrutiny is clearly justified. For these reasons, we have begun a comprehensive study of daytime sleepiness.

Our findings clearly indicate that excessive daytime sleepiness can be objectively described and that it is possible to document the precise degree of amelioration of the symptom achieved by treatment of the underlying disturbance. An

Sleep Apnea Syndromes, pages 23—46

unusual amount of preparatory investigation has been required to develop the methods by which reliable quantification of daytime sleepiness is achieved. Some of this developmental work must be described for purposes of orientation. In addition, the experimental results in sleep apnea patients are from work in progress and therefore should be considered preliminary.

CLINICAL MANIFESTATIONS OF EXCESSIVE DAYTIME SLEEPINESS

Before describing the experimental methods and results, it is important to characterize the clinical nature of the complaint. In essence, the pathologically sleepy patient is distinguished by a markedly increased chronic susceptibility to falling asleep. Therefore, the patient gives a history of falling asleep or becoming extremely drowsy in situations not ordinarily considered soporific. To illustrate, one of our patients was a very enthusiastic football fan. After years of trying, he finally obtained season tickets to the games of his favorite football team (the Oakland Raiders) and slept entirely through every game in a stadium packed with wildly cheering partisans. Another patient, who was a teacher, would actually doze off while standing in front of his class. Another sleep apnea patient, a physician, was extremely drowsy while examining one of his patients, and while listening to breath sounds he had actually fallen asleep with his head cradled against the patient's back. In most instances, careful questioning of patients will elicit similarly unusual examples of falling asleep, such as during sexual intercourse, conversation, eating, and so forth.

Excessive daytime sleepiness can also be inferred from the sheer number of episodes of overwhelming drowsiness. If there are reliable witnesses in the patient's environment, they will usually report many more episodes of dozing than the patient reports. Instances in the first few hours after getting up in the morning are particularly noteworthy.

The problem of excessive sleepiness was further elaborated by Guilleminault et al [5] who suggested an association with complex manifestations of an altered state of consciousness in sleep apnea patients. These manifestations included blackouts, hallucinations and hypnagogic imagery, personality changes, and intellectual deterioration (see also Chapter 1). One of the most common types of experience reported by patients may best be described as automatic behavior. In the typical episode of automatic behavior, the patient first feels that he is not as "awake" as before and usually fights against a feeling of drowsiness. He gradually becomes less aware of his actions and his performance deteriorates. The ability of the patient to express himself in a coherent way is also impaired. Simple answers to simple questions may not indicate the abnormal state of consciousness but attempts at complex answers are abortive and inappropriate. Actions that do not require skill will be performed satisfactorily, albeit in a semiautomatic way; however, if a sudden and well-planned decision is required, the patient will be unable to adapt to the new demand. Amnesia is a very common characteristic of this syndrome. A patient cannot remember what has happened during these episodes although he may have a few disconnected images like a "broken movie."

In addition to the clinical material, Guilleminault et al [5] reported the results of continuous EEG monitoring in sleep apnea patients. They found that patients who had frequent episodes of automatic behavior showed large numbers of "microsleeps," brief instances of sleep waves interrupting ordinary waking patterns. Thus the seemingly bizarre behavior and strange lapses are predictable manifestations of pathological sleepiness. It is very important to appreciate this fact because sleep apnea patients who report these episodes have occasionally been inappropriately treated for temporal lobe epilepsy.

From patient to patient, the variability of the clinical manifestations can be extreme. Socioeconomic status, motivation, and stimulation during the day, as well as severity of the respiratory disturbance during sleep, are factors that obviously influence the overall function of the patient and his ability to resist the relentless sleepiness. Many patients eventually "give up" or may become very depressed, and then the effects of sleepiness inevitably become worse. Certain manifestations of depression may occur as a secondary consequence of pathological sleepiness. For example, a patient who has been prematurely "retired" from his job, has had several auto accidents, and has been divorced as a consequence of his sleepiness may justifiably be somewhat depressed. On the other hand, the remarkable depression seen in other sleep apnea patients may be an intrinsic manifestation of sleep disturbance and/or nocturnal hypoxemia.

Finally, excessive daytime sleepiness is particularly poignant when it afflicts a child [6]. The major effect is failure in school with the cause unrecognized. Over the years, these children may develop serious educational and intellectual impairment that can destroy their chances to lead productive and fulfilling lives. The lost years are all the more tragic because in many cases of childhood sleep apnea a simple tonsillectomy will totally reverse the syndrome.

It is also worth mentioning that the total amount of sleep is not a very important criterion in the diagnosis of pathological sleepiness. Occasionally, patients will say that they sleep as much as 12 to 16 hours a day. However, even in the laboratory, total sleep time per se does not differentiate persons with hypersomnia or excessive daytime sleepiness from normal controls [7].

In most cases, pathological sleepiness develops slowly and insidiously, and the patient cannot pinpoint the onset. Occasionally, however, there appears to be a relatively abrupt onset. One very hypersomnolent patient felt he could date the precise onset of sleepiness to a convention he attended 20 months earlier.

The "Asymptomatic" Patient

As more and more public attention is paid to respiratory problems during sleep and the significance of snoring, there is inevitably an increasing frequency of the diagnosis of sleep apnea in patients who appear to be asymptomatic with regard to hypersomnolence. For example, we report in Chapter 1 that 7 of 50 sleep apnea patients were referred by their wives who had directly observed loud snoring and respiratory pauses and subsequently became aware of the significance of these phenomena through newspaper articles.

Lugaresi et al [8] have reported the existence of a typical upper airway sleep apnea syndrome with hemodynamic abnormalities in adult males who were clinically normal except for a history of heavy snoring. Orr and his colleagues [9] have recently compared a number of sleep-related physiological variables in small groups of "symptomatic and asymptomatic" patients.

It is difficult to know a priori how many so-called asymptomatic patients truly have no impairment of alertness in the daytime. It is not uncommon, however, to see a patient fall asleep literally seconds after he has stoutly maintained that he is "wide awake." It is absolutely clear that some patients deny the existence of severe sleepiness either because it is psychologically repugnant or because they have lost their frame of reference for true alertness. Some patients are simply and honestly unaware of their countless microsleeps and lapses of attention. On the other hand, some sleep apnea patients are clearly less sleepy than others. It is reasonable to assume that many patients may exist who are entirely asymptomatic, at least by comparison with ordinary adults. These considerations are important because they can seriously confound attempts to correlate degree of reported sleepiness with other variables such as PaO_2, weight, duration of illness, and so forth.

From a practical point of view, the most difficult problem in determining whether a patient truly has excessive daytime sleepiness is the language used to state the complaint. Many patients will complain that they are "tired all the time," or that they have "no pep and no energy," of that they never feel like doing anything. Although the overlap of depression, fatigue, and sleepiness is not always clear, the best approach is to suspect pathological sleepiness in any situation of chronically reduced performance.

SOME CONSIDERATIONS OF THE DEFINITION OF NORMAL AND PATHOLOGICAL SLEEPINESS

If we consider sleepiness as a potential attribute of the awake individual, and independent from sleep per se, it is a curious fact that over the past century of sleep research with hundreds of specific studies of prolonged sleep loss, this most consistent consequence of such manipulations has been almost entirely ignored.

Though sleepiness ought to be one of the most important concerns of both basic and clinical sleep research, there is no established tradition of investigative approaches except indirectly through performance testing; there are certainly no widely accepted definitions or sizeable body of knowledge.* As a foundation to our own work on sleepiness, we have adopted two axioms. The first is that sleepiness is an *elemental* feeling state which is accessible to introspection and relatively discriminable from related feeling states such as physical fatigue, depression, and other dysphorias. The second axiom is that sleepiness is essentially a physiological drive state that occurs in response to sleep loss and leads to sleep-seeking behavior as well as an increased tendency to fall asleep [10]. Our first attempts to deal more systematically with daytime drowsiness led to the development of the Stanford Sleepiness Scale (SSS), a seven-point Likert self-rating scale [11], and its cross-validation with performance measures before, during, and after sleep deprivation [12]. This scale rates only the intensity of sleepiness and does not include statements on the associated pleasantness or unpleasantness of the feeling. The Stanford Sleepiness Scale is reproduced in Table I.

Need for an Objective Measure of Sleepiness: Development of the Multiple Sleep Latency Test (MSLT)

Although the SSS has been a useful tool, particularly in ease and cheapness of administration, it has proven to have an important disadvantage in its individual consistency. We have been confronted with patients who are heavy-lidded and

TABLE I. Stanford Sleepiness Scale

Scale	Characteristics
1.	Feeling active and vital; alert; wide awake
2.	Functioning at a high level; but not at peak; able to concentrate
3.	Relaxed; awake; not at full alertness; responsive
4.	A little foggy, not at peak; let down
5.	Fogginess, beginning to lose interest in remaining awake; slowed down
6.	Sleepiness; prefer to be lying down; fighting sleep; woozy
7.	Almost in reverie, sleep onset soon; lost struggle to remain awake
X	Asleep (If you are sleeping during any of the time periods, then write "X" for these periods)

*It is of some interest that all the major books dealing with sleep research, eg, "The Sleeping Brain" (edited by Chase) or "Sleep and Wakefulness" (by Kleitman), do not index "sleepiness" or refer to it explicitly in the text.

falling asleep in front of our eyes while in the act of giving themselves highly alert SSS ratings of 1 or 2. As indicated earlier, we have assumed that some people have been relentlessly and steadfastly sleepy for so long that they no longer have a frame of reference for judging relative alertness, or that there is a simple denial of what is perceived as an extremely negative attribute.

In view of our dissatisfaction with the Stanford Sleepiness Scale and, parenthetically, our concern that the conventional alternative of performance testing would be tremendously confounded by motivational factors, we decided to exploit the basic concept of sleepiness as a state of an increased tendency to fall asleep. Since the exact time of transition from wakefulness to sleep is relatively easy to specify in polygraphic recordings (see Fig 1), it has been possible to design a standard situation in which the momentary sleep tendency of an individual can be measured in terms of the speed of falling asleep, also known as the sleep latency. For a number of years in both our research studies and sleep clinic tests, we have routinely asked patients and subjects to give us an SSS rating before the beginning of an all-night sleep recording or a daytime nap recording. Accordingly, as a first test of the relationship between the subjective feeling of sleepiness and the objective tendency to fall asleep, we compiled all of the data available from tests as mentioned above. In a summary of approximately 1,000 trials over about 50 subjects and patients, we found that a highly significant relationship existed between the sleep latency and the SSS rating prior to "lights out" [10]. These data are displayed in Figure 2. The standard deviations

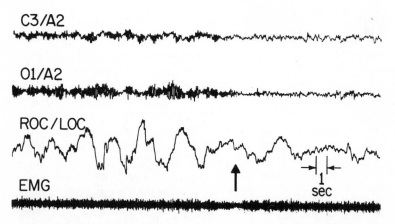

C3/A2

O1/A2

ROC/LOC

EMG

1 sec

Fig 1. Polygraphic tracing of sleep onset. The upper channels are taken from monopolar recordings of central and occipital electroencephalogram. The third tracing is a recording of eye movements from left and right outer canthi using electrooculogram. The bottom tracing is a bipolar surface electromyogram from the chin. Sleep onset occurs at the arrow, which represents a change from relaxed wakefulness (note alpha rhythm in EEG channels) to stage 1 NREM sleep. The tracings were made at a paper speed of 10 mm/sec.

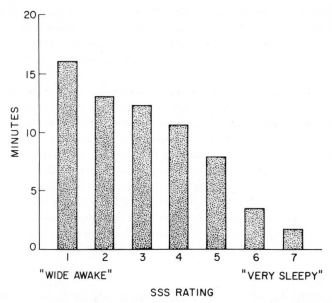

Fig 2. Each bar represents the average latency to sleep onset as a function of the Stanford Sleepiness Scale (SSS) rating given before "lights out." The data include approximately 1,000 trials in a group of 50 patients and subjects.

of the sleep latency means were very large, however, suggesting the expected individual inconsistency.

The next step was to develop the measurement of sleep latency on a repetitive basis throughout the day and to validate such repeated measures against the most predictable cause of extreme subjective sleepiness – namely, total sleep deprivation. In a study by Carskadon and Dement [13], six normal college students (four men and two women) aged 18–20 years were observed before, during, and after total sleep loss. Every two hours during the time they were awake, a sleep latency test (SLT) was administered. For each test, subjects went to bed in individual rooms and were instructed to close their eyes, lie quietly, and try to fall asleep. The beginning of measurement was the moment of "lights out," and the sleep latency test was terminated after one minute of sleep. The definition of sleep onset was, in essence, the end of unambiguous wakefulness. This definition was adopted to avoid the possibility of significant accumulation of sleep time while waiting for unambiguous signs of sleep to appear – namely, spindles and slow waves – and nonetheless represents a fairly unambiguous, easily rated point of functional transition. If subjects remained awake, the sleep latency test was terminated after 20 minutes. The sleep latency score was judged as the interval in minutes between the start of the test and the first 30-second epoch scored as non-rapid eye movement (NREM) stage 1 sleep.

The results were dramatic, as illustrated in Figure 3. The figure shows a decline of sleep latency early in the deprivation period to minimum levels (less than one minute) that were maintained until recovery of sleep was permitted. The sleep latency values returned to baseline levels after the second recovery night.

An additional study of daytime sleepiness in children by Carskadon et al [14, 15] should be mentioned because it combined many of the features of our current studies in patients and provided a further validation of the overall approach. In this study, children aged 10–13 years were observed around the clock with all-night polysomnographic recordings and daytime measures of sleep latency, performance, and subjective sleepiness. In addition to three baseline days, the children were observed after a night of partial sleep loss (sleep allowed only between 4:00 and 8:00 AM). Figure 4 shows the effect of acute partial sleep deprivation on nine children and demonstrates the exquisite sensitivity of multiple sleep latency measurements. By contrast, neither performance tests nor self rating of sleepiness showed any effect of partial sleep loss.

THE MULTIPLE SLEEP LATENCY TEST (MSLT) AND SLEEPINESS INDEX IN NORMAL ADULTS AND IN PATIENTS WITH SLEEP APNEA

The success of the sleep latency test as a measure of normal sleep tendency as well as changes in response to sleep loss encouraged us to design a protocol for

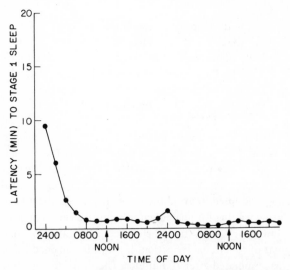

Fig 3. Each dot represents the average sleep latency for a group of six normal college students in a study of sleep loss. Note the decline of sleep latency to minimum values after only one night of sleep deprivation.

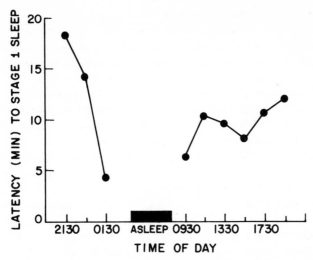

Fig 4. A reduction of nocturnal sleep to four hours resulted in significantly reduced sleep latencies in children (compared to baseline days, when sleep latencies were very close to 20 minutes, or longer). Each dot shows the average sleep latency during and after sleep loss.

the study of clinical populations. The experimental protocol combines all-night sleep recordings and continuous daytime evaluation. The protocol runs for 48 consecutive hours which has the distinct advantage that patients and control subjects can be studied over a weekend. Table II is an outline of the protocol for the measurement of daytime sleepiness. The nocturnal polysomnograms enable us to be sure that daytime results are not due to unusual nocturnal sleep times as well as allowing a replication of the nocturnal respiratory parameters particularly in sleep apnea patients.

It will be noted that the protocol allows for a sleep latency test every two hours through the day, six in all. Collectively, these tests give a continuous evaluation of daytime sleepiness which we now call the Multiple Sleep Latency Test (MSLT). In practice, such a plot will combine the results of both days of the protocol. In addition, from these data we calculate the Sleepiness Index for each day according to the following formula:

$$\text{Sleepiness Index (SI)} = 100 - (5\Sigma SLT/6).$$

We also average the SI for both days to give an overall score for the entire protocol. Thus, the maximally alert subject who does not fall asleep on any of the tests would have a sum of 120 for all SLT scores and, thus, SI = 0. Instantaneous sleep onset on all six tests would give an SI of 100.

The performance testing includes an abridged version of the Wilkinson Addition Test (WAT). In this test, given at six-hour intervals, the subjects add columns

TABLE II. 48-Hour Sleepiness Protocol

Time (hours)	Activity
2100–	(usually Friday evening) – Subject arrives at laboratory, is oriented and prepared for polysomnogram (PSG)
2200–2300	Bedtime and onset of PSG[a]
0800–0900	(usually Saturday morning) – Subject gets up, breakfast
0900–0930	Wilkinson Addition Test (WAT)[b]
1000–1020	Sleep Latency Test (SLT)[c]
1100–1130	Serial Alternation Task (SAT)
1200–1220	SLT
1230–1400	Lunch and free time
1400–1420	SLT
1500–1530	WAT
1600–1620	SLT
1700–1730	SAT
1800–1820	SLT
1830–2000	Dinner and free time
2000–2020	SLT
2100–2130	WAT

[a]The second 24-hour period will be an exact duplicate of the first and the subject will generally leave the laboratory at about 2200 on Sunday night.

[b]All tests begin on the hour. Therefore, the subjects will usually have brief increments of free time between the end of one test and the beginning of the next.

[c]In most instances when the subjects are patients, the SLT will last only a few minutes. It is therefore over well before 20 minutes after the hour. The subject can get out of bed as soon as the SLT is terminated.

of five, two-digit numbers for 30 minutes [16]. Twice a day, subjects perform the Serial Alternation Task (SAT), which consists of alternately pressing two microswitches rhythmically for 30 minutes. The SSS ratings are made every 30 minutes.

Subjects

Twenty-nine adult subjects have completed the sleepiness protocol as part of the current studies of sleep apnea. The total includes a comparison group of seven unselected normal adults, 16 patients with a previously diagnosed unambiguous sleep apnea syndrome, and six "normal" adult males who were selected as age-, sex-, and weight-matched controls for the sleep apnea patients. This report will focus on the latter two groups. Table III presents identifying data on

TABLE III. Identifying Data: 16 Sleep Apnea Patients and Six Matched Controls*

Patient	Age (years)	Weight (lbs)	Height	Type of apnea	Sleep complaint	Condition of recording	Socioeconomic status
FE	42	224	5'10"	Upper airway	EDS	B A	White collar
LB	40	225	5'11"	Upper airway	EDS	B A	Professional
PM	59	232	5'8½"	Upper airway	EDS	B A	Professional
HS	53	200	5'10"	Upper airway	EDS	B A	White collar
AL	56	327	5'8"	Upper airway	EDS+	B A	Disabled
JP	12	149	5'1"	Upper airway	Marginal	B A	White collar
DG	30	255	6'	Upper airway	EDS	B	Blue collar
RS	55	221	5'4½"	Upper airway	EDS	B	Retired
LK	69	180	6'1¾"	Central/mixed	none	B	White collar
AS	74	147	6'1"	Central/mixed	none	B	White collar
MC	58	183	5'9½"	Upper airway	EDS	B	Professional
MB	63	240	6'1"	Upper airway	EDS	B	White collar
AF	45	214	5'9"	Upper airway	EDS	B	Disabled
JB	42	177	5'11"	Upper airway	EDS	A	White collar
AT	59	319	6'	Upper airway	EDS	A	Blue collar
MW	32	360	6'3"	Upper airway	EDS	A	Disabled
Control							
HW	38	186	5'9"				Blue collar
PG	46	190	5'7"				Blue collar
JG	48	180	5'8"				Blue collar
LS	42	275	6'1"				Blue collar
RJ	56	184	5'7"				White collar
EL	44	192	5'9"				Professional

*EDS, Excessive daytime sleepiness; condition of recording: B A, before and after therapy; B, before therapy; A, after therapy only.

the 16 sleep apneic patients and the six matched controls. Six of the 16 sleep apneic patients were studied twice — before and after tracheostomy or tonsillectomy — and three were studied *only* after tracheostomy. It will be noted that 14 of the 16 sleep apnea patients had predominantly upper airway apnea and, of these, one was a child. One adult (AF) had acromegaly and therefore presented a secondary upper airway sleep apnea syndrome. Two subjects had predominantly central or mixed apnea.

RESULTS

Multiple Sleep Latency Tests in Control Subjects

Figure 5 presents the results of the MSLT for the six matched controls. The standard deviations are large, attesting to the intersubject differences; however, the overall pattern of longer sleep latencies toward the beginning and end of the day was consistent across individuals. The mean Sleepiness Indices for the two days ranged from 15 to 70; grand mean was 46. Three of the matched control subjects (PG, JG, LS) seemed unusually sleepy by this test, with SI values of 70, 59, and 59, respectively. However, nocturnal polysomnographic recordings showed no abnormalities in any of the control subjects. Two subjects (PG and LS) also had extremely short sleep latencies (one to two minutes) in the middle

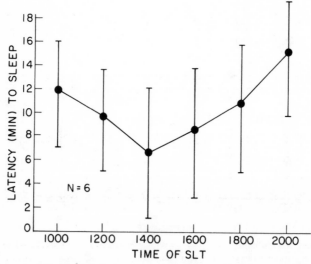

Fig 5. Mean values and standard deviation for age- and sex-matched normal control subjects, sleeping on a regular schedule.

of the day. The comparison group, which included four females and ranged in age from 19 to 44 years (mean = 28), was overall less sleepy than the control group. The individual Sleepiness Indices ranged from 20.4 to 53.2; grand mean was 32.9. No one in the comparison group was overweight.

Multiple Sleep Latency Tests in Untreated Sleep Apnea Patients

The clinical status of all patients was established in prior polysomnographic diagnostic recordings. The types of apnea, their duration, and frequency were unambiguous. Though respiratory variables were recorded in the two-day sleepiness protocol, they were not quantitatively analyzed. All of the sleep apnea patients had hundreds of episodes of apnea in both rapid eye movement (REM) and NREM sleep. Inspection of the nocturnal recordings in the two-day protocol showed no discernable change from previous diagnostic recordings in untreated patients.

The pooled sleep latency scores for the most homogenous group, ten patients with upper airway sleep apnea before treatment, are shown in Figure 6. With the exception of the last test of the day, the mean values are all at about four minutes or less and the standard deviations are relatively small. These data represent the first objective confirmation of pathologically excessive daytime sleepiness in upper airway sleep apnea patients. The two-day means of the Sleepiness

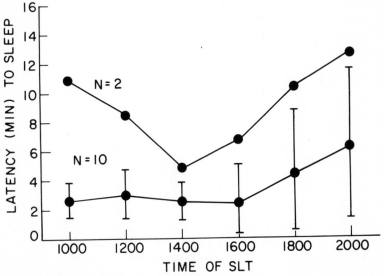

Fig 6. The lower line represents the mean sleep latency values and standard deviations for ten patients with upper airway sleep apnea before they received treatment. The upper graph shows the average sleep latency scores of two patients with central and mixed sleep apnea episodes, whose sleep complaint was insomnia. Note the similarity of the latter to Figure 5.

Index ranged from 60.4 to 99 and the mean for all patients was 82.7, well above the control values. In contrast to the matched control group, short sleep latencies occurred early in the day, as well as in the middle of the day. Though not marked, there was a tendency for longer sleep latencies to occur toward the end of the day. The individual Sleepiness Indices for controls and sleep apnea patients are shown in Figure 7. The difference between the groups is highly significant (P < 0.001) but there is a small degree of overlap.

One unique feature of the sleep latency test in patients with upper airway sleep apnea is very important in terms of assessing daytime sleepiness. In most of the patients, there was a tendency for mild airway obstruction to occur just before polygraphic sleep was evident. This mild obstruction would usually lead to a snore, a snort, or a cough, sometimes with a body movement, that would often produce a clear, though relatively brief delay in the development of the defined sleep onset. Thus, if anything, the MSLT scores in patients are somewhat elevated, with the consequence that the SI values may be spuriously low. Figure 8 shows a polygraphic example of this type of event.

Patient AF, who was tested only before treatment, was the only member of the upper airway sleep apnea group whose problem was almost certainly secondary. A severe excessive daytime sleepiness developed about ten years after an

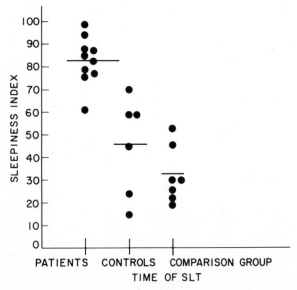

Fig 7. Individual Sleepiness Index values are shown for upper airway sleep apnea patients (left), age- and sex-matched control subjects (center), and subjects in the comparison group (right). Mean differences were significant between each of the two normal groups and the group of patients. The control groups were not significantly different from one another.

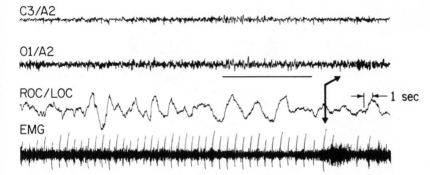

Fig 8. Sleep onset interrupted by an arousal in a patient with upper airway sleep apnea. (Tracings are as described in the legend for Figure 1.) The underlined portion is a ten-second episode of sleep. The arrows indicate a body movement (electromyogram burst) and consequent arousal (alpha rhythm in EEG channels). Although respiratory variables were not recorded at the time, direct observation of the patient showed a respiratory pause during the sleep episode followed by snorting breaths at the arrows. Because the episode of sleep was less than 30 seconds, sleep onset could not be scored.

acromegalic condition had become flagrantly obvious. The sleep-related airway obstruction could be related to pharyngeal and glossal tissue growth caused by excessive secretion of growth hormone. His Sleepiness Index was 87.9, one of the highest.

Two patients (LK, AS) who had predominantly central or mixed sleep apnea were included in this study. They both originally came to the Stanford Sleep Disorders Center complaining of insomnia. Neither complained of falling asleep inappropriately during the day. From the point of view of pathological sleepiness, they were completely asymptomatic. The objective results confirmed that they were a good deal less sleepy during the day than the other patients. Their combined MSLT scores are included in Figure 6, and their two-day mean Sleepiness Indices were 54.6 and 55.7.

Two-Day Stability of Sleepiness Scores

The Sleepiness Indices for day 1 and day 2 in the upper airway sleep apnea patients as well as the six matched controls are plotted in Figure 9. The consistency across the two days is relatively good; however, there was a tendency for some of the patients to have lower scores on the first day which is almost certainly due to anxiety over the procedures. Since the patients were generally quite close to the lower limit for sleep latency, a minute or two prolongation could make a disproportionately large difference in the Sleepiness Index for the day. None of the control subjects showed this effect. Rather, their scores tended to be higher on the first day.

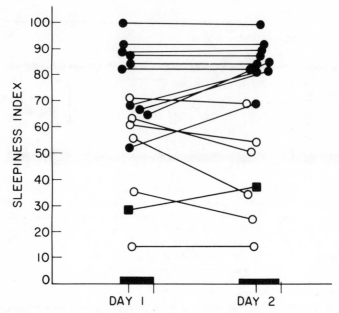

Fig 9. Open circles represent Sleepiness Indices of normal control subjects. Closed circles are Sleepiness Indices for patients with upper airway sleep apnea. The squares represent the Sleepiness Index scores for the one child with sleep apnea. Symbols in the left column show Sleepiness Indices computed from the first day (1) of each experiment: those on the right are from day 2.

Relation of Objective and Subjective Sleepiness Scores

The relation between objective and subjective indices of daytime sleepiness is very important because it involves the concept of the sleep apnea patient who is "asymptomatic" by history. It also confronts the issue of our general reliance on the subjective complaint in making a diagnosis of pathological sleepiness. In Figure 10, we have plotted all of the one-day Sleepiness Indices for the ten untreated upper airway sleep apnea patients against the means of all SSS ratings made by the patients on the same day. The data from the matched controls are also plotted. No correlation between the two measures was present for the sleep apnea patients, whereas a significant correlation was found in the control group.

One patient (HS) was completely asymptomatic. He was evaluated at the Center only because of the repeated urging of his wife who accompanied him and gave testimony about his frequent and repetitive sleep attacks. In spite of this, the patient continued to deny feeling sleepy at any time even when he would fall asleep literally seconds later. His mean SSS on the first day of the protocol was 2.1 with a Sleepiness Index of 73.4. On the second day, the mean

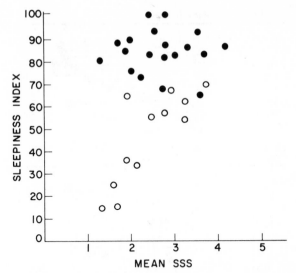

Fig 10. Sleepiness Indices versus average daily SSS ratings in normal control subjects (open circles) and patients with upper airway sleep apnea (closed circles). Sleepiness Indices in patients were uncorrelated with subjective sleepiness ratings. In the control subjects there was a significant direct correlation between objective Sleepiness Indices and the subjective ratings.

SSS was 1.2 and the Sleepiness Index was 80. Even when confronted with his objective performance, the patient remained unconvinced and refused treatment.

Effect of Treatment

Six patients have been studied both before and after treatment for their upper airway sleep apnea syndrome, five adults by tracheostomy and the child by tonsillectomy. Their follow-up evaluation in the sleepiness protocol was carried out at varying durations after the treatment procedure, but all were studied within three months. The before and after two-day mean Sleepiness Indices for all six patients are presented in Table IV and plotted in Figure 11 against mean SSS ratings. In every case, the treatment was successful in totally resolving the sleep-related upper airway problem. Posttreatment sleep was normal in sleep stage configuration and total amount at the time of testing.

All patients showed a sharp decrease in posttreatment objective daytime sleepiness. In every instance the level was reduced below the clearly pathological. Differences in SI values ranged from a low of 32.5 to a high of 75.5. The latter reduction occurred in patient HS whose Sleepiness Index in the posttreatment test was zero. He did not fall asleep on any of the sleep latency tests. Dramatic improvement also occurred in subject LB, whose overall reduction was 72 points

TABLE IV. Sleepiness Indices

Patient	Before treatment	Posttreatment	Change
AL	99	54.3	44.7
LB	94	22.0	72.0
FE	85	46.7	38.3
HS	75.5	0	75.5
PM	87	54.5	32.5
JP	32.7	0	32.7
Mean	78.9	29.6	49.3

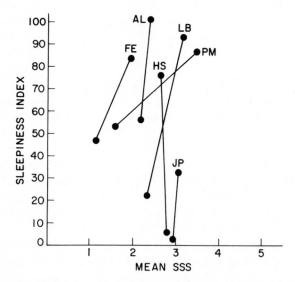

Fig 11. Effects of treatment on Sleepiness Indices and SSS ratings in five adults and one child (JP). In every case, the Sleepiness Index was significantly reduced after treatment, although subjective evaluations (SSS) did not always reflect this improvement.

in the Sleepiness Index. Subjects AL, FE, and PM showed posttreatment SI values of 54.3, 46.7, and 54.5, respectively. All three remained considerably overweight at the time of posttreatment testing. The child (JP), who was 11 years old at the time of testing, showed pathological daytime sleepiness only by comparison with other children. By adult standards, his sleepiness score was well in the normal range. Nonetheless, during the pretreatment testing he fell asleep on every sleep latency test, and in the posttreatment test his Sleepiness Index dropped to zero.

There was essentially no change in the subjective SSS ratings for the groups as a result of treatment. Only one patient (PM) showed a really substantial subjective improvement. It is of interest that this patient was a physician and was uniquely well aware of his intellectual impairment prior to the surgery. The three patients who were studied *only* after tracheostomy were widely variable. Subject AT showed a Sleepiness Index of 68.1 and subject MW showed a Sleepiness Index of 84.4. Subject JB was the least sleepy, with a Sleepiness Index of 45.6. Subjects AT and MW were markedly obese at the time of testing, which is why they were originally selected in spite of the lack of pretreatment data. Subject MW was unique among all posttreatment cases in and out of this study in that he continued to complain of excessive sleepiness in the weeks after the tracheostomy.

Subject AL deserves special mention because he was clearly Pickwickian prior to treatment with very marked obesity (147 kg at the time of testing), polycythemia, cardiomegaly, and pronounced CO_2 retention in the waking state. From the point of view of his sleep apnea syndrome, he was seriously ill, with oxygen saturations reaching zero during apneic episodes and with runs of ventricular tachycardia. Of the entire subject group, he was by far the most impaired by his daytime hypersomnolence. Indeed, his sleepiness level was essentially untestable because he would invariably fall asleep during the calibration procedure before the beginning of every sleep latency test. He could not do any of the other performance tests and it was impossible to keep him fully awake between test sessions even when standing up. He was arbitrarily assigned a Sleepiness Index of 99 for purposes of data analysis, but he was clearly more sleepy overall than other patients who scored in the 90s. His posttreatment results assessed three months after surgery showed a very satisfactory improvement (see Table IV). In addition, the gross clinical impression was excellent in that he was able to remain awake between tests, he could read a book, he could converse, and could do all sorts of things that were impossible for him prior to the treatment.

COMMENT

From a practical point of view, the most important result of our attempts to deal with daytime sleepiness as an objective variable is the clear documentation that chronic tracheostomy or other upper airway surgery which resolves the sleep-related obstruction will also improve the pathological sleepiness. The sample of patients studied to date both before and after treatment is small, however, and larger numbers will be required to establish this conclusion with certainty.

The wide range in Sleepiness Index scores in the posttreatment period is difficult to explain. If we include the three patients who were studied only after treatment, Sleepiness Indices range from 0 to 84.4. There are three major problems in the interpretation of this variability.

In the first place, we do not have any assessment of daytime sleepiness in the patients prior to the development of the sleep apnea syndrome. In other words, we do not know whether they have been restored to their premorbid baseline or not. With one exception, the nine patients who went through the sleepiness protocol following treatment showed scores that were below the highest Sleepiness Index of the matched control group. (Two patients were even below the normal range.)

A second problem is that we cannot be sure patients were tested only after they had achieved maximum improvement in their pathological sleepiness. Longitudinal testing will be needed to clarify this issue. From a subjective point of view, great differences exist in the rate of response to treatment. Some patients report a marked change in the way they feel as early as the day after their first night of posttreatment sleep. Others find the improvement more gradual and are not aware of marked changes in the immediate postoperative period.

Third, there is clearly a ceiling effect in the assessment of daytime sleepiness using the MSLT. Even among patients who fall asleep essentially instantly on every sleep latency test, some are much more impaired (sleepy) than others. Thus, even the patient who had a Sleepiness Index of 84.4 following treatment was substantially improved, as he was little more than a vegetable before his tracheostomy.

Cause of Excessive Daytime Sleepiness in Sleep Apnea Syndrome

A number of factors have been implicated in affecting daytime sleepiness in human beings. Table V lists some of these. Of all these factors, only two have been adequately tested. In sleep apnea patients, the most obvious potential causes of excessive daytime sleepiness are sleep disturbance, chronic sleep loss, and blood gas changes. Obesity may play a role, but is definitely not present in many cases.

The present results are not very helpful in resolving the problem. In the adult upper airway sleep apnea patients, PaO_2 at night, insofar as the continually fluctuating level could be assigned a value, did not predict the daytime Sleepiness Index. Similarly, evidence of alveolar hypoventilation in the waking state was not correlated specifically with daytime sleepiness. Finally, no relationship was apparent between the Apnea Index (number of apneas/hours of sleep) and the Sleepiness Index. A low but significant correlation existed between body weight and Sleepiness Index.

At this point in the study, the number of patients evaluated is far too small to sort out the various possibilities by which sleep apnea might produce pathological sleepiness. However, a few additional comments might be made to under-

TABLE V. Factors Affecting Daytime Sleepiness

Definite

Sleep deprivation (total or partial, depending on amount)
Time of day (biorhythms)

Presumptive

Age (childhood to adulthood)
Sleep interruption
Blood gas changes
  Awake
  Asleep only
  Fluctuating
Sleep stage abnormality
Obesity
Encephalopathy
Low motivation

Other

Sex (hormones)
Diet
High temperature
Low stimulation

score the complexity. For example, though there is no question that sleep is very disturbed in a sleep apnea patient, it is often difficult to evaluate the extent of the disturbance or even to know with certainty what is the best indicator. Figure 12 illustrates the apneic episodes that were typical of the 12-year-old patient (JP). As can be seen, there was absolutely no EEG evidence of arousal or interruption of sleep. Yet, patient JP was definitely excessively sleepy in the daytime as a result of his illness and experienced immediate reversal following resolution of the sleep apnea syndrome by tonsillectomy. In most cases (see Chapter 10), there is considerable sleep disturbance in terms of the many EEG arousals associated with termination of apneic episodes. However, these arousals are typically very brief and often ambiguous in that waking patterns and sleep patterns occur simultaneously. In addition, in the two patients with central sleep apnea (LK, AS), the sleep disturbance was more pronounced and unambiguous; yet, the daytime sleepiness was unremarkable. It is possible that the patients with upper airway sleep apnea were very severely sleep-deprived earlier in their illnesses; although substantial amounts of nocturnal sleep were present at the time of testing, these amounts were not adequate to reverse the chronic pathological sleepiness established earlier. These issues might be clarified by carrying out an experimental sleep disturbance in normal controls which duplicates over a fairly long period of time the hundreds of brief arousals experienced by patients.

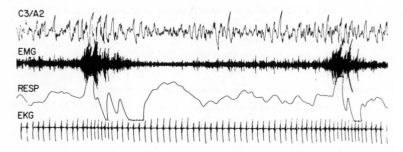

Fig 12. Polygraphic recording in a child (JP) with upper airway sleep apnea. (The EEG and electromyogram tracings are as described in the legend for Figure 1.) Respiration was recorded from a mercury-filled capillary strain gauge attached to the patient's chest. Electrocardiogram was recorded from surface electrodes taped to the chest. The tracing shows that slow-wave sleep was uninterrupted by the respiratory pause.

A major problem in evaluating the role of nocturnal alveolar hypoventilation is the difficulty of measurement. Should one correlate the Sleepiness Index with the lowest PaO_2 values, the average PaO_2, or some overall integrated value? It is well known that emphysema patients with serious hypoxemia are not necessarily hypersomnolent. However, such patients have not been evaluated by means of the MSLT. One final point in favor of nocturnal hypoxemia as the cause of excessive daytime sleepiness is the tendency of the upper airway sleep apnea patients (see Fig 8) to be less sleepy at the end of the day. In all patients except AL, all sleep between sleep latency tests was rigorously prevented. Thus, freedom from sleep-induced hypoxemia during the entire day may have had an ameliorative effect on the daytime sleepiness.

Subject MW, who had the highest Sleepiness Index following tracheostomy, had normal blood gases both awake and asleep. He was, however, markedly obese at the time of testing. Obesity may play a role that is not well understood. It cannot be the only factor, however, because marked reductions in daytime sleepiness occurred after tracheostomy with no weight loss whatsoever in most of the patients. Until more is known, the best formulation is probably that excessive daytime sleepiness is multifactorial with many sources. Tracheostomy alters several of these potential sources simultaneously.

The other side of the coin might be worth stating — that is, to what degree might sleep deprivation and the consequent change in depth of sleep be involved in the apnea process? This, in turn leads to the question of how does upper airway sleep apnea begin in the first place? Is there a vicious circle of heavy snoring, apneas, sleep disturbance, deeper sleep, more apneas, more sleep disturbance, and so on? Such a question might be resolved by observing the effect of experimental sleep deprivation on respiration during sleep in normal or borderline subjects.

Finally, we wish to comment on the value of SSS ratings and other subjective evaluations of daytime sleepiness in the upper airway sleep apnea syndrome. In the first place, subjective sleepiness is clearly unreliable, and from a practical point of view, a physician should place his major reliance on an observer in the patient's environment. In the second place, the unreliability is uniformly in the direction of denying excessive sleepiness. We almost never see a patient who complains of excessive daytime sleepiness who does not show clear objective signs. Finally, we have the clear impression that the patients' ability to give reliable subjective accounts was greatly improved after treatment. It is as if having access to a new experience in alertness gave them the necessary frame of reference for such judgments.

ACKNOWLEDGMENTS

This research was supported by National Institute of Neurological Diseases and Stroke grant NS 10727, National Institute of Child Health and Human Development grant HD 08339, and Institute of Mental Health grant MH 5804 to Dr Dement. This research on children was supported in part by grants from the Spencer Foundation and the William and Flora Hewlett Foundation.

REFERENCES

1. Guilleminault C, Dement WC: 235 cases of excessive daytime sleepiness. J Neurol Sci 31:13–27, 1977.
2. Dement W, Zarcone V, Varner V, Hoddes E, Nassau S, Jacobs B, Brown J, McDonald A, Horan K, Glass R, Gonzales P, Friedman E, Phillips R: The prevalence of narcolepsy. Sleep Res 1:148, 1972.
3. Dement W, Carskadon M, Ley R: The prevalence of narcolepsy. II. Sleep Res 2:147, 1973.
4. Karacan I, Thornby J, Anch M, Holzer C, Warheit G, Schwab J, Williams R: Prevalence of sleep disturbance in a primarily urban Florida county. Soc Sci Med 10:239–244, 1976.
5. Guilleminault C, Billiard M, Montplaisir J, Dement WC: Altered states of consciousness in disorders of daytime sleepiness. J Neurol Sci 26:377–387, 1975.
6. Guilleminault C, Eldridge F, Simmons F, Dement WC: Sleep apnea in eight children. Pediatrics 58:23–30, 1976.
7. Hishikawa Y, Wakamatsu H, Furuya E, Sugita Y, Masaoka S, Kaneda H, Sato M: Sleep satiation in narcoleptic patients. Electroencephalogr Clin Neurophysiol 41:1–18, 1976.
8. Lugaresi E, Coccagna G, Farneti P, Mantovani M, Cirignotta F: Snoring. Electroencephalogr Clin Neurophysiol 39:59–64, 1975.
9. Orr WC, Imes NK: Sleep apnea in symptomatic and asymptomatic groups. Sleep Res 6:177, 1977.
10. Dement W: Daytime sleepiness and sleep "attacks." In Guilleminault C, Dement W, Passouant P (eds): "Narcolepsy." New York: Spectrum, 1976, pp 17–42.

11. Hoddes E, Dement W, Zarcone V: The development and use of the Stanford Sleepiness Scale (SSS). Psychophysiology 9:150, 1972.
12. Hoddes E, Zarcone V, Smythe H, Phillips R, Dement W: Quantification of sleepiness: A new approach. Psychophysiology 10:431–436, 1973.
13. Carskadon MA, Dement WC: Sleep tendency: An objective measure of sleep loss. Sleep Res 6:200, 1977.
14. Carskadon MA, Karvey K, Dement WC: Sleep tendency in children. Sleep Res 6: 91, 1977.
15. Carskadon MA, Harvey K, Dement WC, Anders TF: Acute partial sleep deprivation in children. Sleep Res 6:92, 1977.
16. Wilkinson RT: Sleep deprivation: Performance tests for partial and selective sleep deprivation. In Abt LA, Reiss BF (eds): "Progress in Clinical Psychology," vol 8. New York: Grune and Stratton, 1968.

DISCUSSION

Dr Weil raised the question of what really accounts for the extreme sleepiness of sleep apnea patients. He noted that subjects studied at high altitudes present patterns similar to those described here. Although the total amount of sleep logged and its distribution were good, subjects complained of poor sleep and of fatigue the next day. When sleep records were analyzed, the only impressive finding was a number of short awakenings during sleep. In the high altitude study, sleep had to continue unbroken for certain periods of time to be perceived as satisfying. The high altitude subjects presented nearly normal percentages of stages 3–4 NREM sleep (15 to 20% of total sleep time), whereas these stages are reduced in sleep apnea patients.

Dr Severinghaus asked whether, when someone is deliberately awakened from REM sleep and then from NREM sleep, the time delay before going back to sleep is the same or whether it varies with sleep stage. Dr Dement point out the difficulty of answering this critical question because the time of night is a major factor; someone awakened early in the night tends to fall asleep quickly. The speed of falling asleep is very much a function of the circadian rhythm of sleepiness. Very few (if any) circadian rhythm studies have been done thus far in sleep apneic patients, and information about patterns of variables such as body temperature in sleep apneic patients is not now available.

4
Respiratory Control Mechanisms During NREM and REM Sleep

Eliot A Phillipson and Colin E Sullivan

INTRODUCTION

The mechanisms underlying respiratory disturbances during sleep, including sleep apneas, are unlikely to be defined without knowledge of the normal behavior of the respiratory control system during sleep. Therefore we have examined the components of the respiratory control system in dogs during non-rapid eye movement (NREM) and rapid eye movement (REM) sleep by systematically increasing and decreasing a number of afferent respiratory inputs that are involved in ventilatory regulation. This communication will provide a summary of our investigations, with the detailed data being available in the original reports [1–5]. The general picture that has emerged from these studies indicates clear differences in respiratory control between NREM and REM sleep. In NREM sleep ventilation appears to be regulated by the automatic respiratory control system and breathing movements are principally involved in metabolic homeostatic functions. In contrast, during REM sleep breathing movements appear to subserve nonrespiratory requirements and, with one important exception, are relatively unresponsive to classical respiratory stimuli.

METHODS

A detailed description of the general methods has been published elsewhere [1, 2]. Our studies were performed in five dogs (weight 19–27 kg) that were trained to lie quietly in place and to sleep in the laboratory. Months before the studies the dogs were prepared surgically with a permanent tracheostomy and with exteriorized cervical vagal loops [6]. During the studies the dogs breathed through a cuffed endotracheal tube that was inserted through the tracheostomy and connected to a pneumotachograph and differential pressure transducer for

Sleep Apnea Syndromes, pages 47–64

measurement of respiratory airflow rates and instantaneous respiratory frequency (f). The airflow signal was integrated electronically to provide tidal volume (V_T), and the product of V_T and f gave the instantaneous minute volume of ventilation ($\dot{V}_I$). All volumes were corrected to BTPS conditions. Tracheal gas was sampled continuously through a heated line and drawn through an infrared analyzer for measurement of CO_2 concentration. All transducer signals were recorded on a pen-writing polygraph and were also stored on magnetic tape for later playback at speeds that allowed more accurate analysis of the respiratory variables.

The sleep studies were generally performed during the afternoon, two to four hours following a feeding, a time at which the dogs normally slept. Laboratory temperature was maintained constant at 18–19°C during all studies. We determined the stage of sleep using behavioral and electroencephalographic (EEG) criteria. The EEG was recorded on a polygraph through needle electrodes that were inserted into the scalp over the frontal area. Frequently electrooculograms were also recorded through needle electrodes inserted above and lateral to one eye. For purposes of these studies we were able to define four sleep stages in the dogs [1, 2] : wakefulness (W); drowsiness or light sleep (D); slow-wave sleep (SWS); and REM sleep. During SWS the dogs were unresponsive to external stimuli that elicited responses (eye opening, turning of head, etc) during W or D, and the EEG was dominated by high-voltage waves at 2–4 Hz. This stage of sleep corresponds approximately to stage 3 NREM sleep in man [7]. Rapid eye movement sleep was characterized by a typical low-voltage, high-frequency EEG pattern, frequent bursts of rapid eye movements, and frequent twitching movements of the ears, nose, lips, and limbs. Throughout these investigations measurements during REM sleep were confined to periods in which there were both EEG and behavioral characteristics of REM sleep, since by these criteria REM sleep was easily distinguished from both SWS and W.

INCREASED RESPIRATORY STIMULI

Hypercapnia

We examined ventilatory responses to hyperoxic progressive hypercapnia using the rebreathing method of Read [8]. The dogs rebreathed from a spirometer that was initially filled with 2–3 liters of 6–7% CO_2 in O_2. The precise volume and composition of gas mixture that reliably produced a mixed venous plateau on the CO_2 record at the initiation of rebreathing were determined for each dog in a series of preliminary studies. Following establishment of the mixed venous plateau, the alveolar (end-tidal) CO_2 pressure ($PaCO_2$) increased linearly with time as rebreathing continued and independently of changes in ventilation (Fig 1). Rebreathing was continued until the dog awoke, which usually occurred within three minutes. Arousal from SWS or REM sleep always occurred abruptly and was indicated by either a sudden change in EEG during SWS or a sudden cessation of phasic muscular movements in REM sleep, coincident with which the dogs invariably sat or jumped up. Thus the timing of arousal was easily determined.

As shown in Figure 1, during SWS the ventilatory response to CO_2 consisted of a progressive increase in both V_T and f as $PaCO_2$ increased. When analyzed on a breath-by-breath basis, there was a typical linear relationship between instantaneous $\dot{V}_I$ and $PaCO_2$ (Fig 2) and a high degree of correlation ($r > 0.90$) between the variables [3]. Furthermore, the $PaCO_2$ at arousal was highly reproducible in each dog during SWS (mean of four dogs 55.3 ± 2.7 mm Hg). In contrast, the responses to hypercapnia during REM sleep were markedly different. First, the irregular pattern of breathing typical of REM sleep was essentially unaffected by CO_2 (Fig 1). Secondly there was little increase in $\dot{V}_I$ as $PaCO_2$ increased (Fig 2). Thus the slopes of the $\dot{V}_I/PaCO_2$ response lines were markedly reduced in REM sleep (11–18% of those in SWS), and there was only a weak correlation between the two variables ($r < 0.40$). The response of both V_T and f to CO_2 were similarly affected. Finally the duration of rebreathing before arousal was longer in REM sleep (1.70 ± 0.17 minutes) than in SWS (0.95 ± 0.05 minutes), and the $PaCO_2$ at arousal was significantly higher (61.2 ± 3.1 mm Hg).

These differences in ventilatory and waking responses to CO_2 between SWS and REM sleep occurred despite comparable eucapnic alveolar and mixed venous CO_2 pressures and similar rates of rise of $PaCO_2$ during rebreathing [3]. Thus the differences in response cannot be attributed to differences in the magnitude of chemical stimulus. Similarly, changes in cerebral blood flow, which occur in REM sleep [9], also cannot be implicated since, in the rebreathing method used in these studies, the rate of rise of cerebral CO_2 concentration is independent of cerebral blood flow [10]. Furthermore, the rapidity of change in the responses with changes in sleep stage suggest that neural rather than metabolic mechanisms were responsible. For example, in panel A of Figure 3 a CO_2 rebreathing run was started during REM sleep, but shortly thereafter there was a change to NREM sleep. Coincident with the change in sleep stage was an abrupt change to a regular pattern of breathing and a $\dot{V}_I$ response to CO_2 that was typical of SWS (Fig 4). Arousal occurred at a $PaCO_2$ of 60 mm Hg. Panel B of Figure 3 shows another CO_2 response run in the same dog that was initiated during SWS. Shortly before arousal due to hypercapnia would have occurred (based on previous runs in SWS), there was a change to REM sleep. Coincident with the change in sleep stage was an abrupt change to an irregular pattern of

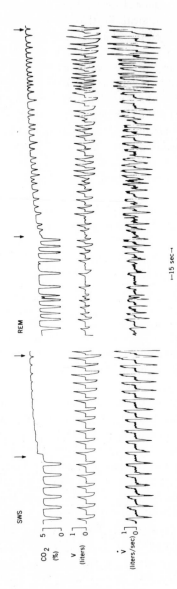

Fig 1. Recorder tracings during hyperoxic progressive hypercapnia in one dog during slow-wave sleep (SWS) and rapid eye movement (REM) sleep. CO_2, concentration of CO_2 in tracheal gas; V, inspired volume (expired volume, below zero line); $\dot{V}$, airflow rate (inspiration upward, expiration downward). First arrow, onset of rebreathing; second arrow, arousal.

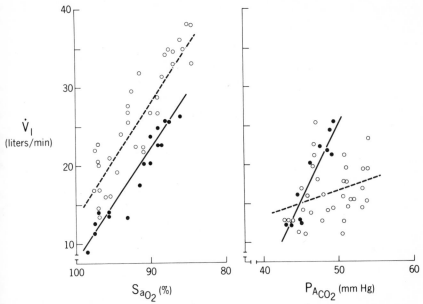

Fig 2. Breath-by-breath response of minute volume of ventilation ($\dot{V}_I$) to decreasing arterial oxygen saturation (SaO_2) or increasing alveolar CO_2 pressure (Pa_{CO_2}; $PaCO_2$ in text) in one dog. •, Slow-wave sleep; ○, rapid eye movement sleep. Lines through data represent calculated linear regressions. (From Phillipson EA: Am Rev Respir Dis 115 (Suppl):217–224, 1977. Reprinted by permission of publisher.)

breathing and an abrupt decrease in $\dot{V}_I$ response to CO_2 (Fig 4). Furthermore arousal was delayed until $PaCO_2$ had reached 68 mm Hg.

Hypoxia

We examined the ventilatory response to isocapnic progressive hypoxia using a modification of the method of Rebuck and Campbell [11]. The dogs rebreathed from a spirometer that was initially filled with 3–5 liters of 8–10% O_2 in N_2. The precise volume and composition of gas mixture selected for each dog were such that arterial oxygen saturation (SaO_2) decreased to 75% in about one minute of rebreathing. The SaO_2 was measured with an ear oximeter whose accuracy was verified in a series of preliminary studies in which oximeter SaO_2 was compared with SaO_2 in carotid arterial blood [4]. The $PaCO_2$ was kept constant at the eucapnic level during hypoxia by drawing a variable amount of the rebreathing gas through a CO_2 absorber and returning it to the spirometer. Rebreathing was continued until the dog awoke, which invariably occurred within three minutes. As in the case of hypercapnia, with arousal from

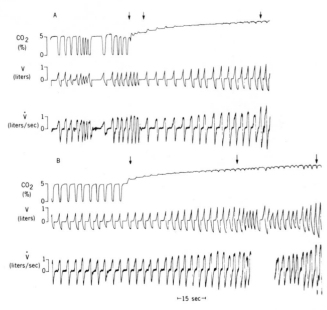

Fig 3. Recorder tracings showing effects of change in sleep stage in response to hyperoxic progressive hypercapnia in one dog. CO_2, V, $\dot{V}$, as in Figure 1. First arrow in each panel, onset of rebreathing; second arrow, EEG and behavioral signs of abrupt change in sleep stage; third arrow, arousal. A) Rebreathing commenced during REM sleep; shortly thereafter, change to NREM sleep. B) Rebreathing commenced during SWS; shortly before arousal from SWS should have occurred, change to REM sleep.

hypoxia there were abrupt changes in EEG and behavior and the dogs invariably jumped up immediately upon awakening.

As shown in Figure 5, during SWS the ventilatory response to hypoxia consisted of a progressive increase in both V_T and f as SaO_2 decreased. When analyzed on a breath-by-breath basis, there was a linear relationship between instantaneous $\dot{V}_I$ and SaO_2 (Fig 2) and a high degree of correlation between the variables ($r > 0.90$). Similar relationships were also found between V_T and SaO_2 and between f and SaO_2 [4]. Furthermore, the SaO_2 at arousal was highly reproducible in each dog during SWS (mean of four dogs, 87.5 ± 2.6%). During REM sleep the pattern of breathing remained irregular despite progressive hypoxemia (Fig 5). Nevertheless, in contrast to the response to CO_2, there was an overall increase in ventilation as SaO_2 decreased, and the slopes of the $\dot{V}_I/SaO_2$ response lines were the same as in SWS (Fig 2; [4]). However, the duration of rebreathing before arousal was longer in REM sleep (1.15 ± 0.16 minutes) than in SWS (0.53 ± 0.07 minutes) and the SaO_2 at arousal was significantly lower (70.5 ± 3.4%).

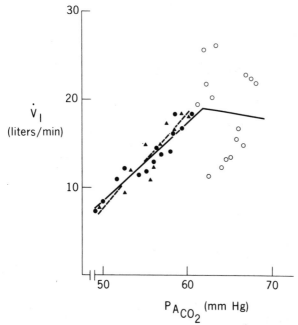

Fig 4. Breath-by-breath response of minute volume of ventilation ($\dot{V}_I$) to increasing alveolar CO_2 pressure ($PaCO_2$) during CO_2 rebreathing tests shown in Figure 3. ▲ — ▲) NREM sleep following REM sleep (Fig 3A); ●—●) SWS (segment between first and second arrows in Fig. 3B); ○—○) REM sleep following SWS (segment between second and third arrows in Fig. 3B).

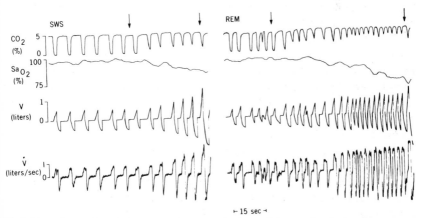

Fig 5. Recorder tracings during eucapnic progressive hypoxia in one dog during slow-wave sleep (SWS) and rapid eye movement (REM) sleep. CO_2, V, $\dot{V}$, as in Figure 1; SaO_2, arterial oxygen saturation. First arrow, onset of rebreathing; second arrow, arousal.

Afferent Vagal Stimulation

We examined the effects on breathing of increasing one type of afferent vagal input, that related to sustained lung inflation (ie, the classical Hering-Breuer inflation reflex). The lungs of the dog were inflated at the onset of a spontaneous inspiration with a measured volume of air, and the endotracheal tube was then occluded to maintain lung inflation [12]. The duration of apnea elicited by the reflex was then measured as the period of time to the first inspiratory effort, indicated by an abrupt decrease in tracheal pressure. As shown in Figure 6, during SWS sustained inflation of the lungs resulted in a long period of apnea, the duration of which was highly reproducible for a given volume of inflation. In addition, the duration of apnea varied directly with the volume of lung inflation [1]. In contrast, during REM sleep inflation of the lungs elicited little or no apneic response, and the irregular pattern of breathing typical of REM sleep was virtually unaffected by the maneuver (Fig 6).

DECREASED RESPIRATORY STIMULI

Vagal Blockade

We examined the effects on breathing of removing all afferent vagal input by cold blocking the cervical vagus nerves [13]. Small radiators were applied snugly to the exteriorized vagal loops and cold alcohol circulated through the radiators by a thermostatically controlled refrigerated circulator. The criteria of complete vagal blockade using this technique have been described previously[14]. Following vagal blockade we waited at least 15–20 minutes before making measurements in order to ensure that a new steady state was achieved. As shown in Figure 7, during SWS vagal blockade had a profound effect on the pattern of breathing with respiratory f decreasing to 3–5 breaths/min. This slowing of f was due to a small prolongation of inspiratory time (resulting in increased V_T), and a marked prolongation of the expiratory pause between breaths. Thus there was a recurrent apnea of 10–18 seconds after cessation of expiratory airflow, during which SaO_2 decreased gradually to approximately 90%. Despite these changes, the pattern of breathing remained very regular during SWS [1]. In contrast, vagal blockade had no effect on the irregular pattern of breathing typical of REM sleep, and coefficients of variation of all the respiratory variables were as high during vagal blockade as when the vagi were intact [1]. Furthermore, because of the increased f and $\dot{V}_1$ during REM sleep [1], there was little fluctuation in SaO_2 between breaths (Fig 7).

Hyperoxia

We examined the effects of transiently decreasing or completely removing afferent input from the peripheral chemoreceptors by having the dogs inspire

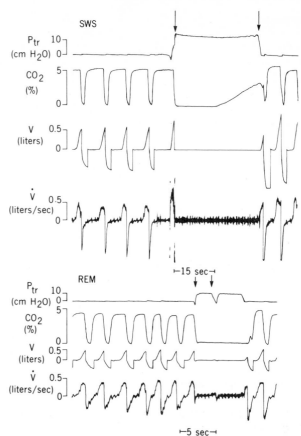

Fig 6. Recorder tracings during sustained lung inflation in slow-wave sleep (SWS) and rapid eye movement (REM) sleep. CO_2, V, $\dot{V}$, as in Figure 1; Ptr, tracheal pressure. First arrow, onset of sustained lung inflation; second arrow, first inspiratory effort. Note differences in Ptr and V calibrations and in paper speed between SWS and REM.

one or two breaths of 100% O_2. When the vagus nerves were intact, respiratory f during SWS was sufficiently rapid that there was little decrease in SaO_2 between breaths. Thus 100% O_2 had only a small effect on f and V_T. However, when the vagi were blocked, resulting in respiratory slowing and significant arterial desaturation during each expiratory pause, inspiration of 100% O_2 had a marked effect. Specifically, instantaneous respiratory f decreased further due to prolongation of the expiratory apnea (up to 24–32 seconds), and the inspiratory flow rate and volume of the subsequent breaths were often less than the pre-O_2 breaths (Fig 7). These results were highly reproducible in each dog [5]. The long apnea following O_2 administration invariably resulted in an elevated alveolar and presumably cerebral pCO_2 (Fig 7). This increased CO_2

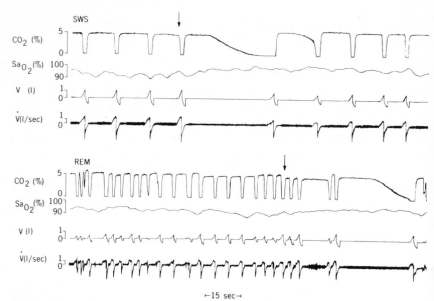

Fig 7. Recorder tracings showing effects of vagal blockade and of hyperoxia in one dog during slow-wave sleep (SWS) and rapid eye movement (REM) sleep. CO_2, SaO_2, V, $\dot{V}$, as in Figure 5. Cervical vagus nerves blocked completely throughout both records. At arrow, dog inspired one breath of 100% O_2.

stimulus probably initiated the post-O_2 breaths since SaO_2 was still well above the normal level.

In contrast to SWS, during REM sleep inspiration of 100% O_2 generally had little effect on the pattern of breathing even when the vagus nerves were blocked (Fig 7). This result is predictable in view of the high levels of SaO_2 generally present during REM sleep. However, there was an important exception to this finding: When spontaneous periods of apnea (which are common in REM sleep) happened to be preceded by inhalation of 100% O_2, some of the apneas continued for durations that were longer (up to 40 seconds) than found during room air breathing (up to 20 seconds). This result is also predictable in view of the intact ventilatory response to hypoxia during REM sleep. Thus, whereas 100% O_2 generally had no effect on the rapid and irregular breathing of REM sleep, it did allow spontaneous apneic periods to continue for a longer duration than normal.

Metabolic Alkalosis

We examined the effect of decreasing the ventilatory stimulating effect of CO_2 by inducing a mild chronic metabolic alkalosis in the dogs [15]. For this purpose they were maintained on a low chloride diet for five to seven days and given an oral diuretic (furosemide, 20 mg daily) which resulted in an arterial pH of 7.45–7.50 (normal pH, 7.34–7.37). During SWS metabolic alkalosis slowed respiratory f (from 11–14 to 7–10 breaths/min). When the vagus nerves were blocked, f became correspondingly slower than it was when pH was normal; and administration of 100% O_2 produced even greater respiratory slowing since it now required a longer period of time for blood and cerebral pCO_2 to increase to levels that would initiate inspiration. Thus the combination of metabolic alkalosis, SWS, vagal blockade, and 100% O_2 slowed breathing to as low as one breath per minute, and resulted in expiratory durations of up to 57 seconds.

In contrast, metabolic alkalosis had little effect on the pattern of breathing during REM sleep. This result is compatible with the earlier observation that hypercapnia had no effect on the pattern of breathing and little effect on $\dot{V}_I$ during REM sleep.

DISCUSSION

Effects on Respiratory Timing of Increased or Decreased Respiratory Stimuli

As a background for discussion of our results in the context of their relevance to sleep apnea, the data for one dog have been summarized into two composite diagrams (Figs 8 and 9) showing the effects on breathing of systematic increases or decreases in afferent respiratory stimuli. During SWS breathing was highly regular; increasing chemical stimuli (either hypercapnia or hypoxia) increased respiratory f (and V_T) progressively; and successive removal or reduction of afferent stimuli (by vagal blockade, hyperoxia, and alkalosis) slowed f progressively, resulting in long periods of expiratory apnea between successive breaths. Not shown here is the fact that during W the effects of removing respiratory stimuli were considerably less, indicating that wakefulness per se is a major source of ventilatory stimulation even in the absence of other respiratory inputs. In contrast to SWS, the irregular pattern of breathing characteristic of REM sleep was virtually unaffected by all of these experimental maneuvers (Figs 8 and 9). However, hypoxia did produce an overall increase in $\dot{V}_I$, and hyperoxia allowed spontaneous apneas of REM sleep to continue for a longer period of time (Fig 7).

Mechanisms of Respiratory Control During Sleep

From these studies in sleeping dogs have emerged clear differences in respiratory control between SWS and REM sleep. In SWS breathing is highly regular with little breath-to-breath variability in f or V_T. In addition, ventilatory responses to classical respiratory stimuli (chemical and vagal) are predictable on the

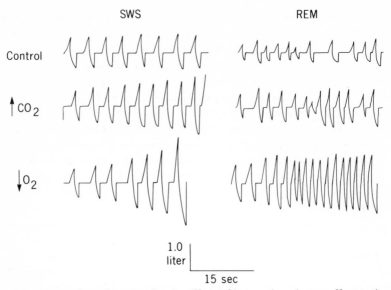

Fig 8. Recorder tracings of one dog showing effects of increased respiratory afferent stimulation during slow-wave sleep (SWS) and rapid eye movement (REM) sleep. Tracings show inspired volumes (above horizontal zero line) and expired volumes (below zero line). $\uparrow CO_2$) Progressive hypercapnia; $\downarrow O_2$) progressive hypoxia. Levels of hypercapnia and hypoxia were comparable in SWS and REM.

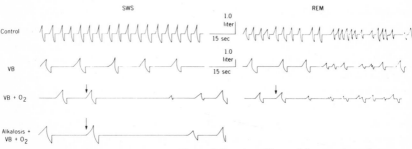

Fig 9. Recorder tracings of same dog as Figure 8 showing effects of decreased respiratory afferent stimulation during slow-wave sleep (SWS) and rapid eye movement (REM) sleep. Tracings show inspired and expired volumes as in Figure 8. VB) Vagal blockade; VB + O_2, one breath of 100% O_2 inspired (at arrow) during vagal blockade; alkalosis + VB + O_2, one breath of 100% O_2 inspired (at arrow) during vagal blockade and chronic metabolic alkalosis. Note change in volume calibration for all records during VB.

basis of traditional concepts of respiratory control. The entire pattern of responses suggests that during SWS breathing is primarily controlled by the automatic (metabolic) respiratory control system [16], consisting of the classical pontomedullary respiratory neurons and their afferent inputs from the central and peripheral chemoreceptors and the vagus nerves. Thus when afferent input was increased by hypercapnia or hypoxia, respiratory f increased; and when afferent input was decreased by vagal blockade, hyperoxia, and alkalosis, f decreased. However, the magnitude of respiratory slowing that followed the reduction of afferent inputs in these otherwise intact healthy dogs was greater than would have been predicted, and indicates the primary importance of these inputs in maintaining respiratory periodicity during SWS. Indeed, as afferent inputs were progressively removed or reduced there were relatively small changes in inspiratory duration, but successively longer expiratory apneas lasting up to 57 seconds between breaths. The conclusion from these observations is that in the absence of sufficient afferent stimulation during SWS there is no initiation of inspiration, but simply prolonged expiratory apnea.

In contrast to SWS, during REM sleep breathing does not appear to be primarily regulated by the automatic control system. This conclusion derives from the fact that the pattern of breathing was highly irregular during REM sleep and was essentially unresponsive to any increase or decrease in classical, automatic system inputs — vagal or chemical. The important exception to this generalization is that hypoxia was capable of increasing $\dot{V}_I$ during REM sleep although the pattern of breathing remained highly irregular. Thus in REM sleep respiration appears to be driven by inputs that are unrelated to the automatic control system, and considered in this context, breathing movements do not appear to be primarily "ventilatory" in origin or purpose. Of interest in this regard is the observation that the degree of respiratory irregularity during REM sleep increases when rapid eye and other phasic muscular movements are increased [4], suggesting that the breathing movements are part of the generalized muscular activity of REM sleep. The origin and purpose of these movements are not clear [17]. However, we have pointed out elsewhere [18] that the irregular pattern of breathing and decreased ventilatory response to CO_2 in REM sleep are reminiscent of ventilatory activity in man under conditions in which the voluntary (behavioral) respiratory control system [16] is active. Therefore, the possibility exists that the voluntary system is involved in respiratory control during REM sleep, but at present direct evidence to support this notion is still lacking.

Implications for Sleep Apnea

Based on the preceding analysis of respiratory control mechanisms during sleep, a scheme can be developed to account for NREM and REM sleep apneas (Table I). This scheme applies primarily to central (diaphragmatic) as opposed to obstructive apneas [19, 20]. However, it may also have relevance to the latter since many of the stimuli that drive the phrenic and intercostal upper motor neurons in the brain stem also increase activity in the closely related neurons that control the muscles of the upper airway.

TABLE I. Possible Mechanisms of Sleep Apnea

Sleep stage	Onset of apnea	Termination of apnea
NREM	Loss of wakefulness stimulus to breathing, plus either: 1) insufficient afferent respiratory inputs; or 2) defects in neurons of "respiratory centers"	Build-up of afferent respiratory inputs during apnea to levels that either: 1) initiate inspiration, or 2) produce arousal
REM	Related to activity in "REM-generating centers." Unrelated to classical respiratory inputs	Related to activity in "REM-generating centers" or development of hypoxemia sufficient to initiate inspiration

As suggested above, in NREM sleep breathing appears to be regulated primarily by the automatic control system, and the initiation of inspiration depends critically upon sufficient afferent respiratory stimuli. Therefore, apneas occurring in this stage of sleep should be attributable to defects in the automatic system. The onset of such apneas could be due, for example, to lack of sufficient afferent input from central or peripheral chemoreceptors, or to defects in the central respiratory neurons of the brain stem that integrate these inputs. These same defects need not produce apnea during W since additional inputs, related to wakefulness and generated outside the automatic system per se, provide sufficient drive to initiate inspiration. The termination of an apneic period in NREM sleep would then result from a gradual build-up of afferent respiratory stimuli (due to hypercapnia or hypoxia) sufficient either to initiate breathing or to produce arousal, which in turn would stimulate breathing. This scheme for the genesis of NREM sleep apneas appears to fit well with clinical experience. For example, adults with NREM sleep apneas typically have decreased chemosensitivity [20]; and both children and adults with central hypoventilation syndromes and prolonged or even fatal sleep apneas typically demonstrate gross impairment of respiratory chemosensitivity [21].

An alternative mechanism that could also produce NREM sleep apnea is an active inhibition of inspiration, rather than a lack of sufficient inspiratory-excitatory stimuli. Such inhibition might be due, for example, to increased inhibitory vagal stimuli in view of the presence of an active Hering-Breuer inflation reflex during SWS (at least in the dog).

If, as suggested earlier, breathing during REM sleep is normally driven by inputs unrelated to and generally unresponsive to the automatic control system, then defects in this system should be of less consequence in REM sleep than in SWS. A striking clinical example of this distinction is the report by Shannon et al [22] of two infants with severely impaired automatic respiratory control who were apneic in NREM sleep but who breathed relatively normally in REM sleep.

Thus it appears likely that the onset of an apneic period in REM sleep is not due to defects in classical respiratory inputs or medullary respiratory neurons, but is probably related to activity in the "REM-sleep-generating centers" that are thought to be located in the pons [23]. The termination of such an apnea would generally be due to a similar mechanism. However, if the apnea were prolonged sufficiently to produce hypoxemia, it would be terminated by stimuli from the peripheral chemoreceptors since hypoxic chemosensitivity is intact during REM sleep. Conversely, if the sensitivity to hypoxia were impaired, then REM sleep apneas could become prolonged. Thus it would seem reasonable to search for impaired hypoxic sensitivity in those individuals who demonstrate prolonged apneas during REM sleep.

ACKNOWLEDGMENTS

This work was supported by Operating grant MA-4606 of the Medical Research Council of Canada. Colin E Sullivan was supported by a Fellowship of the Asthma Foundation of New South Wales, Australia.

REFERENCES

1. Phillipson EA, Murphy E, Kozar LF: Regulation of respiration in sleeping dogs. J Appl Physiol 40:688–693, 1976.
2. Phillipson EA, Kozar LF, Murphy E: Respiratory load compensation in awake and sleeping dogs. J Appl Physiol 40:895–902, 1976.
3. Phillipson EA, Kozar LF, Rebuck AS, Murphy E: Ventilatory and waking responses to CO_2 in sleeping dogs. Am Rev Respir Dis 115:251–259, 1977.
4. Phillipson EA, Sullivan CE, Read DJC, Murphy E, Kozar LF: Ventilatory and waking responses to hypoxia in sleeping dogs. J Appl Physiol (in press).
5. Sullivan CE, Kozar LF, Murphy E, Phillipson EA: Primary role of respiratory afferents in sustaining breathing rhythm. J Appl Physiol (in press).
6. Phillipson EA, Hickey RF, Bainton CR, Nadel JA: Effect of vagal blockade on regulation of breathing in conscious dogs. J Appl Physiol 29:475–479, 1970.
7. Rechtschaffen A, Kales A: "A Manual of Standardized Terminology, Techniques, and Scoring System for Sleep Stages of Human Subjects." Los Angeles: BIS/BRI, University of California at Los Angeles, 1968, pp 4–11.
8. Read DJC: A clinical method for assessing the ventilatory response to carbon dioxide. Aust Ann Med 16:20–32, 1967.
9. Reivich M, Isaacs G, Evarts E, Kety S: The effect of slow wave sleep and REM sleep on regional cerebral blood flow in cats. J Neurochem 15:301–306, 1968.
10. Read DJC, Leigh J: Blood-brain tissue P_{CO_2} relationships and ventilation during rebreathing. J Appl Physiol 23:53–70, 1967.
11. Rebuck AS, Campbell EJM: A clinical method for assessing the ventilatory response to hypoxia. Am Rev Respir Dis 109:345–350, 1974.
12. Phillipson EA, Hickey RF, Graf PD, Nadel JA: Hering-Breuer inflation reflex and regulation of breathing in conscious dogs. J Appl Physiol 31:746–750, 1971.

13. Fishman NH, Phillipson EA, Nadel JA: Effect of differential vagal cold blockade on breathing pattern in conscious dogs. J Appl Physiol 34:754–758, 1973.

14. Phillipson EA, Murphy E, Kozar LF, Schultze RK: Role of vagal stimuli in exercise ventilation in dogs with experimental pneumonitis. J Appl Physiol 39:76–85, 1975.

15. Seldin DW, Rector FC: The generation and maintenance of metabolic alkalosis. Kidney Int 1:306–321, 1972.

16. Mitchell RA, Berger AJ: Neural regulation of respiration. Am Rev Respir Dis 111: 206–224, 1975.

17. Gardner R Jr, Grossman WI: Normal motor patterns in sleep. In Weitzman E (ed): "Advances in Sleep Research," vol 2. New York: Spectrum, 1976, pp 67–107.

18. Phillipson EA: Regulation of breathing during sleep. Am Rev Respir Dis 115 (Suppl): 217–224, 1977.

19. Lugaresi E, Coccagna G, Mantovani M, Cirignotta F, Ambrosetto G, Baturic P: Hypersomnia with periodic breathing: Periodic apneas and alveolar hypoventilation during sleep. Bull Physiopathol Respir 8:1103–1113, 1972.

20. Guilleminault C, Tilkian A, Dement WC: The sleep apnea syndromes. Annu Rev Med 27:465–484, 1976.

21. Mellins RB, Balfour HH Jr, Turino GM, Winters RW: Failure of automatic control of ventilation. Medicine 49:487–504, 1970.

22. Shannon DC, Marsland DW, Gould JB, Callahan B, Todres ID, Dennis J: Central hypoventilation during quiet sleep in two infants. Pediatrics 57:342–346, 1976.

23. Hobson JA: The cellular basis of sleep cycle control. In Weitzman E (ed): "Advances in Sleep Research," vol 1. New York: Spectrum, 1974, pp 217–250.

DISCUSSION FOLLOWING DR PHILLIPSON'S PRESENTATION

Dr Krieger noted that the degree of respiratory slowing induced by vagal blockade in these studies was considerably greater than is generally reported in cats or dogs. Dr Phillipson pointed out that most other studies of vagal blockade or vagotomy had been done in anesthetized or decerebrate animals and that these conditions are by no means comparable to slow-wave sleep (SWS). Thus, although anesthesia and sleep both abolish voluntary conscious influences on breathing, anesthetics also have additional pharmacological effects that influence breathing. More importantly, the degree of respiratory slowing during SWS was also considerably greater than is observed following vagal blockade in awake dogs, pointing out the important stimulating influence of wakefulness on breathing. In the same vein Dr Severinghaus noted the absence of apneustic breathing during SWS when the respiratory frequencies were very slow. Dr Phillipson agreed and pointed out that apneustic breathing may also be an artifact of anesthesia or decerebration. For example, St. John [1] demonstrated that cats with pneumotaxic center lesions and vagotomy had apneustic breathing when anesthetized but not when conscious.

Dr Weil expressed surprise at the lack of effect of metabolic alkalosis on breathing during REM sleep, in view of the intact ventilatory response to hypoxia during REM sleep and the fact that alkalosis should have attenuated this response. Dr Phillipson replied that these observations were not incompatible in that under normoxic conditions ventilation during REM sleep was not being driven by the peripheral chemoreceptors, as evidenced by the general lack of effect of hyperoxia on breathing during this stage of sleep. Furthermore, in one dog surgical denervation of the peripheral chemoreceptors also did not produce any noticeable effect on breathing during REM sleep. It is only during prolonged apneas in REM sleep, during which hypoxia may develop, that peripheral chemoreceptor drive is of importance in that it serves to terminate such apneas.

Dr Weitzman inquired as to whether the dogs increase their respiratory frequency when they awaken from sleep with their vagus nerves blocked. Dr. Phillipson replied that they do, from an average of 3–4 breaths/min during SWS to 8–10 breaths/min during wakefulness. Furthermore, with external stimuli such as sudden noises the respiratory rate may increase further and become irregular, similar to the changes noted during REM sleep with the vagi blocked. In reply to Dr Severinghaus, Dr Phillipson pointed out that vagal blockade also does not prevent panting in the dogs.

Dr Severinghaus wondered whether the dogs could be kept "permanently apneic" in SWS if their pCO_2 levels were kept low and they were given high amounts of O_2. Dr Phillipson replied that this possibility had not been examined in the dogs during sleep, but that the awake dog with intact vagi does demonstrate post-hyperventilation apnea, despite the fact that vagal impulses provide a major respiratory drive in dogs. Thus he concluded that elimination of sufficient afferent respiratory stimuli, whether vagal or chemical, can result in prolonged apnea – ie, a failure to initiate inspiration.

Dr Lugaresi speculated about the neural structures involved in the changes in responses to respiratory stimuli during REM sleep and suggested that the hypothalamus might be involved. Dr Phillipson indicated that homeothermic temperature-regulating mechanisms also appear to be suspended during REM sleep, and these changes do appear to involve hypothalamic integrative mechanisms [2]. Thus a number of autonomic homeostatic mechanisms are suspended during REM sleep. However, there are limits to these changes. For example, in the case of respiratory control, once pCO_2 reaches excessive values, REM sleep appears to be terminated abruptly.

Dr Guilleminault commented on the great increase in respiratory variability coincident with the phasic muscular activity of REM sleep. This phasic muscular activity in cats and dogs is well correlated with bursts of ponto-geniculo-occipital (PGO) waves. He suggested that it would be of interest to implant recording electrodes in the pons or lateral geniculate of the dogs and to correlate changes in respiratory pattern during REM sleep with bursts of PGO waves.

Dr Phillipson concluded by pointing out the broader physiological implications of his studies. Specifically the profound slowing of respiratory frequency to as low as one breath per minute as a result of the combination of SWS, hyperoxia, vagal blockade, and metabolic alkalosis (Fig 9) indicates that afferent respiratory stimuli are of critical importance in the maintenance of respiratory rhythmicity and that the brain stem respiratory centers may not have an intrinsic autorhythmicity.

REFERENCES TO DISCUSSION

1. St. John WM: Rhythmic respiration in awake vagotomized cats with chronic pneumotaxic area lesions. Respir Physiol 15:233–244, 1972.
2. Parmeggiani PL, Franzini C, Lenzi P: Respiratory frequency as a function of preoptic temperature during sleep. Brain Res 111:253–260, 1976.

5
Some Observations on Breathing During Sleep in the Cat

John Orem

INTRODUCTION

This chapter deals with observations which began in 1974 and which originated primarily from William C Dement's and Christian Guilleminault's encouragement that breathing during sleep should be studied in animals as part of an effort to understand the pathophysiology of sleep apnea. In addition to William Dement, who supported the research and in whose laboratory the majority of the work was done, Allan Netick and Jacques Montplaisir initiated and/or participated in various aspects of the research.

In the work to be reported, unanesthetized, nontransected cats implanted with electrodes for chronic recording of sleep-wakefulness parameters [electrooculograms (EOG), electroencephalograms (EEG), electromyograms (EMG)] were subjected to head restraint in a device adapted from a stereotaxic instrument. The restraint was atraumatic and simply involved securing bolts within the skullcap to a head plate on the device. This is illustrated in Figure 1.

Head restraint permitted techniques which would be difficult or impossible otherwise. It allowed single neuron recordings within the brain stem, measurements of airflow rates with a pneumotachograph, simultaneous determinations of breathing and upper airway resistance, and recordings of laryngeal muscle activity in association with breating. The disadvantages can only be imagined since we do not know if restraint produces breathing patterns and neuronal activity in association with breathing. The disadvantages can only be imagined occurs in measures of wakefulness activity. Our wakefulness conditions (adapted restraint) represent a fraction of the spectrum of possible wakefulness conditions. Accordingly, "wakefulness" in the present work should be understood as

Sleep Apnea Syndromes, pages 65–91

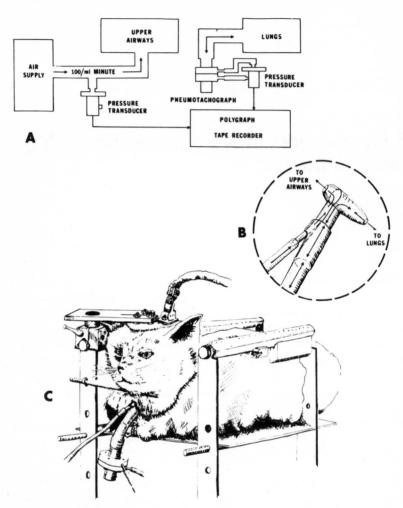

Fig 1. A) Block diagram of the arrangement for recording breathing and upper airway resistance. B) The endotracheal tube which allowed separation of breathing and measurements of upper airway resistance. C) Sketch of the apparatus used for chronic recordings with head restraint.

a condition of central nervous system arousal (desynchronized electroencephalogram) without movements, other than of the eyes, but with a background of tonic electromyographic activity.

The present chapter is generally a description of breathing during sleep in the cat; it is not motivated by any particular theoretical view of the control of breathing. If there is a theme it would be that breathing parameters do not fall along single functions across states but instead describe functions which are unique in each state of consciousness.

BREATHING PATTERNS IN SLEEP AND WAKEFULNESS

Although our interest in breathing during sleep began with recordings of brain stem respiratory neurons [1], as this work progressed it became obvious that a description of breathing patterns was needed. Descriptions of breathing were to come from several sources [2, 3], including ourselves [4]. In our work, the cats were prepared with a chronic tracheal fistula in addition to the other implantation procedures for chronic recordings in the restraint device. The trachea was cannulated through this fistula with a shortened, cuffed endotracheal tube. The tube was connected to a pneumotachograph. Airflow rates, EEGs, EOGs, and EMGs were recorded on a polygraph and on magnetic tape. The pneumotachograph was calibrated with a flow meter, and a CDC 3150 was programmed to determine the frequency of breathing (f), durations of inspiration and expiration (T_I and T_E), peak airflow rate (PF), tidal volume (V_T), and instantaneous minute volume (V_E) for selected episodes of wakefulness (W), non-rapid eye movement (NREM) and rapid eye movement (REM) sleep. The computer also calculated the correlation coefficients between all possible pairs of these variables on a breath-by-breath basis. The study involved seven cats, and a total of 4,735 breaths from wakefulness, 4,493 breaths from NREM, and 4,853 breaths from REM were analyzed.

Frequency of Breathing During Sleep and Wakefulness

Recent reports on the cat [3] and the dog [2] show NREM sleep breathing rates lower than those in W or REM sleep. Early literature on the subject reported that REM sleep involved a more rapid and variable rate of breathing than NREM sleep [5–7]. Human breathing rates purportedly increase [8–10], decrease [11, 12], or are unchanged [8, 13] during sleep.

Our results from the cat are presented in Figure 2. In W, f ranged from 29.9 to 46.0 in the different cats. In NREM, f dropped to average rates 6–18 cycles/min (or 31.2% ± 0.7) less than the W rate. The lowest average rate in NREM was 19.5/min while the highest was 30.2/min. In REM, there was an increase in f to rates which overall exceeded W rates. Mean f in REM varied from 29.6 to 55.9 breaths/min.

The general form of the frequency changes across states corresponds to the data of Phillipson et al [2] and Remmers et al [3], but there is disagreement as to how T_I and T_E change. We found that state-dependent changes in f derived from changes in both T_I and T_E (Fig 3) and that T_I vs T_E relationships across

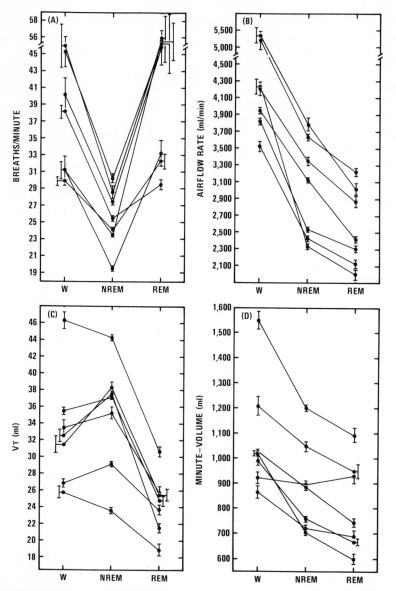

Fig 2. Means and standard errors of the mean for the rate of breathing (A), peak inspiratory airflow rate (B), tidal volume (C) and minute volume (D) for each of seven cats during wakefulness (W), non-rapid eye movement (NREM), and rapid eye movement (REM) sleep.

states did not form a single function. There was a progressive increase in the inspiratory portion of the total cycle (T_I/T_{TOT}) from W to NREM and then to REM. Figure 3 shows regression lines plotted from T_I and T_E relationships in W,

NREM, and REM for one cat. The important thing is that the NREM points lie to the right of the W points on the T_I vs T_E plot and that similarly, the REM points lie to the right of the NREM points on the axis defined by the perpendicular to an isofrequency line. Accordingly, the same frequency was obtained in the different states by different T_I vs T_E combinations. Phillipson et al [2] show a small increase in the T_I/T_{TOT} ratio in REM compared to W, and although Remmers et al [3] report that in REM sleep T_I and T_E are equivalent to wakefulness values, their Figure 3 shows average spirograms which indicate a much higher T_I/T_{TOT} ratio in REM.

Increases and decreases in the rate of breathing during sleep-wakefulness coincide with elevations and declines in body temperature. In NREM there is a decreased hypothalamic and body temperature [14, 15], and in REM hypothalamic temperature increases to near wakefulness levels [15]. Incremented frequencies of breathing in response to elevated body temperatures are well known [16–21], so possibly the changes in the rate of breathing during different states of sleep-wakefulness derive from changes in body temperature or from changes in central mechanisms common to breathing rate and body temperature.

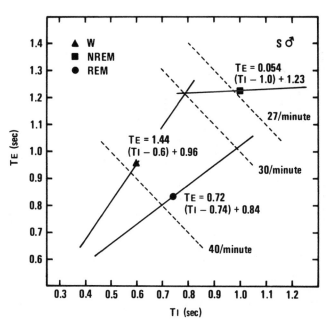

Fig 3. Regressions about the mean for the relationship between T_I and T_E during W (triangle), NREM (square), and REM (circle) sleep. Dotted lines are isofrequency lines. Note that different frequencies were attained in W, NREM, and REM by different T_I vs T_E combinations. The data shown here are from one cat.

Several studies have described V_T vs f, Hering-Breuer curves [19–23]. These curves show a positive relationship between V_T and f which indicates a progressive decrease in the threshold of the inspiratory off switch with time from the onset of inspiration. In an analysis of the relationship between V_T and f within and across states of consciousness, we consistently failed to find a positive V_T vs f relationship (Fig 4). Instead, within each state there was a negative V_T vs f correlation. The average product moment correlation coefficient across all cats in W was –0.47; in NREM it was –0.30, and in REM, –0.62. The effect of the negative relationship between f and V_T was a stabilization of minute volume within each state. A similar relationship has been described for conscious man [24], and Bradley et al [21] have noted that with constant chemical drive the V_T vs T_I relationship is mainly distributed in a direction crossways to the volume-threshold curve.

We attempted to obtain a volume-threshold curve by varying chemical drive during sleep and wakefulness. For this we used a series of added dead spaces and observed ventilation during the sleep-wakefulness cycle (see [4] for details). The

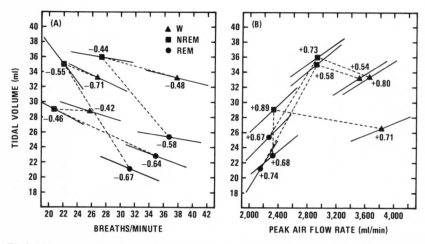

Fig 4. Means, regression lines, and correlation coefficients showing the relationship between tidal volume and rate of breathing (A) and between tidal volume and peak inspiratory airflow rate (B) during W, NREM, and REM sleep. A and B are plots of data from three different cats. The sessions plotted were the same for A and B. The data from the individual cats are connected by the dashed lines. Regression lines are drawn around the mean values (symbols) and the correlation coefficients from a breath-by-breath analysis are shown near the symbols. Note that there is a negative relationship between tidal volume and frequency of breathing (A) and a positive relationship between peak inspiratory airflow rate and tidal volume (B) for breath-by-breath respiration within W, NREM, and REM, but that these relationship do not form monotonic functions across states.

results from two cats are shown in Figure 5. Figure 5A shows a positive relationship between V_T and f during NREM with the 18- to 64-ml dead spaces. In W, up to the 46-ml dead space there was a negative V_T vs f relationship and in REM

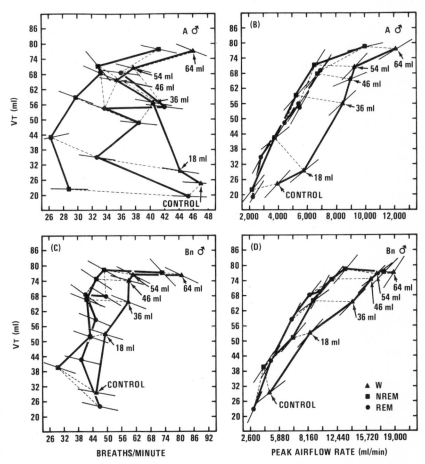

Fig 5. The relationship between tidal volume and rate of breathing (A and C) and between tidal volume and peak inspiratory airflow rate (B and D) under control conditions and with added dead spaces. A and B are data from one cat; C and D are data from another. The wakefulness means under each condition are shown as triangles, the means for NREM sleep are shown as squares, and the means for REM sleep are circles. Regressions around the mean for each state and condition are shown as thin, solid lines. The dashed lines interconnect data from the different states under the same dead space. Note that while the relationship between the rate of breathing and tidal volume is irregular (A and C), there is a consistent and clear positive relationship between peak inspiratory airflow rate and tidal volume both within each state on a breath-by-breath basis and across dead spaces.

there was no systematic relationship between these variables. The negative regression between V_T and f was seen from a breath-by-breath analysis at each level of ventilatory drive. Part C illustrates the V_T vs f relationship across dead spaces for another cat. There is an indication of a positive V_T vs f relationship during W and NREM, but not during REM. The frequency changes are small until tidal volume attained a maximum value. With the 64-ml tube there was a dramatic increase in frequency. In the cat shown in Figure 5C, it was not possible to obtain REM sleep with the 64-ml dead space. With this amount of dead space, a reduction in the amplitude of the EEG and suppression of EMG activity were seen, and there was no indication of sleep. Presumably when there is a dramatic increase in frequency of breathing, with tidal volume at its maximum, the animals are near the point at which sleep is no longer possible, either because of the strategy involved to cope with the dead space or because of a narcosis from hypercapnia and hypoxia.

Phillipson et al [2] and Remmers et al [3] have shown that vagotomy does not alter the frequency changes characteristic of W, NREM, and REM. Both groups have concluded that the frequency changes during sleep derive from central mechanisms rather than vagal reflexes. The nature of the central mechanism is unknown. Cohen and Hugelin [25] and Hugelin and Cohen [26] demonstrated that midbrain reticular stimulation increased the slope, decreased the duration, and increased the overall integrated activity of the phrenic nerve. Andersen and Sears [27], and Pitts et al [28] before them, stimulated the medullary reticular formation and produced inspiratory or expiratory facilitation, depending on the site stimulated. From these experiments, Andersen and Sears propose tonic, presumably reticulospinal, influences on respiratory motoneurons. Recently we have recorded medial medullary reticular neurons which are tonically active only during REM sleep and whose rate of discharge is positively correlated with the rate of breathing in that state [29]. These cells are the first example of possible tonic respiratory neurons, and in view of the influence of state on respiration, it is notable that they are also state specific. The positive correlation between the discharge rate of the medullary neurons and the rate of breathing suggests that they may be part of the neural circuitry which controls the cycle length of the rhythmic generator during REM sleep. A further discussion of these cells is presented in the last section of the chapter.

Peak Airflow Rates During Sleep and Wakefulness

In the factor analyses of breathing during sleep and wakefulness (used to obtain the correlation matrices) a volume and frequency factor consistently emerged from the data. Peak airflow rate (PF) was the most heavily loaded variable of the volume factor, ie, it was most highly correlated with this factor. The PF was highest in W and lowest in REM (Fig 2). In the different cats, mean

PF varied from 3.5 to 5.3 liters/min during W. The NREM PFs averaged 1.3 liters/min less than those in W ($30 \pm 8.3\%$ less). Mean REM PF values were on the average 0.5 liters/min less than the NREM values ($14.8 \pm 4.9\%$ less).

The larger PFs in W derived partially from a late inspiratory effort. This was seen as a sharp peak on the flow curve just at the end of inspiration. In NREM and REM this late inspiratory effort was absent or was substantially reduced.

In contrast to the unpredictable V_T vs f relationship across dead spaces (see above) there was a systematic positive relationship between PF and V_T across dead spaces as well as within each state when computed on a breath-by-breath basis (Figures 4 and 5).

Remmers et al [3] note that the mean inspiratory flow rate during REM was sometimes less than in W and NREM. They found no differences between the patterns of diaphragmatic activation in sleep and wakefulness and concluded that lesser average flow rates in REM may derive from a loss of costal breathing in that state [3]. Remmers and his colleagues interpret the changes in breathing patterns during NREM to be due to "a single fundamental alteration: a delay in the I—E phase transition. This implies that the recruitment pattern of inspiratory motor units is virtually identical in the awake and SWS conditions and that a larger end-inspiratory volume is achieved in SWS because the progressive activation is permitted to evolve over a longer period" ([3], p 236). They continue: "REMS causes by some mechanism a reversal of the action of SWS on I—E phase transition. Here, too, the effect appears to be an isolated one, leaving the diaphragmatic activation patterns and the expiratory flow rate uninfluenced for the most part."

The only point in all of this with which our data agree is that the longer inspiratory pull during NREM (SWS) accounts for the increased tidal volume during that state. Our disagreements are as follows: 1) the T_I vs T_E relationship we see in REM is not a "reversal of the action of SWS on I—E phase transition." As already indicated, the T_I vs T_E relationships are unique in W, NREM, and REM. From W to NREM there is an increase in the T_I/T_{TOT} ratio, and similarly this ratio increases from NREM to REM. 2) Remmers et al [3] contend that the pattern of activation of the diaphragm is equivalent in sleep and wakefulness. In contrast we see systematic changes in the airflow tracings in W, NREM, and REM. In particular there appears a late inspiratory effort which is progressively reduced and lost in NREM and REM (Fig 6). Clark and Euler [23] working with anesthetized cats noted that in the high volume range (range 3) there was sometimes an increase in volume in combination with an increase in T_I exceeding values predicted from range 2. They note: "The extra volume increase could often be observed as a small "bump" on the peak of the volume wave form or as in a few cat experiments, as a sudden increase in phrenic activity just prior to the termination of inspiration" ([23], p 281). From this we would tend to believe that the late inspiratory effort derives from diaphramagic contraction

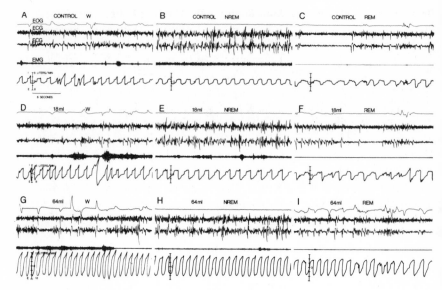

Fig 6. Polygraphic recordings of breathing during W, NREM, and REM sleep under control conditions (A–C) and with an 18-ml (D–F) and a 64-ml (G–I) added dead space. All records are from the same cat. EOG) Electrooculogram; EMG) electromyographic activity from the nuchal muscles. Inspiration is upward on the flow-rate tracings. Note that the large inspiratory peak flows during wakefulness are achieved by a secondary inspiratory effort occurring at the end of inspiration. These secondary efforts which create a late peak on the airflow tracings are generally absent in NREM and REM.

and that the pattern of activation of the diaphragm would differ, at least with respect to a possible late inspiratory activation in W, NREM, and REM.

Our interest in peak flow developed serendipitously. This factor emerged in the correlation matrices as an elemental volume factor which correlated highly with tidal and minute volumes. The average correlation coefficient for peak flow and tidal volume was +0.70 in wakefulness, +0.71 in NREM, and +0.59 in REM. Beyond this, it seemed that the rate of airflow must depend upon the force of contraction of the respiratory muscles (assuming other factors, eg, airway resistances, are constant). The force of contraction of the respiratory muscles in turn depends upon mechanisms of temporal and spatial summation of excitatory and inhibitory inputs to respiratory motoneurons. Accordingly, peak flow appears as an indication of inspiratory effort which declines fairly monotonically from W to REM sleep.

Tidal Volume and Minute Volume During Sleep and Wakefulness

Tidal volume (V_T) depends on the rate of airflow and duration of airflow. In W, airflow rates were high (as judged from PF) but the duration of this flow was short. In NREM, airflow rate decreased, but the duration of the flow was sufficiently long to produce a mean V_T which was slightly greater than that during W. In REM, airflow rate was below NREM levels, and the duration of airflow was shorter. This combination of reduced airflow rates and short airflow duration in REM produced a V_T which was less than those during W and NREM (Fig 2). Minute volume declined during sleep (Fig 2). In all but one case, mean minute-volume was less in REM than in NREM.

Phillipson et al [2] and Remmers et al [3] report similar changes in tidal volume during sleep-wakefulness in the dog and the cat, respectively, but there is controversy regarding changes in V_T during sleep in humans. Some authors argue that sleep involves a reduction in V_T [9, 11, 31] but Duron [10] reports that tidal volume is large in W, smaller in NREM, and large again in REM. Duron contends that it is important to obtain a measure of respiration during relaxed wakefulness to compare to sleeping values. Although we have no basis for stating that our animals were "relaxed" when awake, they were fully adapted to the apparatus at the time recordings were made. In several cases we studied breathing parameters during drowsiness. Drowsiness was classified as a mixture of EEG synchronization and desynchronization with continuing muscle tone and occasional eye movements. In this state breathing parameters had values intermediate between W and NREM values, so it is unlikely that the direction of our results derived from an excited wakefulness state in which there was surplus respiration.

There are major discrepancies in reported instantaneous minute volumes during sleep and wakefulness. Duron [10] reports an increased minute volume during NREM sleep while other authors have reported a decrease [9, 11, 13, 31, 32]. Similarly, we found a decrease in average instantaneous minute volume during sleep with lowest values occurring in REM sleep. In contrast Phillipson et al [2] in dog and Hathorn [33] and Bolton and Herman [34] in human neonates reported increased average instantaneous minute volumes in REM sleep. The contradiction between these studies derives in part from the hypothetical nature of instantaneous minute volume. When average minute volume is calculated as the product of average tidal volume and average frequency (60/mean T_{TOT}) in three of our seven cats, minute volume is larger in REM than in NREM and in all cases the differences between REM and NREM is smaller. However the average over all of the cats shows a minute volume which is less in REM than in NREM while the average over the data of Phillipson et al [2], which we have calculated in the same way (mean tidal volume times 60/mean T_{TOT}), shows a larger minute volume in REM. The real contradiction between the present results and those of Phillipson et al [2] is over the degree of tidal volume and frequency changes during REM and NREM sleep. In their study frequencies were more than twice as high in REM as in NREM, and tidal volume declined only 16% in REM. In our study, frequencies were 1.6 times higher in REM than in NREM, but tidal volume declined 30% in REM. In view of the occurrence of shallow rapid breaths in REM, low end-tidal CO_2 tensions may result from tidal flows insufficient to show true alveolar CO_2 tensions. Blood gas measurements will eventually resolve these discrepancies.

Conclusions

Each breath consists of 1) airflow rates of 2) a certain duration. The combination of these accounts for the tidal and minute volumes. State of consciousness exerts a powerful influence on both flow rate and the duration of this flow. In our experiments, increased ventilatory drive primarily influenced flow rates; the frequency generator seemed primarily determined by state. Indeed, in REM, frequency was essentially immutable.

UPPER AIRWAY RESISTANCE (UAR) AND LARYNGEAL FUNCTION DURING SLEEP AND WAKEFULNESS

The most common clinical sleep apnea is an obstructive apnea in which, despite diaphragmatic contractions, no air flows through the upper airways. Unusual anatomical features of the upper airways, for example enlarged tonsils and adenoids [35–37] or infiltration of fat into the base of the tongue, have been implicated in some cases of obstructive sleep apnea, but these features are neither necessary nor sufficient to produce obstruction in other cases. This implies a functional obstruction somewhere in the upper airways.

We wondered if normal animals showed a tendency for obstruction during sleep. A T-shaped tube was inserted through the chronic fistula into the trachea (see Fig 1). Each arm of the T was hollow, and each was isolated from the other. The base of the T was also hollow and divided. This allowed separation of breathing through one arm and one-half of the T, while the other arm was used to measure UAR. A constant stream of humidified air (100 ml/min) was directed through the upper airways, and the back pressure on this stream (compared to atmospheric pressure) was measured with a Statham pm 97 pressure transducer connected to the bridge circuit of a dc amplifier. The low flow rate was necessitated by the salivation and swallowing elicited at higher flow rates. Following each recording session, the back pressures were calibrated using a manometer. These pressure changes and the known flow rate of 100 ml/min were used to calculate resistance expressed as cm H_2O/liter/sec. In all experiments the mouth was held closed. Prelaryngeal breathing was measured with a pneumotachograph. Eye movements, electrocorticograms, nuchal EMG activity, breathing, and upper airway pressure were recorded simultaneously on a polygraph and an FM tape recorder. For data analysis, episodes of W, NREM, and REM were played back and digitized at a 20-millisecond sampling rate. A computer calculated the mean level of UAR and the amplitude of the UAR changes during each respiratory cycle. A complete account of this work presented elsewhere [38].

The results of these experiments are shown in Figure 7. In W, the average level of upper airway resistance was low. With the onset of drowsiness and sleep, baseline UAR increased. The average increase in baseline UAR over wakefulness levels varied from 6.8 to 21.7 cm H_2O/liter/sec. During REM sleep, baseline resistance was variable but remained at high levels.

Figure 7 also shows that there are fluctuations in UAR during each respiratory cycle. During inspiration, UAR decreases, and these drops in resistance were

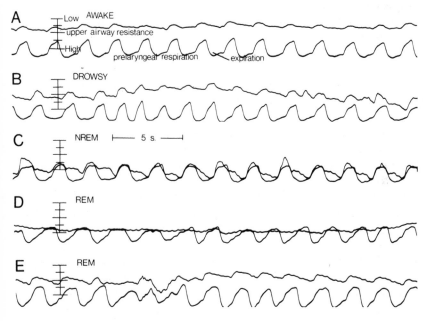

Fig 7. Tracings of upper airway back pressure (resistance) and breathing during wakefulness (A), drowsiness (B), NREM (C), and REM sleep (D and E). In wakefulness UAR was low (tracings are in the upper portion of record) and modulations with each respiration were small. In drowsiness (B), there were fluctuations in the level of UAR. Changes in level generally occurred as small changes over several successive expiratory phases. In NREM sleep, UAR was at high levels (tracings are situated at lower portions of the record), but modulations with each respiration were large. In REM, baseline UAR remained at generally high levels although there was variability (D and E), and respiratory modulations were absent (D) or small (E).

larger in NREM (when baseline resistance was high) than in W (when baseline resistance was low). In REM, the modulations with inspiration were small and were intermittently absent.

Several factors can contribute to UAR changes. Changes in the head-on-neck angle can influence the patency of the upper airways. This was held constant in our study. Engorgement of the nasal tissues with blood may increase UAR during sleep. Nasal resistance represents the greater portion of human UAR with the mouth closed [39] and blood pressure decreases during sleep [7, 40, 41]. However blood pressure changes cannot account for respiratory-modulated UAR changes, and it seems likely that other factors are involved.

Hyperventilation and CO_2 administration produce an increased dilation of the glottis in humans [42] and anesthetized cats [43]. In unanesthetized cats there is a drop in UAR with CO_2 administration. It seemed possible that the changes in UAR during wakefulness and sleep involved similar dilations and contractions at pharyngeal, laryngeal, and nasal levels. The similarity of the pressure changes during increasing hypercapnea (see [43], Fig 3) to those in going from sleep to wakefulness was striking. In wakefulness, modulations with each respiratory cycle were small, such as those seen during hypercapnia; in NREM there was a large inspiratory drop in pressure similar to the drop from high expiratory levels seen in normocapnia in the anesthetized cat. The decreased UAR during hypercapnia was associated with prolongation of intrinsic laryngeal abductor EMG activity (from the posterior cricoarytenoid muscles) into expiration [43, 44].

To test the hypothesis that changes in laryngeal function account for the changes in UAR, the electromyographic activity of the posterior cricoarytenoid muscles was recorded in six adult cats. A transglottic approach was used for placement of the electrodes. Electrode wires were inserted through the barrel of a 25 gauge needle and the exposed tips were bent back away from the beveled point of the hypodermic needle. The needle was inserted through the ventral face of the cricoid cartilage, across the glottis, and through the dorsal aspect of the cricoid cartilage. The hypodermic needle was then withdrawn leaving the exposed wire in the posterior cricoarytenoid muscle. Electrodes were also placed in expiratory laryngeal muscles by puncturing the thyroid cartilage. All electrode wires were led subcutaneously to the head cap. Posterior cricoarytenoid activity during W, NREM, and REM was electronically integrated. The durations of inspiration and expiration were measured and posterior cricoarytenoid activity was determined as activity per unit time during expiration and inspiration. A summary of the data is presented in Figure 8.

The posterior cricoarytenoid (PCA) muscles are inspiratory. They serve to open the glottis just prior to and during inspiration to allow unimpeded influx of air into the trachea and lungs. *During wakefulness,* the EMG activity from the PCA muscles shows intense bursts of activity beginning about 90 milliseconds before the onset of inspiratory airflow and continuing through inspiration. In addition during wakefulness there is a substantial amount of activity persisting during expiration. At the end of expiration, PCA activity is minimal; the activation prior to inspiration occurs and the cycle repeats. *During NREM sleep,* there is a decrease in both inspiratory and expiratory PCA activity. The relative decrease in expiratory activity is greater than the decrease in inspiratory activity.

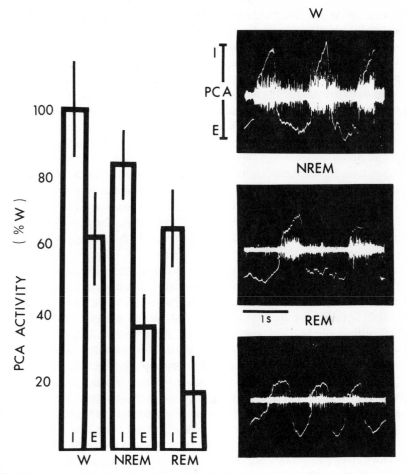

Fig 8. Posterior cricoarytenoid muscle activity during sleep and wakefulness. The histogram provides a summary of PCA activity from nine separate muscle groups during W, NREM, and REM. The data were normalized and expressed as a percentage of wakefulness inspiratory (I) levels. The photographs on the right show PCA muscle activity and breathing during W, NREM, and REM. Inspiration is indicated by an upward deflection of the airflow tracing. I) Inspiration; E) expiration. Note that both tonic or expiratory PCA activity and phasic, inspiratory PCA activity decline during sleep.

In recordings from nine PCA muscle groups in the six cats, the average, integrated wakefulness expiratory activity was 61% of the inspiratory activity. *In NREM,* the inspiratory PCA activity was 84% of wakefulness levels and the expiratory activity was 34% of wakefulness inspiratory activity. *In REM* sleep inspiratory activity averaged 66% of wakefulness levels and expiratory activity was 16% of wakefulness inspiratory levels.

These results show a progressive reduction in laryngeal activity from wakefulness to NREM, and from NREM to REM, and they are consistent with a narrowing of the glottic aperture during sleep. We noted two other features of laryngeal activity which could account for increases in UAR during sleep. First, there was a tendency for the early onset of PCA activity to be delayed during sleep. This, in combination with the weaker abduction during sleep, could lead to a relative obstruction as the weakened larynx works against the developing negative pressure of inspiration. Second, recordings of expiratory laryngeal muscles (adductors) revealed that during NREM *adductor activity sometimes increases.* Accordingly, in NREM as opening efforts are reduced, closing efforts may be increased.

The relationship of these results on the larynx to the pathophysiology of obstructive sleep apnea is uncertain. There is currently much interest on the source of the upper airway obstruction in these cases. Sauerland and Harper [45] recorded a loss of genioglossal activity during sleep. The genioglossus muscle protrudes the tongue and dilates the pharynx. Loss of activity accordingly promotes obstruction. There is a recent report in the literature on fibroscopic observations of a patient with obstructive apnea [46]. The authors report a vocal cord collapse with subsequent complete obstruction of the glottis. This corresponds to the observation that provision of an oropharyngeal airway down to the level of the larynx does not eliminate obstructive episodes [F Eldridge and C Guilleminault, personal communication]. Alternatively, at a recent meeting of the Association for Psychophysiological Study of Sleep, Weitzman and his colleagues [47] presented fibroscopic and fluoroscopic evidence that the obstruction occurs within the pharynx. To quote from the abstract of these authors: "The superior lateral pharyngeal walls are partially or completely closed at the end of an expiration. If partial, a snore will ensue with the next inspiration; if total, the patient will be silent but obstructed and a respiratory effort produces no airflow. At the end of an apnea (eg, 40 sec) and after 10–15 respiratory efforts the lateral pharyngeal walls will open partially and a loud snoring noise and deep respiratory movements will occur with a transient arousal."

The mechanism of upper airway obstruction, whether it be in the larynx as proposed by Krieger et al [46] or in the pharynx as proposed by Weitzman et al and others [47–49] is likely to involve both inactivation of some muscles and activation of others. In the larynx, we sometimes saw an increase in expiratory activity in association with decreased inspiratory activity during NREM sleep.

The increased adductor activity (expiratory) consisted of both an increase during expiration and a tendency for this activity to overlap into inspiration. Similarly, obstruction of the pharynx may involve an imbalance in dilator and constrictor actions. We have observed in anesthetized cats that the pharyngeal constrictors show an activation which augments throughout expiration and halts abruptly at the onset of inspiration. This corresponds with Weitzman's observation that the pharyngeal walls are partially or completely closed at the end of expiration. With the pharynx maximally closed at the end of expiration, the negative pressure of a beginning inspiratory effort, in the absence of activation of the dilators (eg, stylopharyngeus, genioglossus, thyreohyoideus), may close the upper airway.

RECORDINGS OF BRAIN STEM RESPIRATORY NEURONS DURING SLEEP AND WAKEFULNESS

Our interest in breathing during sleep arose primarily from the fortuitous observation of respiratory neurons which lost totally or intermittently their respiratory activity during sleep (Fig 9) [1]. The identity of the neurons was and still is unknown. Their anatomical distribution suggests that they may be related to the accessory respiratory muscles of the upper airways. This would be consistent with inactivation of some of these muscles during sleep (see above).

Action potentials occurring consistently within one or the other phase of the respiratory cycle, or spanning these phases, have been recorded from cells in various regions extending from the caudal medulla to the hypothalamus. Only a small percentage of these respiratory neurons derive their rhythmicity from vagal afference [50]. Some are motoneurons to the laryngeal muscles and the accessory respiratory muscles; and some are involved with efferent transmissions to phrenic and intercostal motoneurons. The latter, projecting axons down the ventrolateral and ventromedial cord, are located caudally in the ventrolateral medulla and in the region of the nucleus of the solitary tract [50–54]. However, it is safe to say that most respiratory neurons oriented as a column extending through the ventrolateral medulla and in the region of the solitary tract, the region of the pontile medial parabrachial and Kolliker-Fuse nucleus and within isolated clusters in pontile and medullary reticular formation, represent systems of unknown interactions whose participation in the respiratory act is uncertain.

In spite of the identification problem, recordings of brain stem respiratory neurons during sleep have provided some interesting information. Our recordings in the normal cat have revealed three distinct mechanisms which produce intermittent, irregular respiration or apnea during sleep [1, 55]. The first, appearing generally in wakefulness and NREM and only rarely in REM sleep, is continuous firing by expiratory neurons following a deep inspiratory effort. This would appear to be a sigh, and it is commonly seen at the transition from W to NREM. The expiratory, apneic phase can last up to ten seconds. The second and third

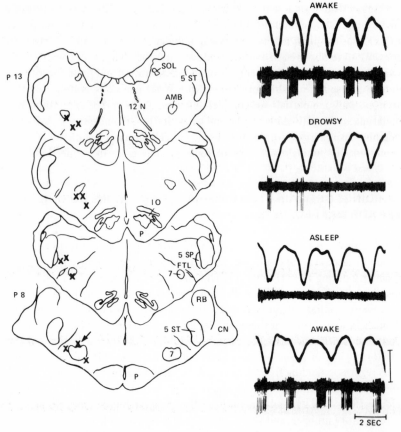

Fig 9. Locations of 12 sleep-sensitive respiratory neurons. Arrow marks the location of the cell whose activity is illustrated on the right. AMB, n. ambiguus; CN, cochlear nucleus, FTL, lateral tegmental field; IO, inferior olive; P, pyramidal tract; RB, restiform body; SOL, solitary tract; 5 SP, nucleus of the spinal tract of V; 5 ST, spinal tract of V; 7, facial nucleus; 12N, hypoglossal nerve.

mechanisms, appearing almost exclusively in REM sleep, are a radical alteration in respiratory rhythmicity and a complete cessation of respiratory effort. The defect in rhythmicity was manifested by erratic bursts associated with irregular breathing. The failure of respiratory drive was inferred from periods of essentially complete neuronal silence. Erratic discharges often alternated with episodes of neuronal silence to produce lengthy episodes of ataxic breathing and apnea.

It has been suggested that supraspinal reflexes derived from intercostal afferents account for the variability in breathing which is often seen in REM [56]. A

reflex role in the irregular and rapid breathing during REM is a matter of empiri-
cal determinations, but it seems unlikely that such reflexes contribute significantly to the breathing patterns of REM. The episodes of irregular breathing
appear as part of a constellation of events deriving from intense central nervous
excitation. They are associated with bursts of eye movements, facial twitches,
and other phasic REM events. Cellular recordings show that REM specific neurons are intensely activated during the irregular breathing episodes (Fig 14)
[29]. Finally, even if there is involvement of a supraspinal reflex, the initiating
events must be central.

A curious finding in our recordings of respiratory neurons involved the
stereotyped respiratory pattern of purring in which laryngeal and diaphragmatic muscle activation occurs in bursts separated by 20–30 milliseconds. The
mechanisms of purring have been described by Remmers and Gautier [57].
Figure 10 shows a single respiratory neuron within the brain stem which showed

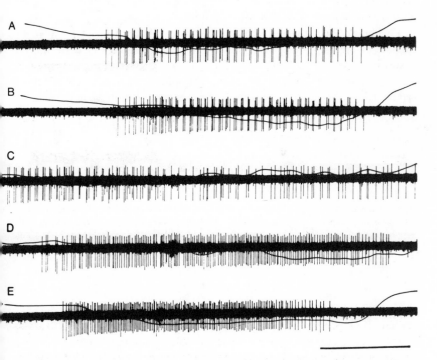

Fig 10. Transition from purring (A–C) to nonpurring (D, E) during NREM sleep. In each
section airflow as measured by a pneumotachograph and the activity of a brain stem respiratory neuron are shown. Downward deflection of the airflow tracing signifies inspiration. The
neuron discharged just before and during inspiration. A–E are consecutive breaths. Note the
transition from a chopped pattern during purring to a more regular pattern during nonpurring. Time calibration: 300 milliseconds.

a chopping of its activity during purring. The neuron was inspiratory and the onset of activity prior to inspiratory airflow suggests that it may be related to the posterior cricoarytenoids which are activated about 90 milliseconds before the diaphragm begins to contract. This figure illustrates a transition from purring to nonpurring, in which A—E represent consecutive breaths. Although it is claimed that purring does not occur in sleep [3], the activity recorded in Figure 10A and B occurred during NREM sleep. We have found that purring can occur throughout NREM sleep, but that at the NREM—REM transition purring stops. The transition to nonpurring illustrated in Figure 10 occurred as the animal was about to enter REM. Breathing was disorganized for approximately two breaths (C and D) as the activity reverted from the chopped pattern (A—C) to the regular pattern of nonpurring. Other neurons were recorded which showed the chopping during purring throughout the respiratory cycle (Fig 11). It would be premature to conclude that the latter represent the central purring oscillatory mechanism proposed by Remmers and Gautier [57] but they are at least consistent with this notion.

Finally, we have observed REM-specific, tonic neurons which were related to the rate of breathing [29]. The characteristics of these neurons were the following:

1) They were observed while recording respiratory neurons between the caudal pole of the facial nucleus and nucleus ambiguus. They were in regions

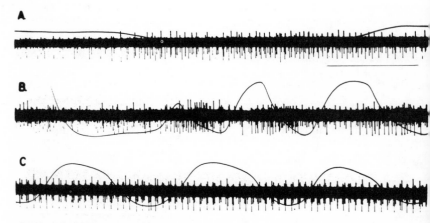

Fig 11. Transition from nonpurring to purring. In each of A, B and C there is an airflow tracing and cellular respiratory activity in the brain stem. A) Nonpurring; inspiratory activity (downward deflection of the airflow tracing) is apparent. B) The animal begins the hyperventilation characteristic of purring and unit activity continues to be phase-locked primarily to inspiration. C) Purring is established, and unit activity is continuous and synchronized into bursts separated by about 30 milliseconds. Time calibration: 300 milliseconds.

medial and dorsal to the retrofacial nucleus which correspond to the medullary region of the lateral and gigantocellular tegmental field. Their action potentials were larger than those of the respiratory neurons.

2) They were silent or only intermittently active during the deep NREM periods preceding REM. At the onset of REM, they began discharging at a gradually accelerating rate for the first few seconds of the REM period. They then reached a level of tonic activity which continued, with modulation through the REM period.

3) Sherman's omega statistic revealed that their pattern of discharge was regular. That is, the variations of the individual interspike intervals from the mean interspike interval were sufficiently small to conclude that the discharges were more evenly spaced in time than if they occurred at random.

4) The rhythmic activity of the cells was modulated throughout the REM periods. Discharge frequencies during each respiratory cycle were positively correlated with the frequencies of the cycles (Figs 12 and 13).

5) The highest discharge rates were associated with bursts of eye movements and the irregular breathing associated with these (Fig 14). This irregular respiration at times consisted of rapid swings of small amplitude around zero airflow. These rapid swings during intense firing of the neurons in part contributed to the positive correlations between rate of respiration and rate of discharge of the neurons.

The REM specificity and tonic regularity of discharge with accelerations during phasic events raise issues of REM generation beyond the scope of this chapter. The important point here is that these cells are in a sense "respiratory." Their tonic discharge rate is positively related to the rate of breathing. Andersen

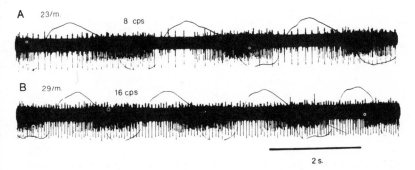

Fig 12. Relationship between the discharge frequency of a REM-specific neuron and rate of respiration. A) The respiration rate is approximately 23/min, and the neuron discharged at a rate of 8 cycles/sec. B) The neuronal discharge rate was 16 cycles/sec, and respiration rate was approximately 29/min. The REM-specific neuron appeared at the onset of REM while recording the phase-spanning expiratory-inspiratory neuron shown in the figure. Downward deflections of the respiration tracings signify inspiration.

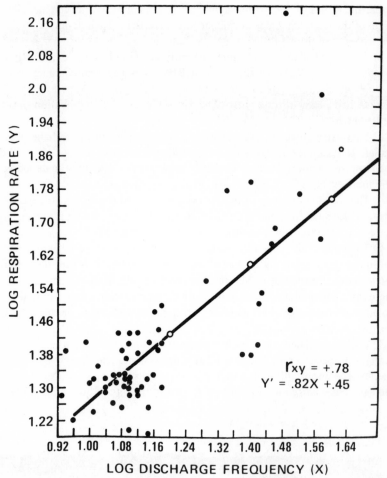

Fig 13. A log-log plot of the rate of breathing against the rate of discharge of a REM-specific neuron. Discharge rate and respiration rate are positively correlated. The presence of two clusters, one at the lower values and one at the higher values, suggests that the positive correlation may derive from a discrete rather than a continuous process.

and Sears [27] and Pitts et al [28] had demonstrated respiratory effects from stimulation of the regions from which these cells were recorded, and tonic influences were postulated to arise from them [27]. In Cohen's theory of the generation of respiratory rhythmicity (for example, Cohen [58]) tonic influences have been proposed, but the present neurons are the first possible example of tonic respiratory neurons. Their state specificity is consistent with the state specificity of breathing patterns.

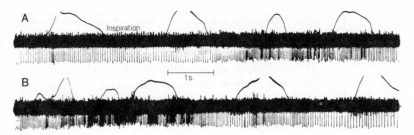

Fig 14. A REM-specific neuron and its relationship to rate of breathing and episodes of irregular or ataxic breathing. A) Discharge rate of the neuron accelerates at the end of the record and breathing rate increases. B) At the beginning, intense activity is associated with irregular breathing.

CONCLUSION

The changes in the central breathing programs as a function of state of consciousness are qualitative. In general, breathing parameters in sleep and wakefulness are not distributed along continua. Instead the central program in each state is distinct, and these programs are evident regardless of the level of ventilatory drive. The respiratory activity of the upper airways is also state-determined.

Although some respiratory neurons are decruited during sleep, there is no clear evidence that a different population of respiratory neurons, each unique in its characteristics, becomes active during W, NREM, and REM. So given that the same population of respiratory neurons is active during sleep and wakefulness, how can the qualitatively different breathing patterns be accounted for?

It has been hypothesized that reticular deactivation is a prerequisite to the appearance of active sleep mechanisms [59]. Reticular deactivation may be equivalent to what has been called the "loss of the wakefulness stimulus" [60]. Fink and his colleagues [60] noted that awake human subjects rendered hypocapnic by overventilation continued to breathe rhythmically with a minute volume one-half to two-thirds of normal. This reduced ventilation persisted unchanged in the presence of a recovering $PaCO_2$ until the latter rose above the CO_2 response theshold. However if the subject fell asleep while the $PaCO_2$ was below threshold, he stopped breathing. The authors concluded "The stimulus for the persistent rhythmic respiration is evidently not CO_2 and it has been provisionally designated the wakefulness stimulus." Experimental support of this notion came from the demonstration that stimulation of midbrain and diencephalic regions which elicit patterns of cortical arousal decreased the duration of expiration and increased the slope and amplitude of integrated phrenic activity [25, 26]. The slower breathing rates and lesser peak flows of

NREM may represent breathing with reticular deactivation (the loss of the wakefulness stimulus). A similar interpretation of the changes in upper airway function is possible. We have found that stimulation of the midbrain reticular formation in anesthetized cats converts laryngeal activity from patterns characteristic of sleep to patterns equivalent to those seen in wakefulness (unpublished observations). The details of the mode of action of the reticular activating system on respiration are unknown. Their elucidation will certainly explain much about the nature of breathing during sleep and wakefulness.

There are aspects of breathing during sleep which cannot be accounted for by a reticular deactivation. In particular the increased rate of breathing in REM, and the ubiquitous irregularities during this state, seem to derive from processes peculiar to REM. Possibly the tonic neurons which discharged specifically in REM at rates positively correlated with the rate of breathing [29] represent this active influence of REM on respiration.

ACKNOWLEDGMENTS

This research was supported by National Institute of Neurological and Communicative Diseases and Stroke grant NS 10727, National Institute of Child Health and Human Development grant HD 08339 and Texas Tech University School of Medicine and the Institute of Biomedical Research grant 12 A501 400000.

REFERENCES

1. Orem J, Montplaisir J, Dement WC: Changes in the activity of respiratory neurons during sleep. Brain Res 82:309–315, 1974.
2. Phillipson EA, Murphy E, Kozar LF: Regulation of respiration in sleeping dogs. J Appl Physiol 40:688–693, 1976.
3. Remmers JE, Bartlett D, Putnam MD: Changes in the respiratory cycle associated with sleep. Respir Physiol 28:227–238, 1976.
4. Orem J, Netick A, Dement WC: Breathing during sleep and wakefulness in the cat. Respir Physiol 30:265–289, 1977.
5. Aserinsky E: Periodic respiratory pattern occurring in conjunction with eye movements during sleep. Science 150:763–766, 1965.
6. Jouvet MF, Michel F, Mounier D: Analyse électroencéphalographique comparée du sommeil physiologique chez le chat et chez l'homme. Rev Neurol 103:189–205, 1960.
7. Snyder F, Hobson JA, Morrison DF, Goldfrank F: Changes in respiration, heart rate, and systolic blood pressure in human sleep. J Appl Physiol 19:417–422, 1964.
8. Reed CI, Kleitman N: Studies on the physiology of sleep. IV. The effect of sleep on respiration. Am J Physiol 75:600–608, 1926.
9. Magnussen G: "Studies on the Respiration during Sleep: A Contribution to the Physiology of Sleep Function." London: Lewis, 1944.

10. Duron B: La fonction respiratoire pendant le sommeil physiologique. Bull Physiopathol Respir 8:1031–1057, 1972.
11. Ostergaard T: The excitability of the respiratory center during sleep and during Evipan anesthesia. Acta Physiol Scand 8:1–15, 1944.
12. Cathala HP, Guillard A: Activité au cours du sommeil physiologique de l'homme. Pathol Biol 9:1357–1375, 1961.
13. Robin ED, Whaley, RD, Crump CH, Travis DM: Alveolar gas tensions, pulmonary ventilation and blood pH during physiological sleep in normal subjects. J Clin Invest 37: 981–989, 1958.
14. Euler C von, Soderberg U: Coordinated changes in temperature thresholds for thermoregulatory reflexes. Acta Physiol Scand 42:112–129, 1958.
15. Parmeggiani PL, Agnati LF, Zamboni G, Cianci T: Hypothalamic temperature during the sleep cycle at different ambient temperatures. Electroencephalogr Clin Neurophysiol 38:589–596, 1975.
16. Haldane JS: The influence of high air temperatures. Int J Hyg Camb 5:494–513, 1905.
17. Cotes JE: The role of body temperature in controlling ventilation during exercise in one normal subject breathing ozygen. J Physiol (London)129:554–563, 1955.
18. Cunningham DJC, O'Riordan JLH: The effect of a rise in the temperature of the body on the respiratory response to carbon dioxide at rest. Q J Exp Physiol 42:329–345, 1957.
19. Hey EN, Loyd BB, Cunningham DJC, Jukes MGM, Bolton DPG: Effects of various respiratory stimuli on the depth and frequency of breathing in man. Respir Physiol 1: 193–205, 1966.
20. Euler C von, Herrero I, Wexler I: Control mechanisms determining rate and depth of respiratory movements. Respir Physiol 10:93–108, 1970.
21. Bradley GW, Euler C von, Marttila I, Roos B: Steady state effects of CO_2 and temperature on the relationship between lung volume and inspiratory duration (Hering-Breuer threshold curve). Acta Physiol Scand 92:351–363, 1974.
22. Grunstein MM, Younes M, Milic-Emili J: Control of tidal volume and respiratory frequencies in anesthetized cats. J Appl Physiol 35:463–476, 1973.
23. Clark FJ, Euler C von: On the regulation of depth and rate of breathing. J Physiol (London) 222:267–295, 1972.
24. Priban IP: An analysis of some short-term patterns of breathing in man at rest. J Physiol (London) 166:425–434, 1963.
25. Cohen MI, Hugelin A: Suprapontine reticular control of intrinsic respiratory mechanisms. Arch Ital Biol 103:317–334, 1965.
26. Hugelin A, Cohen MI: The reticular activating system and respiratory regulation in the cat. Ann N Y Acad Sci 109:586–603, 1963.
27. Andersen P, Sears TA: Medullary activation of intercostal fusimotor and alpha motoneurones. J Physiol (London) 209:739–755, 1970.
28. Pitts RF, Magoun HW, Ranson SW: Localization of the medullary respiratory centers in the cat. Am J Physiol 126:673–688, 1939.
29. Netick A, Orem J, Dement W: Neuronal activity specific to REM sleep and its relationship to breathing. Brain Res 120:197–207, 1977.
30. Parmeggiani PL, Sabattini L: Electromyographic aspects of postural, respiratory and thermoregulatory mechanisms in sleeping cats. Electroencephalogr Clin Neurophysiol 33:1–13, 1972.
31. Birchfield RI, Sieker HO, Heyman A: Alterations in blood gases during natural sleep and narcolepsy. Neurology 8:107–112, 1958.
32. Reed DJ, Kellogg RH: Changes in respiratory response to CO_2 during natural sleep at sea level and at altitude. J Appl Physiol 13:325–330, 1958.

33. Hathorn MKS: The rate and depth of breathing in new-born infants in different sleep states. J Physiol (London) 243:101–113, 1974.
34. Bolton DPG, Herman S: Ventilation and sleep state in the newborn. J Physiol (London) 240:67–77, 1974.
35. Menashe V, Farrehi C, Miller M: Hypoventilation and cor pulmonale due to chronic upper airway obstruction. J Pediatr 67:198–203, 1965.
36. Luke M, Mehrizi A, Folger G, Rowe R: Chronic nasopharyngeal obstruction as cause of cardiomegaly, cor pulmonale, and pulmonary edema. Pediatrics 37:762–768, 1966.
37. Levy A, Tabakin B, Hanson J, Narkewicz R: Hypertrophied adenoids causing pulmonary hypertension and severe congestive heart failure. N Engl J Med 277:506–511, 1967.
38. Orem J, Netick A, Dement WC: Increased upper airway resistance to breathing during sleep in the cat. Electroencephalogr Clin Neurophysiol 43:14–22, 1977.
39. Ferris BG, Mead J, Opie JH: Partitioning of respiratory flow resistance in man. J Appl Physiol 19:653–658, 1964.
40. Candia O, Favale E, Giussani A, Rossi GF: Blood pressure during natural sleep and sleep induced by electrical stimulation of the brain stem reticular formation. Arch Ital Biol 100:216–233, 1962.
41. Kanzow E, Krause D, Kühnel H: Die vasomotorik der Hirnrinde in den Phasen desynchronisierter EEG-Aktivat im natürlichen Schlaf der Katze. Pflüg Arch Ges Physiol 274:593–607, 1962.
42. Hyatt RE, Wilcox RE: Extrathoracic airway resistance in man. J Appl Physiol 16:326–330, 1961.
43. Bartlett D, Remmers JE, Gautier H: Laryngeal regulation of respiratory airflow. Respir Physiol 18:194–204, 1973.
44. Murakami Y, Kirchner JA: Respiratory movements of the vocal cords. An electromyographic study in the cat. Laryngoscope 82:454–467, 1972.
45. Sauerland EK, Harper RM: The human tongue during sleep: Electromyographic activity of the genioglossus muscle. Exp Neurol 51:160–170, 1976.
46. Krieger J, Kurtz D, Roeslin N: Observation fibroscopique directe au cours des apnées hypniques chez un sujet pickwickien. Nouv Presse Med 42:2890, 1976.
47. Weitzman ED, Pollak C, Borowiecki B, Burack B, Shprintzen R, Rakoff S: The hypersomnia sleep-apnea syndrome (HSA): Site and mechanism of upper airway obstruction. Sleep Res 6:182, 1977.
48. Schwartz B, Escande J: Etude cinematrographique de la respiration hypnique Pickwickienne. Rev Neurol 116:667–678, 1967.
49. Guilleminault C, Hill M, Simmons FB, Dement WC: Fiberopticscope studies in obstructive sleep apneic patients. Abstract presented at APSS, Houston, 1977.
50. Euler C von, Hayward JN, Marttila I, Wyman R: Respiratory neurons of the ventrolateral nucleus of the solitary tract of cat: Vagal input, spinal connections and morphological identification. Brain Res 61:1–22, 1973.
51. Merrill EG: The lateral respiratory neurons of the medulla: Their associations with nucleus ambiguus, nucleus retroambigualis, the spinal accessory nucleus and the spinal cord. Brain Res 24:11–28, 1970.
52. Bianchi AL: Localization et étude des neurones réspiratoires bulbaires. Mise en jeu antidromique par stimulation spinale ou vagale. J Physiol (Paris) 63:5–40, 1971.
53. Euler C von, Hayward JN, Marttila I, Wyman RJ: The spinal connections of the inspiratory neurons of the ventrolateral nucleus of the cat's tractus solitarius. Brain Res 61:23–33, 1973.

54. Hukuhara T, Takeda E, Sakai F: Antidromic response of respiratory neurons to electrical stimulation of the spinal cord in relation to their location in the reticular formation of the cat. Proc Int Union Physiol Sci 7:204, 1968.
55. Orem J, Dement WC: Neurophysiological substrates of the changes in respiration during sleep. In Weitzman ED (ed): "Advances in Sleep Research," vol 2. New York: Spectrum, 1975, pp 1–42.
56. Knill R, Bryan AC: An intercostal-phrenic inhibitory reflex in human newborn infants. J Appl Physiol 40:352–356, 1976.
57. Remmers JE, Gautier H: Neural and mechanical mechanisms of feline purring. Respir Physiol 16:351–361, 1972.
58. Cohen ME: The genesis of respiratory rhythmicity. In Umbach W, Koepchen HP (eds): "Central-Rhythmic and Regulation." Stuttgart: Hippokrates-Verlag, 1974, pp 15–35.
59. Moruzzi G: The sleep-waking cycle. Ergeb Physiol 64:1–165, 1972.
60. Fink BR, Hanks EC, Ngai SH, Papper EM: Central regulation of respiration during anesthesia and wakefulness. Ann N Y Acad Sci 109:892–900, 1963.

6
Depression of Intercostal and Abdominal Muscle Activity and Vulnerability to Asphyxia During Active Sleep in the Newborn

David J Henderson-Smart and David JC Read

To the sleep physiologist, irregularity of the breathing rhythm is a useful criterion for the classification of sleep state. To the clinician, this irregularity can be cause for concern, when associated with sleep apnea and its sequelae.

In the preterm baby, recurrent central apnea is a problem commonly encountered [1]. In contrast, the problem of central and obstructive sleep apnea in adults, although well recognized as an entity by the sleep specialist [2], is often overlooked by physicians, possibly due to misleading clinical presentations. Some investigators now believe that disturbances of breathing in sleep also may be important in the genesis of the Sudden Infant Death syndrome [3].

The research we wish to discuss impinges on several of these areas, but particularly focuses on the regulation of breathing in healthy, sleeping babies. In particular, we have investigated the depressed respiratory activity of intercostal and abdominal muscles in active sleep. The consequences of this depression will be examined in relation to lung volume, O_2 stores, and the efficiency of the ventilatory pump, in both normal and impeded breathing.

PARADOXICAL MOTION OF THE RIB CAGE IN THE BABY

We began by simply measuring the rib cage and abdomen/diaphragm movements with mercury-in-rubber strain gauges strapped to the trunk at the level of the nipples and umbilicus respectively. Thirty-eight normal, mature babies in the first 12 weeks of life were studied when supine, clothed, and recently fed. Sleep states were classified as quiet or active from clinical observation, supplemented by records of the extraoculogram in nine babies, using criteria standardized for the newborn [4]: Active and quiet sleep were defined by the

Sleep Apnea Syndromes, pages 93–117

presence or absence, respectively, of limb, facial, or rapid eye movements, irregular breathing, and electrical evidence of rapid eye movements in the extraoculogram. Our respiratory studies were focused on these two states and, in general, were not analyzed for the indeterminate or transitional sleep state.

Similar results were obtained in all babies. Throughout quiet sleep, rib cage expansion and the abdomen/diaphragm descent occurred synchronously during inspiration (Fig 1). With onset of active sleep, asynchronous or paradoxical rib cage movements developed and persisted to a variable degree throughout that sleep phase.

Paradoxical motion of the rib cage, with collapse during inspiration, was known to occur when intrapleural pressure becomes very negative in sick babies with stiff lungs. In our healthy babies a similar state could have arisen from upper airway obstruction developing in active sleep. To assess such a possibility the intrapleural pressure was estimated from an intraesophageal balloon catheter in nine babies. In all babies with these measurements rib cage paradox could be documented when pleural pressure was unchanged, or even diminished (Fig 1). This excluded obstruction and suggested that there must be some change in the rib cage itself, possibly due to loss of muscle tone which is characteristic of postural muscles during active sleep.

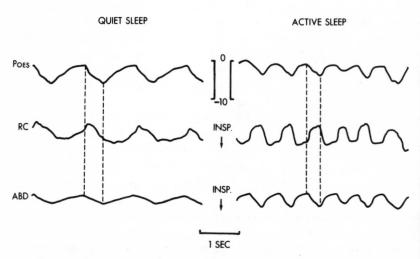

Fig 1. Typical recordings of esophageal pressure (POES), rib cage motion (RC), and abdomen/diaphragm movement (ABD) during quiet and active sleep in a normal baby. Dashed lines have been added to facilitate alignment and show the synchronous movements of rib cage and abdomen/diaphragm in quiet sleep, in contrast with the asynchronous, paradoxical motion of the rib cage in active sleep. Rib cage paradox occurred in active sleep when the negative swings of esophageal pressure were diminished, thus excluding upper airway obstruction as the mechanism.

In order to investigate the dependence of these paradoxical rib cage movements on age, we have commenced a study of older infants and children. So far, we have studied 11 infants between 4 and 9 months old, and two children aged 3 and 5 years; each study examined at least two cycles of active sleep. In contrast to our findings in babies, some of these studies in this older age group showed no rib cage paradox in active sleep; the paradox was absent in both children, and in 2 of the 11 infants. These preliminary results suggest that rib cage paradox may become less prominent with age.

ALTERED RESPIRATORY MUSCLE ACTIVITY RESPONSIBLE FOR RIB CAGE PARADOX IN NEWBORN LAMBS

To obtain direct electromyographic (EMG) recordings of the diaphragm, intercostal, and abdominal muscles, we studied 14 newborn merino lambs. Lambs delivered normally at term were difficult to study because they spent little time asleep and then only very brief periods in active sleep. In contrast preterm lambs proved to be ideal because, when hand-fed and reared by the investigator, they cooperated by sleeping, unsedated, in the laboratory. Like the babies, they spent a considerable part of their sleep time in active sleep. Studies of preterm lambs have only become possible since the discovery that procedures such as corticosteroid administration prior to delivery accelerate maturation of lung surfactant and thereby avoid fatal lung disease. We are indebted to Dr George Alexander for providing 11 such preterm lambs delivered at 132 days, and three delivered at term (149 days).

Bipolar EMG recordings were obtained with wires implanted under local cutaneous anesthesia into the sternal slip of the diaphragm and into the abdominal wall near the level of the umbilicus. The intercostal recordings were obtained by a technique specifically devised for this study. Each set of electrodes consisted of two 26-gauge stainless steel needles passed through a flat piece of rubber. The latter acted as a guard to precisely limit entry depth so the needles could be passed through the intercostal muscles without penetrating the pleura. The method also stabilized the electrodes during respiratory and body movements and thus facilitated holding the same group of muscle units throughout the sleep recording. Because of the small gauge of these needles they could be inserted with little disturbance of the animal and without anesthesia. In view of the findings of Duron [5], our later studies included recordings from both the lateral and the anterior interchondral parts of the intercostal muscles.

Sleep state was recorded clinically in all lambs in a way similar to that used for the babies. In addition, in seven lambs, bipolar recordings of movements of one eye were recorded. The change from quiet to active sleep was easily detected in these lambs because of the many limb, eye, and mouthing movements.

The three term and 11 preterm lambs showed similar results. In quiet sleep, inspiratory changes of the eosphageal pressure, rib cage expansion, and the diaphragm EEG all occurred synchronously (Fig 2). The intercostal EMG recordings revealed activity which was either 1) phasic, being present during inspiration or 2) phase-spanning, usually with more activity during inspiration (Fig 2), but sometimes with little if any respiratory modulation (see Figure 4, upper panel, and Figure 5). Phase-spanning activity occurred most commonly in the lateral intercostals. Abdominal muscle EMG activity also was either 1) phasic, being present during expiration, or 2) phase-spanning or "tonic," with or without augmentation during expiration.

During active sleep all lambs developed rib cage paradox which was similar to that seen in the babies. Intercostal and abdominal muscle activity was depressed throughout active sleep and, in all cases, this occurred at the same time as the rib cage paradox. An example of the change in intercostal activity and the associated rib cage paradox is shown in Figure 2. As in the babies, the para-

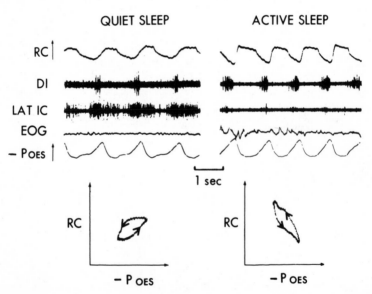

Fig 2. Records from a lamb showing rib cage movements (RC, inflation up), diaphragm (DI) and lateral intercostal EMG activity (LAT IC), eye movements (EOG), and esophageal pressure (POES, negative swings upwards). In quiet sleep the rib cage inflates during inspiration and the intercostal shows both phasic inspiratory and phase-spanning activity. During active sleep, phasic inspiratory intercostal EMG activity is depressed and phase-spanning activity abolished; this is associated with paradoxical rib cage movements. The lower two panels obtained by x-y plots on an oscilloscope from typical breaths in each of the top panels shows the phase change in rib cage movements.

doxical movements occurred under circumstances of unchanged esophageal pressure swings, showing that the paradox was not due to airway obstruction, but to a change in rib cage stability.

At the start of our investigations in the lamb, the major question was: Why did rib cage collapse during inspiration occur in active sleep? When we established that this was related to depressed activity of the intercostals and abdominal muscles rather than to airway obstruction, we decided to examine the activity of these muscles in more detail. Two related questions seemed interesting at this stage. Was there any difference between the control of the lateral and the anterior interchondral portions of intercostal muscles? Were there changes in both the phasic respiratory activities and in phase-spanning or "tonic" activities? These secondary questions were formulated when we became aware of the important observations of Duron on this subject [5].

We have attempted to summarize our current data in relation to these secondary questions in Figure 3, with some illustrative recordings in Figures 4 and 5. Figure 3 is based on our somewhat arbitrary classification of the results obtained from the EMG recordings of 57 sites in the 14 lambs. The method of plotting is presented in the figure legend.

For quiet sleep, comparison of the first and third column of Figure 3 (phasic and phase-spanning) reveals that 1) in general, the anterior intercostals were similar to the diaphragm, showing phasic activity confined to inspiration, and 2) most lateral intercostals and abdominal recordings showed some phase-spanning activity. The phase-spanning activity of the lateral intercostals and the abdominal muscles commonly had inspiratory and expiratory modulation, respectively; such recordings appear as entries on the same line in both columns 1 and 3 of Figure 3.

The depressant effects of active sleep were most marked for abdominal and lateral intercostals; in all cases the phase-spanning activity was lost (column 2 of Fig 3), commonly resulting in the absence of all activity, but occasionally leaving a minor degree of activity in the phase corresponding to the respiratory modulation (column 4, Fig 3; in expiration for abdominals; in inspiration for lateral intercostals). In contrast, the anterior intercostals, although depressed, continued to show some activity in inspiration. The diaphragm activity, although irregular breath by breath, was, in general, unchanged or more active during this sleep phase.

The overall pattern for the pooled results discussed above cannot be attributed to the known gradations of activity at different levels of the rib cage (eg, Fig 5). In five of the lambs, presented in Figure 3, the comparison of activities of anterior and lateral intercostals was based on recordings in the same space; typical traces for two of these lambs are shown in the upper two panels of Figure 4.

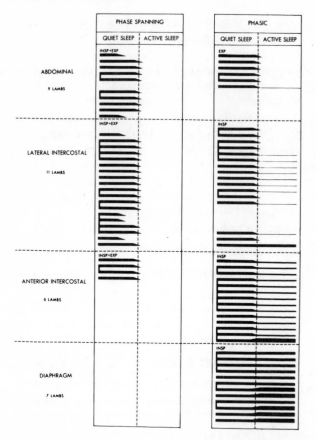

Fig 3. Summary of EMG activities from 57 sites in 14 lambs, comparing quiet and active sleep. The activity of each of the 57 records was classified in quiet sleep as phase-spanning when activity was present either throughout both inspiration and expiration, or for an extended overlap as judged from the records of the rib cage pneumogram or esophageal pressure. When obvious respiratory modulation was present, the site also was classified as phasic. A recording with phase-spanning activity and obvious respiratory modulation appears as bars on the same horizontal line in both panels. Bars representing multiple sites in the same lamb are tied together. The width of each bar provides a crude indicator of changes of activity. The findings are discussed in the text.

ALTERED MUSCLE ACTIVITY ALSO RESPONSIBLE FOR OVERALL DEFLATION OF RIB CAGE

From the viewpoint of our primary interest in the possible vulnerability to asphyxia during sleep, a more important question arose from our observation that there was an overall deflation of the rib cage during the transition from quiet to active sleep. Illustrative recordings are depicted in Figure 5 and discussed in detail in the legend. With overall rib cage collapse, could the lung be similarly deflated? This is discussed later.

DEPRESSED RESPIRATORY RESPONSES TO NASAL OCCLUSION IN THE LAMB

Perhaps the most important question from our viewpoint was whether the depression of intercostal muscles in active sleep persisted during impeded breathing. To answer this we initially occluded the nose of two unanesthetized preterm lambs during repeated sleep cycles.

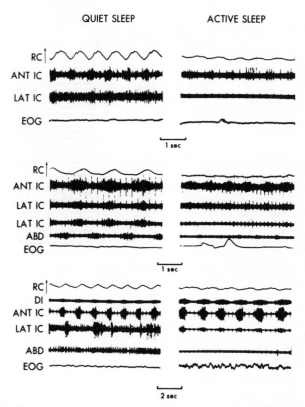

Fig 4. Records from three lambs in which recordings from anterior (ANT IC) and lateral intercostals (LAT IC) were made from the same space. The upper trace shows the typical, more marked depression of lateral intercostals and the loss of all phase-spanning activity in both EMGs in active sleep. The middle panel shows a similar disparity between anterior and lateral intercostals. In this case the phasic lateral intercostal is markedly depressed and resembles the abdominal record (ABD) in this regard. In the lower trace an unusual record is shown to illustrate the increased diaphragm and anterior intercostal EMG activity which occurred. At this time the phasic lateral intercostal activity continues while all its phase-spanning activity ceases along with that in the abdominal EMG. Note the altered rib cage (RC) motion during active sleep in each record.

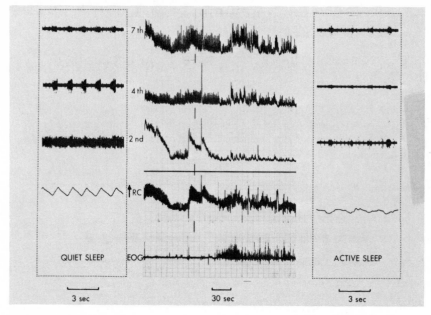

Fig 5. Transition from quiet to active sleep in a newborn lamb with overall rib cage deflation. From the top, recordings of: anterior intercostal EMG in seventh, fourth, and second spaces, rib cage pneumogram (inflation upward), and extraoculogram (EOG). Center panel shows recordings with time compressed by a slow chart speed, the EMG signals having been rectified and processed by a "leaky" integrator. The lateral panels illustrate representative breaths photographed from an oscilloscope on a faster time base; EMG signals as directly recorded. Note the sequence of overall rib cage deflation; reinflation, and subsequent deflation with corresponding changes in the overall activity of the second intercostal; this muscle initially showed phase-spanning "tonic" activity. The marked depression of activity seen in all three muscles with onset of active sleep can be related not only to deflation but to rib cage paradox.

In each of the 21 tests of nasal occlusion for three to ten seconds in quiet sleep, the intercostal EMG activity recorded laterally was greatly augmented from the first impeded breath (Figure 6), and a generalized arousal occurred on 12 occasions, often after only a few occluded breaths (lower panel, Fig 6).

In contrast, during active sleep when the intercostal activity was markedly depressed, no reflex augmentation occurred on any of the 31 tests of nasal occlusion (Fig 6). During the 5 to 12 seconds of each occlusion no attempt was made by the lamb to breathe through the mouth. In only 2 of the 31 tests in active sleep did arousal occur, one at 10 seconds and the other at 12 seconds. One occlusion was maintained for 30 seconds without arousal or return of intercostal muscle activity.

More recent experiments in four preterm lambs confirmed this lack of augmentation of intercostal activity from the first obstructed breath and the delayed arousal during active sleep. However, they indicated a difference between lateral and anterior intercostals in the breath-by-breath augmentation. Whereas the lateral intercostals showed no augmentation at all, the anterior group, like the diaphragm, did at times show breath-by-breath augmentation (Fig 7, upper panel). This variability can be seen when comparing the diaphragmatic responses in the upper and lower panels of Figure 6 and the anterior intercostals in Figure 7.

OVERALL RIB CAGE COLLAPSE DURING ACTIVE SLEEP IN BABIES

In our initial studies of newborn babies we noted that not only did the rib cage move paradoxically in active sleep, but that it deflated overall. In 35 of our

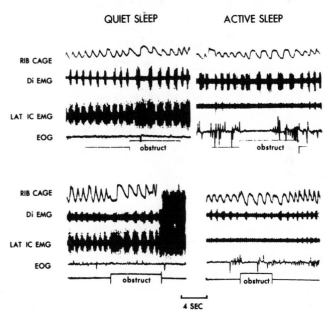

Fig 6. Impaired reflex defense against complete nasal obstruction during active sleep in a newborn lamb. Two tests in quiet sleep, two in active sleep; rib cage pneumogram, inflation upwards. During quiet sleep, lateral intercostal (LAT IC) EMG activity was augmented at the first impeded breath; the test of the lower left panel shows an arousal which frequently occurred in quiet sleep. In active sleep, no reflex, or breath-by-breath augmentation of the intercostal activity occurred; the response of diaphragm activity (Di) to obstruction was variable, sometimes being increased as in quiet sleep, sometimes being reduced. Note increased rib cage (RC) collapse during obstruction in active sleep.

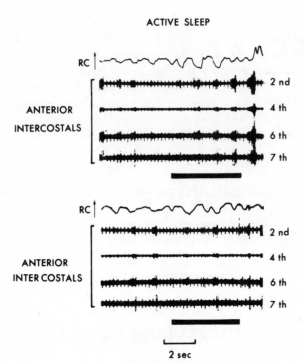

Fig 7. Variable responses of anterior intercostal EMGs to two nasal occlusion tests in the same newborn lamb. Solid horizontal bar marks obstruction. Upper panel shows breath-by-breath augmentation, attributed to chemoreceptors, which was seen at times in this muscle group. No reflex augmentation was apparent at the first obstructed breath.

38 healthy term infants, technically satisfactory records allowed comparisons of the relative rib cage position in the two sleep states. On every occasion the overall resting position diminished.

In ten of these babies, aged between 1 and 16 weeks, we specifically followed the rib cage position and phase relationships throughout the sleep cycle by x-y plotting the rib cage and abdomen/diaphragm movements on an oscilloscope. Typical results in a 10-week-old baby are shown in Figure 8. In addition to the marked looping of the traces in active sleep, it can be seen that the overall inflation of the rib cage decreased at the onset of quiet sleep and then more markedly in active sleep.

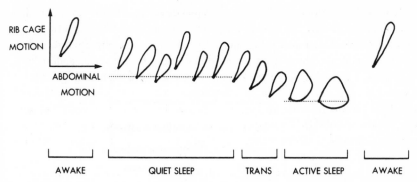

RIB CAGE
MOTION

ABDOMINAL
MOTION

| AWAKE | QUIET SLEEP | TRANS | ACTIVE SLEEP | AWAKE |

Fig 8. Typical breaths traced from an oscilloscope throughout a sleep cycle in a 10-week-old baby showing changes in overall rib cage position and phase relationship. The x-y plots of rib cage and abdominal motion were separated by manual adjustment of the horizontal and intensity controls of the oscilloscope; the rib cage calibration was not altered in any way. The records demonstrate increased looping and rib cage paradox in active sleep and more marked overall deflation of the rib cage at that time. Recovery of the rib cage position on awakening confirms that the changes were not due to any instrumental artifact.

LUNG DEFLATION AND REDUCED OXYGEN STORES DURING ACTIVE SLEEP IN BABIES

These findings of overall rib cage deflation suggested that the lungs could also be deflated in active sleep, leading to reduced oxygen stores and to increased vulnerability to asphyxia. This concept fitted out previous work [6] in which we found increased fluctuations in arterial oxygen saturation and extremely rapid falls in these levels during even brief apnea in active sleep. However, by observation of the rib cage alone, we could not be confident that lung volume changed, because compensatory diaphragm descent might offset any rib cage collapse; examination of previous records in 31 term babies showed that the amplitude of abdomen/diaphragm movements was increased in 29 and unchanged in 2, and the resting position was largely unchanged or varied in its direction of change.

In our most recent work we resolved this question by measuring thoracic gas volume (TGV) directly by occlusion plethysomography in six healthy term babies between 2 and 17 days old. We used the oscilloscope method of Dubois [7] with a nasal mask of silicone putty which limited dead space to 4 ml. Three measurements of thoracic gas volume were obtained in each sleep phase; periods of active or quiet sleep were determined from clinical observation and from the presence of asynchronous or synchronous pen deflections of the rib cage and abdominal pneumograms. The latter also were recorded on FM-magnetic tape, for later playback at a slow paper speed. This produced a compressed record to which was added a phase score for motion of the rib cage versus abdomen/ diaphragm; a five-point score was obtained by inspecting the breath-by-breath x-y plot of rib cage and abdominal movements on an oscilloscope (Fig 9) and transferred to the recorder by a stepping switch. During this scoring the observer was unaware of the sleep state or the nature of the compressed recording being produced. A typical record is shown in Figure 10, which is discussed in detail in the legend.

In each baby, there was a highly significant change in TGV in active sleep (Fig 11). The average reduction was 31% and for the pooled data there was a highly significant difference between active and quiet sleep ($P < 0.001$). The change in lung volume did not appear to be related to the duration of sleep in this brief one- to two-hour period, because the order of testing was random, and, in addition, three babies had measurements in three consecutive sleep states and a similar alteration in TGV occurred with each state change.

The increased abdomen/diaphragm excursion shown in Figure 10 occurred in each baby during active sleep and indicated increased diaphragm shortening in that sleep phase, confirming our earlier experiments in babies.

ASSESSING THE INFLUENCE OF ABDOMINAL MUSCLE TONE DURING SLEEP IN BABIES

With depression of tonic and phasic activity in intercostal muscles it is not difficult to understand how paradox could develop in the intrinsically compliant rib cage which is characteristic of early postnatal life.

On first consideration, it is less obvious that a loss of abdominal muscle tone during active sleep may play a role in the overall deflation and paradoxical motion of the rib cage. However, Goldman and Mead [8], in a study of the relaxation pressure/volume relationships in conscious adult man, concluded that there is an inflating effect of the diaphragm on the rib cage. Abdominal strapping in these experiments could be inferred to increase the resting diaphragmatic tension and to exert an upward pull on the lower rib cage, producing rib cage inflation. Their analysis indicated that abdominal pressure was a major factor determining rib cage position under these special circumstances.

Loss of abdominal muscle tone during active sleep in our babies thus might partly explain the overall collapse and paradoxical motion of the rib cage. These changes might be expected if diaphragm descent was unimpeded, abdominal pressure was reduced, and the upwards pull on the lower rib cage was lost.

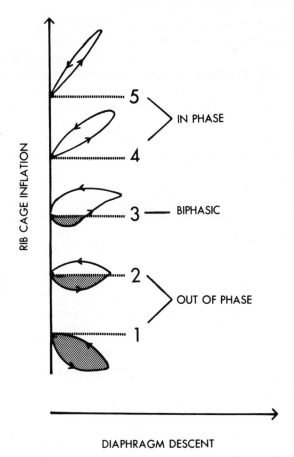

Fig 9. Scoring system for phasic rib cage movements in relation to diaphragm descent in the baby. Typical records traced from an oscilloscope.

To examine this proposition, seven babies were studied during sleep to determine the relationship between rib cage collapse and abdominal pressure. During active sleep abdominal muscle tone was simulated by inflating a 4-cm-wide blood pressure cuff, previously placed around the lower abdomen with care being taken to avoid the rib cage. Responses were assessed from the rib cage pneumogram and the abdominal and intrapleural pressures, as assessed from intragastric and intraesophageal balloon catheters; sleep state was defined clinically, with an extraoculogram in three babies.

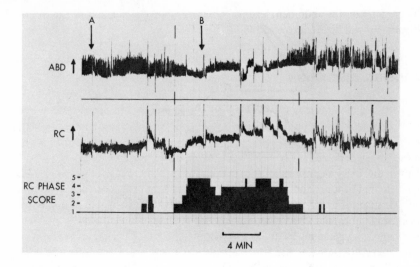

Fig 10. Illustration of the experimental conditions in which thoracic gas volume was measured during active sleep (A) and quiet sleep (B). These records of the abdomen/diaphragm (ABD) and rib cage (RC) pneumograms were played back from FM tape and simultaneously assigned a five-point phase score (see Fig 9) from inspection of an x-y oscilloscope display. These records confirmed the sleep state classification made at the time of testing. Note also the correspondence between the phase score and the changes in the pneumogram records.

On each of 45 occasions in seven babies, inflation of the pressure cuff around the abdomen resulted in an increase in the resting rib cage position to a level similar to that seen in quiet sleep. the rib cage remained in this state until deflation of the cuff, when it returned to its previous collapsed position. There was no observable alteration in sleep state during any of the tests analyzed; on three occasions arousal occurred and these tests were discarded.

The abdominal pressure, which was recorded in 20 tests on four babies, increased on all occasions during abdominal strapping; the range of pressure increment was $0-5$ to 5, with a mean of 3 cm H_2O. Esophageal pressure was recorded during ten tests in three babies and revealed no significant change of intrapleural pressure, thus excluding change of pressure across the rib cage as the basis for the change. The rib cage expansion thus can be attributed to an increased transdiaphragmatic pressure and associated upward pull of the diaphragm on the lower rib cage. These findings are illustrated in Figures 12 and 13, and the technical details are discussed in the legends.

Our experiments suggest that abdominal muscle tone and abdominal pressure may have important roles in stabilizing the rib cage. Under normal circumstances it is possible that, in the prone position, the rib cage could be similarly stabilized by pressure on the abdomen, leading to improved mechanical advantage to the diaphragm and maintenance of lung volume.

GENERAL DISCUSSION

Our studies in healthy newborn babies and lambs were initiated when we observed paradoxical deflation of the rib cage during active sleep. The recording of esophageal pressure in both babies and lambs excluded sudden onset of upper airway obstruction in active sleep as the cause of this rib cage paradox. In the lambs, the EMG recordings established that the rib cage paradox was associated with depressed tonic and phasic activity of intercostal and abdominal muscles. To our surprise this depression persisted when inspiration was prevented by nasal occlusion during the active sleep state; in other states, powerful load-compensating reflexes augmented by the chemoreceptors, with reflex arousal. These chemoreceptor defenses also were depressed in active sleep. Overall, active sleep would seem to lead to increased vulnerability to asphyxial conditions since it was associated with inefficient ventilation due to rib cage paradox, with overall lung deflation and reduced O_2 stores and with depressed proprioceptive and chemoreceptive reflexes.

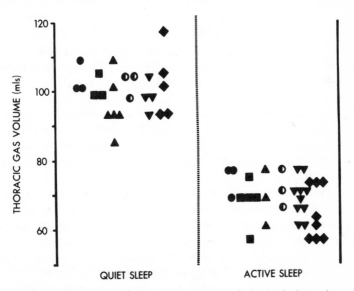

Fig 11. Individual measurements of thoracic gas volume in six babies during active and quiet sleep, showing the variability of measurements in each baby and the overall marked difference between the two sleep states. A different symbol is used for each baby.

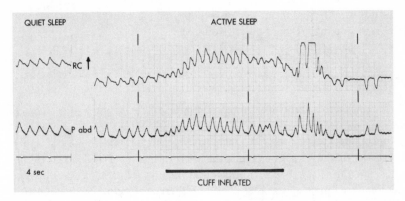

Fig 12. Restoration of overall rib cage to the position of quiet sleep when abdomen was strapped in active sleep in a healthy newborn baby. Rib cage pneumogram (RC) inflation upwards; abdominal pressure recorded by intragastric balloon catheter, -0 to $+20$ cm H_2O, full scale deflection. Note the rib cage deflation and development of paradoxical motion with the change from quiet sleep (left panel) to active sleep (beginning of traces in right panel), and the subsequent sequence of reinflation and deflation of the rib cage when abdominal pressure was changed by the cuff.

Our various findings will now be discussed in relation to the possible underlying mechanisms and to other studies in the literature. Many of our observations can be linked to both historical and current reports. Rib cage paradox in babies has been widely recpgnized in the past in association with lung disease [9]. A few authors such as Howard and Bauer in 1949 [10] and Miller and Behrle in 1952 [11] have described intermittent, paradoxical rib cage motion in a variety of babies, many of whom were probably normal. These early papers do not relate the findings to different sleep phases.

In the current literature, the association between active sleep and rib cage paradox in healthy babies has been observed by Knill et al [12] and by Frantz et al [13]. In the paper by Knill et al [12] the published x-y recordings of "rib cage/abdominal" motion for quiet and active sleep are similar to those obtained in our studies [14].

In animals, several studies have analyzed the EMG changes of respiratory muscles in various sleep states. In adult cats, Duron [5] has previously demonstrated EMG changes very similar to those obtained in our newborn lambs: In active sleep, EMG activity disappeared in the external intercostals recorded laterally, whereas the diaphragm and anterior interchondral muscles showed no change. Duron's study emphasized postural roles for the lateral intercostals, and phasic respiratory roles for the anterior interchondral muscles. He related these differing roles to a higher density of muscle spindles in the lateral intercostals.

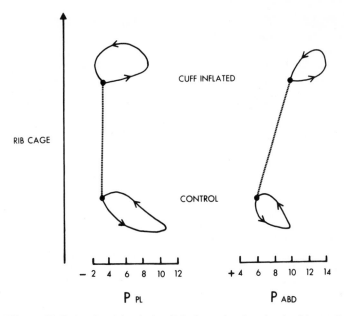

RIB CAGE

CUFF INFLATED

CONTROL

- 2 4 6 8 10 12

P PL

+ 4 6 8 10 12 14

P ABD

Fig 13. Effects of inflating the abdominal cuff during active sleep in a healthy newborn baby. The interrelationships between the rib cage pneumogram, intrapleural (P PL), and intraabdominal (P ABD) pressures are depicted for a typical control breath (lower traces) and for a typical breath with the abdominal cuff inflated (upper traces); P PL and P ABD recorded simultaneously by intraesophageal and intragastric balloon catheters – in centimeters H_2O – in relation to atmospheric pressure. Note that rib cage inflation was associated with more positive abdominal pressures, minimal changes of pleural pressures, and therefore more positive transdiaphragmatic pressures. Arrows indicate the sequence inspiration to expiration and the abolition of rib cage paradox with the use of the abdominal cuff.

Parmeggiani and Sabattini [15] have also reported similar studies in adult cats, for high and low environmental temperatures and for thermoneutral conditions. Active sleep altered hypothalmic unit activity and suppressed both panting and shivering.

Recently, recordings of surface EMG activity of the respiratory muscles of babies have been obtained showing changes in active sleep similar to those found in the cat and lamb [16].

The mechanisms underlying the inhibition of intercostal and abdominal EMG activity during active sleep are likely to be similar to that shown for other non-respiratory spinal motoneurons. In view of the complexity of the mechanisms a detailed review would be unrealistic in the context of the present paper. Elegant accounts by Pompeiano [17] outline the roles of the vestibular projections to both motor and sensory cortex and the changes mediated by parallel pathways descending to spinal levels. These pathways modify the activity of α and γ motoneurons and also the sensory activity, through presynaptic depolarization and inhibition of spinal interneurons. In the present context, the important mechanisms are likely to be the tonic postsynaptic inhibition of spinal motoneurons and the phasic presynaptic inhibition of muscle and cutaneous afferents.

Many, but not all, of the mechanisms associated with active sleep in animals appear to be operating in newborn babies. Prechtl [18] showed that proprioceptive spinal reflexes were tonically depressed in active sleep and phasically abolished during bursts of rapid eye movements. These reflexes showed enhanced activity in quiet sleep, above that in wakefulness.

Our detailed studies of the responses to nasal occlusion in different sleep phases reflected our interest in the vulnerability to an asphyxial death in sleep. This interest was based on Naeye's autopsy evidence for an asphyxial mode of death and for unrecognized asphyxial episodes prior to death in the Sudden Infant Death syndrome [19]. The autopsy studies of Tonkin had focused attention on anatomical obstruction of the upper airways [20]. Nasal obstruction seems particularly important in the newborn period: Swift and Emery [21] pinched the nostrils of sleeping healthy babies and young infants and showed that the switch from nose to mouth breathing was accomplished only with difficulty and delay, at this age. This change to mouth breathing seemed particularly difficult in active sleep.

Other studies in babies confirm the depression of the load-compensating responses during active sleep. Observations were reported by Cross and Lewis [22] when they produced obstruction accidently during plethysmography, by Purcell [23] with unilateral nasal obstruction, by Knill et al [12] with elastic loading and by Frantz et al [13] with occlusion of a face mask.

In the adult dog, Phillipson et al [24] defined the airway pressure and tidal volume responses to elastic loads with and without vagal block, in the awake state and in quiet sleep, but no data were reported for active sleep.

We are unaware of EMG studies of the effects of sleep state on the responses to impeded breathing, in either the adult or newborn, for comparison with our results. An extensive literature, however, exists on the general problem of respiratory reflexes in loaded breathing, which is summarized in several recent monographs and reviews [25–27]. Unfortunately, most of the neurophysiologic studies have been undertaken in anesthetized or decerebrated animals, so little direct information is available on the influence of differing sleep states on the control of respiratory muscles. In the present context, it is possible to highlight only a few points. The intercostal muscles and diaphragm, although subjected to the same central respiratory drives, have rather different proprioceptive controls. The intercostal muscles are richly innervated with muscle spindles and tendon organs; fusimotor drive is strong and involves both tonic and rhythmic units with powerful influences, at least in adult animals. In the newborn animal, these systems seem immature and less powerful, and the vagal system based on pulmonary mechanoreceptors is more prominent at this stage of life [28]. In contrast, the diaphragm has few muscle receptors, with an unusually high proportion of tendon organs; load-compensating reflexes are strongly dependent on vagal mechanisms, and these are well developed at birth. Several other points deserve mention. The excitability of the spinal motoneurons of respiratory muscles is controlled by separate descending pathways from higher centers, as well as by additional intersegmental influences. This allows for the possibility of raising or depressing the overall excitability, independently of the descending central respiratory drive. With overall depression, the alternating respiratory phases of excitation and inhibition detected by intracellular recording [29] may no longer reach the threshold for motoneuron firing or perhaps may reach threshold only for a brief interval in one phase of respiration; with overall excitation, the firing threshold is exceeded throughout all phases of respiration. Such mechanisms presumably account for our observed EMG patterns of phasic and phase-spanning units, and the associated changes in different changes in different sleep states.

The breath-by-breath progression of EMG activity that we observed following nasal occlusion can be attributed to the chemoreceptor responses to progressive asphyxia rather than to varying responses of the proprioceptive systems [30]. The modification of this EMG progression and of the threshold for arousal in active sleep similarly might be attributed to alterations of chemoreceptor systems in different sleep states. Phillipson et al [31] have shown that active sleep depresses the ventilatory responsiveness to hypercapnia in the sleeping adult dog. More recent work from the same laboratory indicates that the ventilatory responsiveness to hypoxia in his adult dogs is not depressed in active sleep, although a greater degree of hypoxemia is required to produce arousal in this sleep state [Phillipson et al, personal communication].

The overall rib cage collapse which we observed in active sleep does not seem to have attracted previous attention. This could possibly be explained by the different recording methods: In our studies we used circumferential mercury in rubber strain gauges strapped to the chest, whereas others [12, 13] have used magnetometers which are prone to drift.

The reduction of lung volume and oxygen stores that we have demonstrated would lead to conditions in which arterial oxygen levels are unstable and liable to fall rapidly during even brief central or obstructive apnea. This is likely to have marked effects in the newborn who already has a low functional residual capacity in relation to metabolic rate [32]. In active sleep, this would be further accentuated by the increased oxygen consumption of that sleep state [33].

Our findings also have important implications for the testing of respiratory reflex responses in different sleep states. In a widely used technique, the pressures and timing of inspiration are recorded following nasal occlusion and used to quantitate reflexes in active and quiet sleep [34]. The interpretation of such tests, however, depends on the assumption that lung volume is unchanged and that the associated mechanical characteristics of the respiratory pump are unaltered. We have shown that these assumptions are incorrect. With the overall change of lung volume, the intrinsic, nonreflex characteristics of the respiratory pump will be altered since the tension developed by a muscle for any level of excitation depends on its initial length, and the pressure developed by the diaphragm at any level of tension depends upon the radius of curvature and thus upon its initial position [35].

Implications for Sleep Apnea

Our results highlight the vulnerability to asphyxia in the newborn baby and young infant during active sleep: Rib cage collapse leads to inefficiency in the ventilatory pump, overall lung volume and O_2 stores are reduced, proprioceptive and chemoreceptive reflex defenses are depressed. The possible relevance of such changes in the genesis of sudden asphyxial death is summarized in Figure 14.

Since all the work is based on normal babies and animals, what missing factor changes a situation of general vulnerability into a fatal episode in an individual baby? Viewed in this way, our work might account for some of the circumstances in which some crib deaths occur, but not the basic defect.

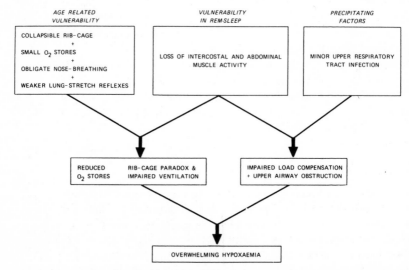

Fig 14. Hypothesis proposed to explain the vulnerability of babies to respiratory failure and overwhelming hypoxemia during sleep and as a possible explanation of the age distribution of crib deaths. (Reprinted with permission: Henderson-Smart DJ, Read DJC: Aust Paediatr J 12:261–266, 1976.)

From our results it could be predicted that apnea in newborn babies would occur most commonly in active sleep, particularly during maximum spinal inhibition. Furthermore, either central or obstructive apnea would be more likely to result in severe hypoxemia because of reduced O_2 stores and delayed arousal in that sleep state. In studies on preterm babies by Gabriel et al and by Schulte and co-workers, this expected result has been found [37, 38]. In our babies, prolonged apneas with cyanosis and bradycardia and all apneas lasting more than ten seconds occurred most commonly in active sleep and particularly at the time of maximal spinal inhibition.

In addition to the direct spinal inhibition of respiratory motoneurons in active sleep documented in our study, a more important mechanism responsible for central apnea is likely to be the inhibition of spinal excitatory afferents [17] to the brain stem reticular formation. Cohen [39], in a study of the high frequency oscillations in the activity of brain stem inspiratory neurons, has emphasized the part played by tonic excitatory input in maintaining the inspiratory burst activity. We have previously shown that the characteristics of the brain stem respiratory oscillator may be altered in the newborn animal [40], and this could explain a dependency on excitatory afferents to initiate and maintain inspiratory activity.

To our knowledge there are no studies in the adult that relate intercostal muscle activity to rib cage movements or oxygen stores. The excessive rates of oxygen desaturation in adult sleep apnea, discussed by Weil in Chapter 7 of this volume, suggest to us that decreases in lung volume may occur. This could be due to sleeping in the supine position [41] or obesity [42], both common findings in sleep apnea patients.

Our results have focused on the differences between quiet and active sleep; however, we have noted overall rib cage collapse (Fig 8) and decreased tonic intercostal EMG activity [unpublished] during the transition from wakefulness to quiet sleep. Lung volume could be decreasing at this time: This should be tested in both the newborns and adults.

ACKNOWLEDGMENTS

We wish to thank the parents of our subjects, and Consultant Staff of King George V Hospital and the Royal Alexandra Hospital for permission to undertake the baby studies. DJ Henderson-Smart is in receipt of an NH & MRC Research Studentship and that body, the Asthma Foundation of New South Wales, the Postgraduate Medical Foundation of Sydney, and Burnard Sunley Charitable Foundation, London, provided the equipment. Dr E Burnard made available the infant plethysmograph and the Division of Animal Production, CSIRO, provided the lambs.

REFERENCES

1. Kattwinkel J; Neonatal apnea: Pathogenesis and therapy. J Pediatr 90:342–347, 1977.
2. Guilleminault C, Tilkian A, Dement WC: The sleep apnea syndromes. Annu Rev Med 27:465–484, 1976.
3. McGinty DJ, Harper RM: Sleep physiology and SIDS: Animal and human studies. In Robinson RR (ed): "SIDS 1974." Toronto: The Canadian Foundation for the Study of Infant Death, 1974, pp 201–229.
4. Anders T, Emde R, Parmelee A (eds): "A Manual of Standardized Terminology, Techniques and Criteria for the Scoring of States of Sleep and Wakefulness in Newborn Infants." Los Angeles: BIS, UCLA, 1971.
5. Duron B: Postural and ventilatory functions of intercostal muscles. Acta Neurobiol Exp 33:355–380, 1973.
6. Henderson-Smart DJ, Storey B, Read DJC: Recurrent apnea and cyanosis in newborn babies. Aust Paediatr J 12:205, 1976.
7. DuBois AR, Botelho SY, Bedell GN, Marshall R, Comroe JH Jr: A rapid plethysmographic method for measuring thoracic gas volume: A comparison with the nitrogen washout method for measuring functional residual capacity in normal subjects. J Clin Invest 35:322–326, 1956.
8. Goldman MD, Mead J: Mechanical interaction between the diaphragm and rib-cage. J Appl Physiol 35:197–204, 1973.
9. Avery ME, Fletcher BD: "The Lung and Its Disorders in the Newborn Infant," vol I. Philadelphia: WB Saunders, 1974.
10. Howard PJ, Bauer AR: Irregularities of breathing in the newborn period. Am J Dis Child 77:592–609, 1949.
11. Miller HC, Behrle FC: Respiratory patterns in newborn infants as determined by airflow and pneumographic studies and their possible relationship to a deficient vagal mechanism. Pediatrics 10:272–284, 1952.
12. Knill R, Andrews W, Bryan AC, Bryan MH: Respiratory load compensation in infants. J Appl Physiol 40:357–361, 1976.
13. Frantz ID III, Adler SM, Abroms IF, Thach BT: Respiratory response to airway occlusion in infants: Sleep state and maturation. J Appl Physiol 41:634–638, 1976.
14. Henderson-Smart DJ, Read DJC: Depression of respiratory muscles and defective responses to nasal obstruction during active sleep in the newborn. Aust Paediatr J 12: 261–266, 1976.
15. Parmeggiani PL, Sabattini L: Electromyographic aspects of postural, respiratory and thermoregulatory mechanisms in sleeping cats. Electroencephalogr Clin Neurophysiol 33:1–13, 1972.
16. Hagan R, Bryan AC, Bryan MH, Gulston G: The effect of sleep state on intercostal muscle activity and RC motion. Physiologist 19:214, 1976.
17. Pompeiano O: Vestibular influences during sleep. In Kornhuber H (ed): "Handbook of Sensory Physiology," vol VI/1. Berlin: Springer-Verlag, 1974, pp 583–622.
18. Prechtl HFR: Patterns of reflex behavior related to sleep in the human infant. In Clemente CD, Purpura DP, Mayer FE (eds): "Sleep and the Maturing Nervous System." New York: Academic Press, 1972.
19. Naeye RL, Fisher R, Ryser M, Whalen P: Carotid body abnormalities in the sudden infant death syndrome. Science 191:567–569, 1976.
20. Tonkin S: Sudden infant death syndrome: Hypothesis of causation. Pediatrics 55: 650–660, 1975.

21. Swift PGF, Emery JL: Clinical observations on response to nasal occlusion in infancy. Arch Dis Child 48:947–951, 1973.
22. Cross KW, Lewis SR: Upper respiratory obstruction and cot death. Arch Dis Child 46: 211–213, 1971.
23. Purcell M: Response in the newborn to raised upper airway resistance. Arch Dis Child 51:602–607, 1976.
24. Phillipson EA, Kozar LF, Murphy E: Respiratory load compensation in awake and sleeping dogs. J Appl Physiol 40:895–901, 1976.
25. von Euler C: The role of proprioceptive afferents in the control of respiratory muscles. Acta Neurobiol Exp 33:329–341, 1971.
26. Remmers JE, Marttila I: Action of intercostal muscle afferents on the respiratory rhythm of anesthetized cats. Respir Physiol 24:31–41, 1975.
27. Davis JN: Control of the muscles of breathing. In Widdicombe JG (ed): "MTP International Review of Science Physiology, Series One," vol 2. Baltimore: University Park Press, 1974, pp 221–245.
28. Schwieler GH: Respiratory regulation during postnatal development in cats and rabbits and some of its morphological substrate. Acta Physiol Scand (Suppl) 304:1–123, 1968.
29. Sear TA: The slow potentials of thoracic respiratory neurones and their relation to breathing. J Physiol 175:404–424, 1964.
30. Callanan D, Read DJC: The role of arterial chemoreceptors in the breath-by-breath augmentation of inspiratory effort in rabbits during airway occlusion or elastic loading. J Physiol 241:33–44, 1974.
31. Phillipson EA, Kozar LF, Rebuck AS, Murphy E: Ventilatory and waking responses to CO_2 in sleeping dogs. Am Rev Respir Dis 115:251–259, 1977.
32. Cook CD, Cherry RB, O'Brien D, Karlberg P, Smith C: Studies of respiratory physiology in the newborn infant. 1. Observations on normal premature and full-term infants. J Clin Invest 34:975–982, 1955.
33. Scopes JW, Ahmed I: Minimal rates of oxygen consumption in sick and premature newborn infants. Arch Dis Child 41:407–416, 1966.
34. Finer NN, Abrams IF, Taeusch HW: Ventilation and sleep states in newborn infants. J Pediatr 89:100–108, 1976.
35. Marshall R: Relationships between stimulus and work of breathing at different lung volumes. J Appl Physiol 17:917–921, 1962.
36. Steinschneider A: The concept of sleep apnea as related to SIDS. In Robinson RR (ed): "SIDS 1974." Toronto: The Canadian Foundation for the Study of Infant Death, 1974, pp 177–190.
37. Gabriel M, Albani M, Schulte FJ: Apneic spells and sleep states in preterm infants. Pediatrics 57:142–147, 1976.
38. Schulte FJ, Busse C, Eichhorn N: Rapid eye movement sleep, motoneurone inhibition and apneic spells in preterm infants. Pediatr Res 11:709–713, 1977.
39. Cohen MI: Synaptic relations between inspiratory neurons. In Duron B (ed): "Respiratory Centres and Afferent Systems." (Abstracts of a Symposium sponsored by INSERM 59:19–29, 1976.) In Bull Eur Physiopathol Respir 12(4):65–100, 1976.
40. Suthers GK, Henderson-Smart DJ, Read DJC: Postnatal changes in the rate of high frequency bursts of inspiratory activity in cats and dogs. Brain Res (in press).
41. Agostoni E, Mead J: Statics of the respiratory system. In Fenn WO, Rahn H (eds): "Handbook of Physiology. Section 3: Respiration," vol I. Washington, DC: American Physiological Society, 1964, pp 387–409.
42. Bedell GN, Wilson WR, Seebolm PM: Pulmonary function in obese persons. J Clin Invest 37:1049–1060, 1958.

DISCUSSION

Dr Phillipson asked about the abdominal cuff experiment, referring to the fact that the rib cage in babies is "floppy," particularly in REM sleep, rather than rigid. Under this condition, he expressed surprise that inflation of the cuff altered the paradoxical motion of the rib cage at all. Dr Henderson-Smart noted that his report dealt with cuff inflation only at the level of the nipples and that measurements with the cuff at a higher level might well show different results. Dr Phillipson also remarked that all the various reasons the infant is vulnerable (developmental, REM-related, etc) lead to overwhelming hypoxemia, but that infants have only very transient ventilatory response to hypoxia and then get outright cerebral depression. Dr Henderson-Smart noted that our knowledge of ventilatory response to hypoxia in the infant is very limited, in fact virtually nonexistent in relation to sleep.

Dr Guilleminault stressed the importance of the developmental issue regarding REM and NREM apnea. In adults REM apnea generally is the worst, but in infants studied by the Stanford group, although there were more periodic breathing and short stop-breathing episodes during REM sleep, the longest and most severe problems occurred during NREM sleep. Dr Henderson-Smart emphasized that although we don't know why apnea occurs in one state or another, it is apparent that the sudden occurrence of an apneic episode while the infant is in a specific state may lead to more rapid development of hypoxemia, vascular changes, and so on. Dr Weitzman agreed that the state of sleep may affect the impact of a apneic episode on other physiological variables. He mentioned that the SIDS research group at Columbia University has reported infants who do not breathe at all during NREM sleep. He added that REM sleep breathing patterns are influenced by a "REM sleep program" and that this superimposed control system makes a long and dangerous apnea less likely despite the inhibition of muscle activity during REM sleep. This supported Dr Phillipson's earlier comments; the hypoxic cerebral depression that develops after a short and transitory response to hypoxia may then interfere with the "REM sleep central program."

Dr Severinghaus commented on the recordings of intercostal muscles that demonstrated a decreased activity during REM sleep. He questioned if these changes had been correlated with other muscle events during sleep such as jaw or leg movements, which would indicate a link to a motor rather than a respiratory center. Dr Henderson-Smart and Dr Read both replied that the intercostal muscle activity fluctuates during REM sleep. Overall, there is a general depression of all intercostal muscles, but if a specific intercostal group, such as the anterior intercostals, is selected, the recorded activity is definitely respiratory. They noted that it would be misleading to link intercostal muscle activity to a motor program unrelated to respiration.

Dr Read remarked how simple it had been a few years ago to teach medical students that the external intercostals were inspiratory and the internals expiratory, but that when an attempt was made to link electrical events to the mechanics, such statements were not clearly valid. Aeronautical engineers studying stress and tensions are challenging the concept of different muscle layers. Many questions remain unanswered at this time.

7
Sleep and Breathing at High Altitude

John V Weil, Meir H Kryger, and Charles H Scoggin

INTRODUCTION

Studies of man at high altitude have enabled physiologists to probe mechanisms of adaptation and maladaptation to hypoxia, both acute and chronic. With few exceptions the focus has been on study of mechanisms in wakefulness with little attention to events during sleep. It has long been known that subjective sleep disturbance is frequent following acute ascent to high altitude, and recent observations which we will describe below led us to suspect that breathing may be abnormal during sleep in long-term high-altitude dwellers. In this paper we describe studies of breathing and hypoxemia during sleep in man following acute ascent to high altitude and in long-term residents of high altitude during sleep at their native altitude. We shall review the background and findings of these acute and chronic studies separately, following which there will be a discussion of both.

ACUTE HIGH ALTITUDE EXPOSURE

Sleep disturbance is one of the most common features of the syndrome of acute mountain sickness, which regularly occurs during the first day or two following ascent to high altitude [1]. Subjectively, one is aware of frequent awakenings throughout the night related to the sensation of not having breathed. This is followed by several deep breaths and resumption of sleep. Indeed, sleep studies confirm the subjective impressions and show an increased frequency of arousals, usually associated with marked periodic breathing and apneic spells [2]. These effects are generally found to be most marked during the first night at altitude, a

Sleep Apnea Syndromes, pages 119–136

period which corresponds with the most severe changes in blood chemistry, suggesting that the two phenomena may be related. Ascent to high altitude leads to hypoxia, which in turn stimulates an increase in ventilation and this promptly produces hypocapnic alkalosis. Over the next few days, renal compensation leads to increased urinary excretion of bicarbonate and the gradual correction of the alkalosis. Prior to compensation, alkalosis exerts a significant inhibitory effect on breathing, and perhaps even more important, has been shown to attenuate the ventilatory responsiveness to hypoxia [3]. A transient attenuation of hypoxic ventilatory drive, attributable to hyperventilation-induced alkalosis could play a permissive role in the development of hypoxemia during sleep. No studies have yet defined the effect on arterial oxygenation of the sleep apneas seen in normal subjects at high altitude, nor has the role of alkalosis in producing these abnormalities been assessed.

The carbonic anhydrase inhibitor acetazolamide, when administered prior to high altitude ascent, promotes a bicarbonate diuresis, with resulting metabolic acidosis. This largely prevents the alkalosis of ascent to high altitude [4], and is associated with augmented breathing and decrease in symptoms including disturbed sleep [4, 5]. The influence of such treatment on the quality of sleep and breathing during sleep has not been studied.

Progestational agents such as medroxyprogesterone acetate (MPA) are effective ventilatory stimulants, and are probably responsible for the hyperventilation of pregnancy and the luteal stage of menstruation [6, 7]. Such agents in normal subjects enhance ventilatory responsiveness to hypoxia and hypercapnia [8], and thus might reduce the severity of sleep apnea at altitude. This paper describes our experience with both of these agents in a study of breathing and sleep in normal man at high altitude.

Methods

Six healthy subjects between the ages of 26 and 41 years were studied during sleep on the summit of Mt Evans (elevation 4,300 m). They were studied in pairs on three occasions separated by intervals of three weeks. Prior to each study, subjects received in randomized sequence placebo capsules, acetazolamide (250 mg every eight hours for 36 hours), or medroxyprogesterone acetate (20 mg every eight hours for seven days). Medication was dispensed to the subjects each day for seven days — in the case of acetazolamide, the subjects received placebo for five days and the active drug for the remainder. All capsules were identical in appearance so that neither the subjects nor the investigators knew what was being administered until the study was completed and all data analyzed.

On the day of the study, the subjects arrived on the summit of the mountain between 3:00 and 4:00 PM, and within an hour measurements were made of ventilatory responsiveness to hypoxia and hypercapnia, following which arterial blood samples were taken for baseline high-altitude values. Ventilatory responses to hypoxia were measured with progressive isocapnic hypoxia [9] starting at an alveolar oxygen tension (PAO_2) of 140 mm Hg, and gradually lowering the oxygen tension by addition of nitrogen to the inspired gas until a final PAO_2 of 40 mm Hg was reached. Carbon dioxide was added to the inspired gas in amounts sufficient to prevent the development of hypocapnia. Values are expressed as the shape parameter A which describes the steepness of the increase in ventilation as PAO_2 is decreased. Ventilatory responses to hypercapnia were measured with a hyperoxic rebreathing method as previously described [10], and results were expressed as the slope S of the V_E vs $PACO_2$ relationship.

By 10:00 PM the subjects had been prepared with EEG electrodes, using the international 10-20 system, placed at C3, A2, O2, P4, F3, and F4 locations. Three electrooculogram (EOG) electrodes were attached, one lateral to each eye, and one near the nasion, and three electromyogram (EMG) electrodes were placed under the chin. A circumthoracic transducer was used to record respiratory movement. Physiological data were recorded on a pair of eight-channel Grass model 6 EEG machines at a paper speed of 15 mm/sec. Arterial oxygen saturation (SaO_2) was monitored with a fiber-optic ear oximeter (Hewlett-Packard) previously calibrated with human blood. Using in vitro techniques, we have shown this device to be linear to oxygen saturations as low as 50%. Oximetry and respiratory pattern were recorded both on the EEG machines and on analog magnetic tape. Sleep records were scored following the completion of the study by a reader who did not know the treatment regimen code. Sleep scores were developed for each page (20 sec/page) using conventional criteria [11]. Each awakening was counted as an arousal even if it were less than half a page (ten seconds) in duration. To count as an arousal, EMG activation, eye movements, and alpha activity had to be present. Each page was also scored for the presence or absence of apneas, and, if present, for their duration. In addition, mean arterial oxygen saturations were measured for each page as well as minima and maxima for oxygen saturation when swings were present. Respiratory pattern and SaO_2 were read independently of EEG scoring and before breaking the treatment code. Respiration and SaO_2 were measured for one page (20 seconds) out of every nine (180 seconds), and mean SaO_2 as well as maximum and minimum were recorded. The presence of periodic breathing and duration of apneas were also noted. Statistical analyses were carried out by two-way analysis of variance with Dunnet's test for multiple comparisons.

Results

Following ascent, the untreated (placebo) subjects developed hypoxemia (PaO_2 42.6 ± 1.4 mm Hg) and hypocapnic alkalosis ($PaCO_2$ 31 ± 0.07 mm Hg, pH 7.458 ± 0.004). Hypoxic ventilatory responses were normal by low-altitude standards [2] (parameter A = 187 ± 35) and were uninfluenced by treatment. Hypercapnic response was also normal by low altitude standards (S = 3.5 ± 0.04) and uninfluenced by treatment. Acetazolamide lowered arterial pH (7.369 ± 0.009 vs 7.458 ± 0.004) and moderately raised arterial oxygen tension (47.4 ± 2.1 vs 42.6 ± 1.4 mm Hg). Surprisingly, there was no associated decrease in $PaCO_2$ as is commonly reported [4, 5] — a discrepancy for which we have no obvious explanation. We were also surprised to find no augmentation of hypoxic ventilatory response as would have been anticipated with the removal of the depressant effect of alkalosis [3]. Administration of MPA was associated with a slight lowering of arterial pH (7.425 ± 0.007 vs 7.458 ± 0.004) with no other changes of note.

The most striking abnormality of breathing during sleep at high altitude was episodic sleep apnea seen frequently in five out of the six subjects (see Fig. 1). The majority of these apneas lasted between 8 and 15 seconds, and were associated with oscillations in arterial oxygen saturation, often of greater than 10%. On the average, periodic breathing was noted during 35% of sleep time in the placebo phase, while treatment with acetazolamide and MPA reduced it to 18 and 5%, respectively — both reductions were statistically significant ($P < 0.05$). When arterial oxygen saturation was averaged by sleep stage (Fig 2), hypoxemia was seen to be consistently more severe during placebo, and was improved for all stages during acetazolamide ($P < 0.01$). A lesser but consistent improvement was also seen with MPA ($P < 0.05$). Oscillation of arterial oxygen saturation was greatest during placebo administration in all stages of non-rapid eye movement (NREM) sleep, and was reduced to levels comparable to awake values in rapid eye movement (REM) sleep (Fig 2). Treatment with MPA produced impressive reductions in SaO_2 oscillations for all sleep stages except REM ($P < 0.01$), while acetazolamide had a small but consistent effect ($P < 0.05$). Sleep time with an arterial oxygen saturation of less than 80% was taken as an arbitrary index of the duration of severe hypoxemia, and is shown in Figure 3. This

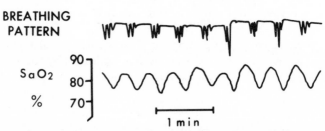

Fig 1. Breathing pattern (circumthoracic strain gauge) and arterial oxygen saturation (ear oximeter) in a typical subject during sleep at high altitude (4,300 m). This pattern seen in five of six subjects included apneic intervals of 8 to 15 seconds duration which were associated with oscillation of arterial oxygen saturation.

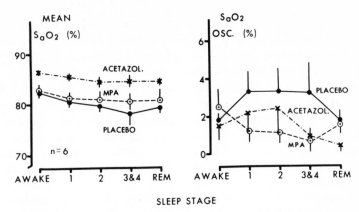

SLEEP STAGE

Fig 2. The left-hand panel shows average arterial oxygen saturation at acute high altitude in relation to sleep stage. During wakefulness and all stages of sleep, arterial oxygen saturation was lowest when the subjects were untreated, and highest following acetazolamide ($P <$ 0.01). MPA had a smaller but consistent effect ($P < 0.05$). The right-hand panel plots oscillation of SaO_2. During all stages this was greatest for placebo and lowest for MPA ($P <$ 0.01) with a smaller but consistent effect noted for acetazolamide ($P < 0.05$).

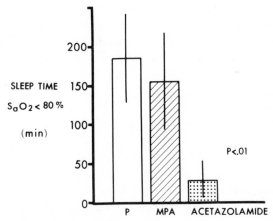

Fig 3. The length of time during which SaO_2 was less than 80% is used as an arbitrary index of the duration of severe hypoxemia. This was slightly and nonsignificantly reduced by MPA, while acetazolamide markedly reduced it ($P < 0.01$).

index was dramatically reduced by acetazolamide ($P < 0.01$) with MPA having no effect. Thus the two drugs had rather different effects on sleep oxygenation. Acetazolamide raised mean arterial oxygen saturation and had a small effect on oscillations, while MPA had a small effect on mean saturation but markedly reduced the amplitude of oscillation. In terms of preventing severe hypoxemia, the effect on mean oxygen saturation appears to be of greater importance than the abolition of oscillations. Neither mean SaO_2, SaO_2 oscillations, nor number or duration of apnea were correlated with hypoxic and hypercapnic ventilatory responses between subjects or between treatments.

No direct comparison was made in this study of the characteristics of sleep at low and high altitude; however, we have previously reported the results of such a comparison and found that ascent to high altitude increases the number of arousals [2]. In the present study an average of 36 arousals per night occurred in the untreated subjects compared with 20 per night at sea level in our previous study. Treatment with MPA did not influence the occurrence of arousals, but acetazolamide reduced them significantly (from 5.2 ± 0.5 to 3.7 ± 0.34 per hour) ($P < 0.01$) to a value similar to that observed previously in subjects of similar age at sea level [2]. There were no other significant changes in sleep stage.

In summary, during acute high-altitude exposure, periodic breathing was found in the majority of subjects and was associated with increased amplitude of oscillation of arterial oxygen saturation and a decrease in average arterial oxygen saturation in all sleep stages. Acetazolamide moderately reduced the amount of periodic breathing, improved average arterial oxygen saturation, and decreased the number of arousals. These changes occurred in the absence of augmentation of ventilatory responsiveness to hypoxia or hypercapnia. While MPA was the most effective agent in reducing periodic breathing, it had much less effect on mean arterial oxygen saturation and no effect on the number of arousals.

CHRONIC HIGH ALTITUDE EXPOSURE

A minority of individuals who have lived for long periods at high altitude develop a syndrome known as chronic mountain sickness, or chronic mountain polycythemia (CMP) [1]. The most prominent manifestations are a markedly elevated hematocrit, lethargy, and inability to think clearly. Some of these patients have very mild lung disease, while in others cardiac or pulmonary function is normal [12]. The elevated hematocrit is a response to excessive hypoxemia [13], which in turn reflects relative hypoventilation — an absence of the usual hyperventilatory response to the hypoxemia of high altitude. In most high-altitude subjects there is a clear correlation between the elevation in hematocrit and the depression in arterial oxygen saturation, but in recent unpublished studies we have been impressed that in some individuals the severity of the polycythemia is disproportionate to the depression of arterial oxygen saturation as measured when these patients were awake. This led to the suspicion that severe hypoxemia may be occurring during sleep. We also wondered about the role of depressed hypoxic ventilatory drive. It is known that prolonged hypoxic exposure leads to a marked attenuation in ventilatory responsiveness to hypoxia and to a lesser extent to hypercapnia. This has been seen in chronic residents of high altitude [14–17], and in individuals with prolonged hypoxemia due to cyanotic congenital heart disease [18, 19]. Thus studies in long-term residents of high altitude offer the opportunity to investigate the relationship between decreased ventilatory drives and breathing disturbances during sleep. In this situation we again made use of the ventilatory stimulant effects of MPA [8, 20] to determine the influence of this agent on drives to breathe and on the hypoxemia of sleep at high altitude.

Methods

The subjects were ten men who were all long-term residents (greater than 20 years) of Leadville, Colorado (elevation 3,100 m). Five had repeatedly documented chronic mountain polycythemia, with hematocrits greater than 60% at some time in the past. Because of recent treatment with phlebotomy by their local physicians, the hematocrit at the time of study was slightly reduced from its peak in most of the subjects. Their average age was 44 years. The other five were normal controls of similar age (46 years) and duration of high-altitude residence. All of the controls were in excellent health and all had repeatedly documented normal hematocrits. Sleep measurements were made on two consecutive nights, with the first night discarded to minimize lab effect. This two-night sequence was done once with each control subject, and twice for each subject with CMP. For the polycythemic patients, a randomized placebo-controlled, double-blind trial was carried out to compare placebo with MPA in a dosage of 10 mg every eight hours for eight days. The placebo and MPA studies were separated by an interval of one month. In all subjects, the sleep studies were preceded by measurement of arterial blood gases and ventilatory response to hypoxia and hypercapnia, as outlined above. The recording and analysis of full-night EEG, respiratory pattern, and oximetry data are described above.

Results

Compared to controls, patients with CMP had elevated hematocrits ($55 \pm 1\%$ vs $48 \pm 1\%$ in controls) ($P < 0.01$) and more severe hypoxemia (PaO_2 44 ± 1.8 mm Hg vs 55 ± 3.0 in controls) ($P < 0.01$). Ventilatory responsiveness to hypoxia was similar for the two groups (parameter A = 71 ± 22 in CMP and 70 ± 20 in controls) and was reduced when compared to normal low-altitude values [10]. Hypercapnic response slopes (S) averaged 1.95 ± 0.46 for CMP and 1.78 ± 0.06 for controls. During sleep, three types of breathing dysrhythmias were seen: undulating respirations of varying amplitude but without true apnea (see Fig 4), periodic breathing with short apneic spells lasting 8–12 seconds, and episodes of gross irregularity of both frequency and amplitude. Of these, the undulant pattern was the most common in both the control and CMP subjects. Breathing dysrhythmia was present during a similar proportion of sleep for both groups (22.6 ± 5% for controls and 25.0 ± 6% for the CMP patients). Despite the similarities in the type and duration of breathing dysrhythmia, there were striking differences in arterial oxygenation during sleep (Fig 5). The differences were of two types: First, mean arterial oxygen saturation was higher in the control subjects than in the polycythemics and, second and more dramatic, the frequent occurrence of brief, but severe, episodes of desaturation in the majority of CMP

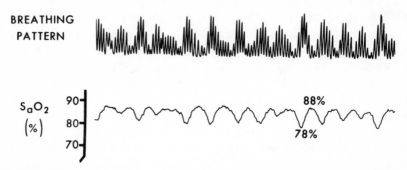

Fig 4. Breathing pattern and arterial oxygen saturation in a subject with chronic mountain polycythemia (CMP) during sleep at his native altitude of 3,100 m. In contrast to the findings at acute high altitude, the breathing pattern was one of undulating depth of breathing, which in the typical CMP subject was associated with oscillation of arterial oxygen saturation.

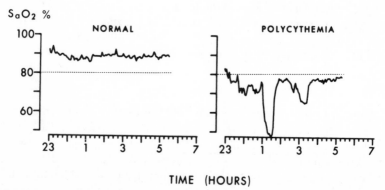

TIME (HOURS)

Fig 5. Arterial oxygen saturation during a whole night's sleep as shown for a control subject and a CMP subject during sleep at high altitude (3,100 m). In the normal subject a high SaO_2 is maintained and is stable, while in the CMP subject, average arterial oxygen saturation is considerably lower and there are episodes of very severe hypoxemia. The dashed line is a reference point drawn at 80% SaO_2 to facilitate comparison.

patients. Mean arterial oxygen saturation (Fig 6) fell during sleep, especially in stages 3 + 4 and REM in both the normal and CMP subjects, but started at a lower value and fell more precipitously in CMP. The duration and distribution of sleep stages were identical for the two groups.

Effects of MPA Administration

Medroxyprogesterone acetate improved daytime arterial oxygenation in association with a decrease in $PaCO_2$ but with no apparent augmentation of ventilatory responsiveness to hypoxia or to hypercapnia. It did not alter the proportion of sleep time with breathing dysrhythmia, which was $25 \pm 6\%$ with placebo compared to $23 \pm 6\%$ during MPA treatment. There was, however, significant improvement in arterial oxygen saturation during sleep stages 2, 3 + 4, and REM (Fig 6). More impressive was the striking abolition of episodes of severe desaturation seen during placebo tests (Fig 7). This may be seen by examining the duration of time spent below a certain level of SaO_2. For this analysis we have chosen an arbitrary SaO_2 value of 80% to make the point that the patients treated with MPA logged much less time with severe hypoxemia (Fig 8). While on placebo, the CMP patients totaled 201 minutes with SaO_2 below 80%, while on MPA this was reduced to 38 minutes ($P < 0.01$). Treatment with MPA altered sleep pattern by reducing stage 3 + 4 sleep from 46± to 27± minutes ($P < 0.05$), and significantly increased stage 2 sleep from 187± to 222± minutes ($P < 0.05$). There were no effects on other aspects of sleep, including sleep efficiency, REM latency, or the amount of REM sleep.

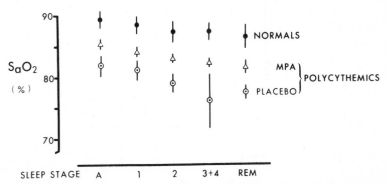

Fig 6. Average arterial oxygen saturation is shown for normal controls and CMP subjects during sleep at 3,100 m. During sleep SaO_2 decreased slightly but significantly when compared to awake values, and was lowest during REM sleep. In untreated CMP subjects, arterial saturation was markedly lower for all stages, especially 3 + 4 and REM. Treatment with MPA produced substantial improvement but left significant residual hypoxemia when compared to the controls.

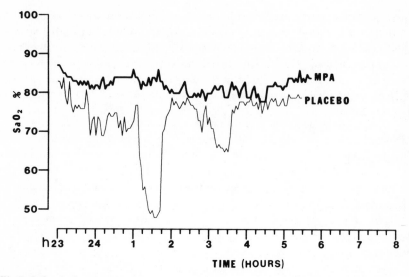

Fig 7. SaO_2 during sleep in a CMP subject before and after treatment with MPA. MPA significantly increased mean arterial oxygen saturation, but more impressive was the complete abolition of the episodes of severe hypoxemia seen without treatment.

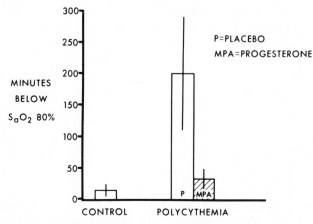

Fig 8. Duration of severe hypoxemia expressed as the time spent with SaO_2 below 80%. There was much more severe hypoxemia in CMP patients than in controls ($P < 0.01$), and this was largely corrected by the administration of MPA ($P < 0.01$).

In summary, both control and CMP patients spent about one-quarter of each night's sleep in breathing dysrhythmia, predominantly of an undulant rather than apneic type. This breathing abnormality had only small effects on arterial oxygenation in the normal subjects, but resulted in marked hypoxemia and oscillations in arterial oxygenation in the CMP subjects. Despite these differences in oxygenation, sleep duration and distribution remained similar for the two groups. Administration of progestational agents improved average oxygenation during sleep, but more strikingly abolished the severe episodes of desaturation. These effects occurred with no associated changes in the pattern or extent of breathing dysrhythmia.

DISCUSSION

In sleep during acute exposure to high altitude, periodic breathing with apneas is common as is severe hypoxemia. The periodic breathing occurred mainly in sleep stage 2 and was virtually absent during REM sleep. Neither hypoxemia nor breathing dysrhythmia could be related to hypoxic or hypercapnic ventilatory responsiveness. Treatment with acetazolamide prevented the alkalosis of high altitude and resulted in moderate reductions in periodic breathing with a large improvement of arterial oxygenation, and decrease in number of arousals. On the other hand, MPA had little effect on blood chemistry and produced a marked decrease in the amount of periodic breathing, with only a modest effect on arterial oxygen saturation.

In the studies of sleep in chronic residents of high altitudes, undulant periodic breathing without true apneas was the characteristic pattern and was most marked during REM sleep. While similar periodicity of breathing occurred in CMP and control subjects, periodicity led to severe arterial hypoxemia in only the CMP subjects. Hypoxic ventilatory response was reduced in these subjects, but this was true in both groups and thus could not be related to nocturnal hypoxemia. Treatment with MPA had little effect on periodic breathing, but markedly improved arterial oxygenation especially by preventing the brief but very severe episodes of hypoxemia seen in the untreated subjects. The discussion will focus on two central questions: first, the possible etiologies of periodic breathing at high altitude, and second, the mechanistic link between periodic breathing and hypoxemia.

The cause of periodic breathing in normal man acutely at high altitude has never been clear. Two major schools of thought on the subject emphasize on the one hand the potential importance of hypoxemia, with the other focusing on the attendant hypocapnic alkalosis. Some provocative clues relevant to this controversy come from the extensive studies of respiration in sleep of normal sea level man conducted by Bülow [21]. He found, as have others, that periodic breathing during sleep is common in normal man especially with increasing age [22]. Apnea also occurs, but less commonly. His work provides several points in favor of the idea that hypocapnia rather than hypoxia is importantly related to periodic breathing. First, apnea, when it occurred, commonly followed an episode of decreased $PaCO_2$. Second, periodic breathing was relieved by CO_2 administration, and third, the amount of periodic breathing was closely correlated with the extent to which hypercapnic ventilatory response was decreased during sleep. This led to the conclusion that stable sleep required an elevated and constant $PaCO_2$. In contrast, PaO_2 seemed unimportant. It was shown that periodic breathing was neither decreased by oxygen administration nor exaggerated by hypoxia. However, it was shown that mild hypoxia (P_IO_2 = 100 mg Hg) did in some individuals exaggerate the depression in hypercapnic ventilatory response found in normoxic sleep.

The relative importance of depressed ventilatory responses to hypoxia and to hypercapnia in the pathogenesis of periodic breathing is unclear. It seems reasonable that decreases in these responses could play a permissive role in the occurrence and continuation of episodes of apnea or decreased tidal volume. Such episodes might either be prevented or shortened in patients with high drives and prolonged in those with low drives. Indeed, sleep apneas tend to occur in situations in which decreased ventilatory responses to hypercapnia and hypoxia are found, including normal man [21], obesity-hypoventilation syndrome [23], idiopathic hypoventilation [24, 25], children with upper airway obstruction [26], and infants with sleep apnea [27]. However, we could find no relationship at high altitude between the occurrence and duration of apneic spells and measurements of ventilatory drives during wakefulness. However, Bülow [21] has emphasized the importance of making such measurements during sleep, which unfortunately was not possible in the present study. The elegant studies of Phillipson et al [28] have shown that during NREM sleep ventilatory responses to hypercapnia are reduced, and to a striking degree during REM sleep, while, in contrast, hypoxic responses are well preserved, suggesting that hypoxic drive may assume an especially important role in maintenance of breathing during REM sleep in health. Reed and Kellogg in studies of man at high altitude found that ascent to high altitude and sleep had opposing effects on hypercapnic ventilatory response such that during sleep at high altitude this response was relatively little altered. They also found that hypoxic response remained intact during sleep at high altitude [29–31].

In our study the effect of acetazolamide tends to support the conclusions of Bülow [21] in that this drug improved alkalosis with only slight effects on pO_2 and impressively reduced periodic breathing. It would also suggest that the effect of $PaCO_2$ on periodic breathing is actually related to hydrogen ion concentration rather than to $PaCO_2$ per se. If hypocapnic alkalosis is an important factor in producing periodic breathing, there are at least two categories of possible mechanism. First, it may be as suggested above that decreased hydrogen ion stimulation of chemoreceptors is important. However, it is also possible that there is an element of upper airway obstruction. Peltier [32] has shown that in normal individuals hyperventilation, which produces hypocapnic alkalosis, leads to apneas associated with obvious stridor and upper airway obstruction. Remmers et al [33] have shown that carbon dioxide is an important regulator of upper airway caliber and resistance and that in the presence of hypocapnia pharyngeal muscles actively increase airway resistance. While our subjects at high altitude did not appear to be obviously obstructed during sleep, we are aware of no studies in which the role of obstruction has been investigated in the periodic breathing of acute high altitude.

Next we will consider potential mechanisms whereby periodic breathing leads to hypoxemia, and particularly the vexing question of why periodic breathing sometimes induces hypoxemia and at other times does not. At the outset there would seem to be at least three possible mechanisms: hypoventilation, increased cardiac output, and abnormal ventilation perfusion balance.

The most obvious explanation of hypoxemia during periodic breathing or apnea is hypoventilation, but several lines of evidence make this an unattractive explanation. First, in preliminary studies carried out in a high altitude chamber at a simulated altitude of 4,300 m, we measured blood pCO_2 and pH in arterialized venous samples which has been shown to be an accurate estimate of arterial values [34]. We were impressed that the severe hypoxemia noted at the nadir of the SaO_2 oscillations during periodic breathing was not associated with an increase in pCO_2 as would have been expected if hypoventilation had caused the hypoxemia. Others have also commented on the observation that hypoxemia in sleep apnea seems disproportionate to the hypercapnia [35]. At high altitude PaO_2 falls on the steep portion of the dissociation curve so that a decrease in PaO_2 causes a greater fall in SaO_2 than at sea level. Yet it is clear that even at high altitude one cannot mimic the hypoxemia of periodic breathing or apnea by simple breath holding. In both our acute and chronic high-altitude studies, decreases in arterial oxygen saturation during periodic breathing averaged 1% decrease in SaO_2 per second. In several studies in awake man during breath holding at altitude, the maximum rate of fall is calculated to be 0.3–0.5%/sec, about one-third to one-half the rate of fall observed during sleep [36–38]. Precipitous declines in SaO_2 greater than anticipated from breath holding alone are also evident in tracings published in reports of obstructive apneas at sea level [35].

How does periodic breathing or apnea differ from a breath hold in such fashion as to accelerate the rate of development of hypoxemia? One theoretical possibility would be an increase in cardiac output as this would accelerate the uptake of oxygen and hence the drop in pO_2 within a static alveolar volume. However, there is no evidence that cardiac output is increased; in fact, at both high altitude and at sea level, sleep apnea is associated with impressive decreases in heart rate [2, 35]. It is unlikely that stroke volume could rise sufficiently to elevate cardiac output in the face of profound bradycardia.

Another possible explanation could be the development of ventilation-perfusion imbalance, specifically a shunt or perfusion of underventilated areas of lung. It is probable that regional atelectasis or underventilated lung develops during sleep and it is presumed that local constriction of small pulmonary arteries normally operates to produce parallel decreases in perfusion, thus preventing hypoxemia. It has been demonstrated in dogs that alkalosis or increased pulmonary vascular pressures dramatically attenuate such local hypoxic pulmonary vasoconstriction [39]. Both are relevant to the present study. Alkalosis is prominent in the acute high-altitude studies, while pulmonary hypertension is known to be common among long-term residents of high altitude [40] and in patients with the sleep apnea syndrome at low altitude [35].

Another factor of potential importance which has remained largely unexplored is the possible role of changes in intrathoracic pressure. Because the most severe hypoxemia during sleep apnea is associated with inspiratory obstruction [41], we measured arterial oxygenation (ear oximeter) in 20 high-altitude subjects (3,100 m) during positive and negative pressure breath holds. This was accomplished by asking the subjects to blow into or inspire against a manometer to produce respective pressures of plus and minus 20 cm H_2O. The results shown in Figure 9 indicate a striking increase in hypoxemia during negative pressure

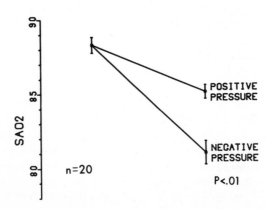

Fig 9. Influence of positive vs negative pressure during breath holding on the development of arterial hypoxemia in 20 subjects at an altitude of 3,100 m. Positive pressure breath holds (+ 20 cm H_2O) produced only small decrements in SaO_2, while negative pressure breath holds (−20 cm H_2O) produced much greater decrements (P < 0.01). This effect of negative pressure could contribute to the development of hypoxemia during inspiratory obstructive apneas.

breath hold. This effect which might contribute to the severe hypoxemia of obstructive apneas could be attributable to high intravascular pressure because negative intrathoracic pressure increases the pressure gradient across pulmonary vascular walls. It is also possible that it relates to increased transmural left atrial pressure or to alteration of cardiac output. In any event it constitutes another factor which potentially contributes to the development of hypoxemia during apnea.

The major problem in relating ventilation-perfusion defects to hypoxemia at high altitude is that venous admixture influences arterial oxygenation less during hypoxia than in normoxia or hyperoxia. Thus very severe $\dot{V}/\dot{Q}$ abnormalities would have to be invoked to explain the observed decreases in arterial oxygen saturation at high altitude. The answer may be to consider the combined effects of $\dot{V}/\dot{Q}$ disturbance and decreased cardiac output. As mentioned above, bradycardia accompanies sleep apnea at high altitude and at sea level. While stroke volume has not been measured, such bradycardias suggest that cardiac output is reduced during apnea. If this occurred, the oxygen content of mixed venous blood would be reduced and the effects of venous admixture on arterial oxygenation would be augmented. Thus, the hypoxemia of sleep apnea might reflect the combined effects of an increase in venous admixture and a decrease in venous oxygen content consequent upon a decrease in cardiac output.

ACKNOWLEDGMENTS

This work was supported by a Program Project grant (HL 14985) from the National Heart and Lung Institute.

REFERENCES

1. Monge CM, Monge CC: In "High Altitude Diseases: Mechanism and Management." Springfield, Illinois: CC Thomas, 1966.
2. Reite M, Jackson D, Cahoon R, Weil JV: Sleep physiology at high altitude. Electroencephalogr Clin Neurophysiol 38:463–471, 1975.
3. Gabel RA, Weiskopf RB: Ventilatory interaction between hypoxia and [H+] at chemoreceptors of man. J Appl Physiol 39:292–296, 1975.
4. Cain SM, Dunn JE II: Low doses of acetazolamide to aid accommodation of men to altitude. J Appl Physiol 21(4):1195–1200, 1966.
5. Forwand SA, Landowne M, Follansbee JN, Hansen JE: Effect of acetazolamide on acute mountain sickness. N Engl J Med 279(16):839–845, 1968.
6. Goodland RL, Reynolds JG, Pommerenke WT: Alveolar carbon dioxide tension levels during pregnancy and early puerperium. J Clin Endocrinol Metab 14:522–530, 1954.
7. Doring GH, Loeschcke HH: Atmung und Saure-Basengleichgewicht in der Schwangerschaft. Pflüg Arch Ges Physiol Menschen Tiere 249:437–451, 1947.

8. Zwillich CW, Natalino MR, Weil JV: The influence of a progestational agent on the control of breathing in man. Clin Res 23:353A, 1975.

9. Weil JV, Byrne-Quinn E, Sodal IE, Friesen WO, Underhill B, Filley GF, Grover RF: Hypoxic ventilatory drive in normal man. J Clin Invest 49:1061–1072, 1970.

10. Hirshman CA, McCullough RE, Weil JV: Normal values for hypoxic and hypercapnic drives in man. J Appl Physiol 38:463–471, 1975.

11. Rechtschaffen A, Kales A (eds): "A Manual of Standardized Terminology, Techniques and Scoring System in Sleep Stages of Human Subjects." Washington DC: Public Health Service, US Printing Office, 1968.

12. Kryger M, McCullough R, Collins D, Scoggin C, Weil J, Grover R: Treatment of chronic mountain polycythemia (CMP) with respiratory stimulation. Am Rev Respir Dis 115: 345, 1977.

13. Weil JV, Jamieson G, Brown DW, Grover RF: The red cell mass-arterial oxygen relationship in normal man. J Clin Invest 47:1627–1639, 1968.

14. Weil JV, Byrne-Quinn E, Sodal IE, Filley GF, Grover RF: Acquired attenuation of chemoreceptor function in chronically hypoxic man at high altitude. J Clin Invest 50: 186–195, 1971.

15. Sorenson SC, Severinghaus JW: Respiratory sensitivity to acute hypoxia in man born at sea level living at high altitude. J Appl Physiol 25:211–216, 1968.

16. Sorenson SC, Severinghaus JW: Irreversible respiratory insensitivity to acute hypoxia in man born at high altitude. J Appl Physiol 25:217–220, 1968.

17. Lahiri S, Kao FF, Velasquez T, Martinez C, Pezzia W: Irreversible blunted respiratory sensitivity to hypoxia in high altitude natives. Respir Physiol 6:360–374, 1969.

18. Sorenson SC, Severinghaus JW: Respiratory insensitivity to acute hypoxia persisting after correction of tetralogy of Fallot. J Appl Physiol 25:221–223, 1968.

19. Blesa MI, Lahiri S, Phil D, Rashkind WJ, Fishman AP: Normalization of the blunted ventilatory response to acute hypoxia in congenital cyanotic heart disease. N Engl J Med 296:237–241, 1977.

20. Sutton FD Jr, Zwillich CW, Creagh CE, Pierson DJ, Weil JV: Progesterone for outpatient treatment of Pickwickian syndrome. Ann Intern Med 83:476–479, 1975.

21. Bülow K: Respiration and wakefulness in man. Acta Physiol Scand 59(Suppl M209): 1–110, 1963.

22. Webb P: Periodic breathing during sleep. J Appl Physiol 37:899–903, 1974.

23. Zwillich CW, Sutton FD, Pierson DJ, Creagh EM, Weil JV: Decreased hypoxic ventilatory drive in the obesity-hypoventilation syndrome. Am J Med 59:343–348, 1975.

24. Kafer ER, Leigh J: Recurrent respiratory failure associated with the absence of ventilatory response to hypercapnia and hypoxemia. Am Rev Respir Dis 106:100–106, 1972.

25. Moore GC, Zwillich CW, Battaglia JO, Cotton EK, Weil JV: Respiratory failure associated with familial depression of ventilatory response to hypoxia and hypercapnia. N Engl J Med 295:861–865, 1976.

26. Ingram RH, Bishop JB: Ventilatory response to carbon dioxide after removal of chronic upper airway obstruction. Am Rev Respir Dis 102:645–647, 1970.

27. Shannon DC, Marsland DW, Gould JB, Callahan B, Todres ID, Dennis J: Central hypoventilation during quiet sleep in two infants. Pediatrics 57:342–346, 1976.

28. Phillipson EA: Regulation of breathing during sleep. Am Rev Respir Dis 115:217–225, 1977.

29. Reed DJ, Kellogg RH: Changes in respiratory response to CO_2 during natural sleep at sea level and at altitude. J Appl Physiol 13(3):325–330, 1958.

30. Reed DJ, Kellogg RH: Effect of sleep on hypoxic stimulation of breathing at sea level and altitude. J Appl Physiol 15(6):1130–1134, 1960.
31. Reed DJ, Kellogg RH: Effect of sleep on CO_2 stimulation of breathing in acute and chronic hypoxia. J Appl Physiol 15(6):1135–1138, 1960.
32. Peltier LF: Obstructive apnea in artificially hyperventilated subjects during sleep. J Appl Physiol 5:614–618, 1953.
33. Remmers JE, Gautier H, Bartlett D Jr: Factors controlling expiratory flow and duration. In Pengelly LD, Rebuck AS, Campbell EJM (eds): "Loaded Breathing." London: Churchill-Livingstone, 1974, pp 122–129.
34. Forster HV, Dempsey JA, Thomson J, Vidruk E, doPico GA: Estimation of arterial PO_2, PCO_2, pH, and lactate from arterialized venous blood. J Appl Physiol 32:134–137, 1972.
35. Tilkian AG, Guilleminault C, Schroeder JS, Lehrman KL, Simmons FB, Dement WC: Sleep induced apnea syndrome: Hemodynamic studies during wakefulness and sleep. Ann Intern Med 85:714–719, 1976.
36. Otis AB, Rahn H, Fenn WO: Alveolar gas exchange during breath holding. Am J Physiol 157:445–462, 1949.
37. Rahn H, Bahnson HT, Muxworthy JF, Hagen JM: Adaptation to high altitude: Changes in breath-holding time. J Appl Physiol 6:154–157, 1953.
38. Ferris EB, Engel GL, Stevens CD, Webb J: Voluntary breathholding (III). J Clin Invest 25:734–743, 1946.
39. Benumof JL, Wahrenbrock EA: Blunted hypoxic pulmonary vasoconstriction by increased lung vascular pressures. J Appl Physiol 38(5):846–850, 1975.
40. Reeves JT, Grover RF: High-altitude pulmonary hypertension and pulmonary edema. In Yu PN, Goodwin JF (eds): "Progress in Cardiology." Philadelphia: Lea & Febiger, 1975, pp 99–111.
41. Guilleminault C, Tilkian A, Dement WC: The sleep apnea syndromes. Annu Rev Med 27:465–484, 1976.

DISCUSSION

Dr Phillipson observed that progesterone eliminates the occasional profound drop in oxygen saturation but has little or no effect on periodic breathing. He questioned whether these severe drops in saturation were related to hypersomnolence and whether progesterone could prevent obstructive sleep apnea. Unfortunately, obstruction was not assessed during Dr Weil's experimental protocol. Dr Severinghaus remarked that polycythemics are known to have diminished ventilatory response to hypoxia and asked about the hypoxic response in the two groups — control and polycythemic — studied. Dr Weil stated that hypoxic response was reduced (and virtually identical) in both cases and also that progesterone did not lead to any important changes. Mean pCO_2 values decreased with hormonal ingestion, but no pH changes were observed. The greatest desaturations were seen in stages 3–4 and REM sleep, in contrast to observations in acute high altitude experiments. At acute high altitude, Dr Weil's group observed periods during sleep when no periodic breathing occurred and felt that REM sleep triggered these periods. In 1961, Bülow pointed out that apneas during sleep were dramatically pCO_2 dependent, and that periodic breathing was often preceded by a period of decreasing pCO_2. A similar pattern was noted intermittently in acute high altitude experiments.

Dr Weitzman remarked that the high hematocrit reported during high altitude studies was unusual. Dr Weil expressed confidence that altitude itself plays a role as polycythemia seems to be frequent in sleep apnea patients at Denver's altitude, whereas it is seen only infrequently in sleep apnea patients studied at sea level. Questions concerning the role of polycythemia were raised – especially concerning its possible deleterious effects. A blind, randomly distributed phlebotomy study was done in polycythemic patients with chronic obstructive lung disease. Subjects could invariably determine if blood had or had not been withdrawn (venous puncture was maintained for 30 minutes in all cases) and there was consistent subjective improvement after phlebotomy. Interestingly, Dr Meir Kryger has found that polycythemic subjects tested at high altitude showed considerable intellectual deficiency. Eight polycythemic subjects and five controls matched for age and education were given four-hour psychometric batteries; all of the polycythemic subjects were within the demented range. In comparison, all of the controls were normal except for one in whom a mild memory deficit was found. This could reflect decreased cerebral oxygen delivery due to increased hematocrit.

Dr Severinghaus reported results from his studies of cerebral blood flow in high altitudes in Bolivia. Cerebral blood flow was found to be a linear function of hematocrit; at normal hematocrit the cerebral blood flow at high altitude was almost normal, but in polycythemic subjects it became considerably below normal, while in anemic patients it was above normal. Dr Severinghaus also remarked that Dr Weil's presentation implied that the process of desaturation lasts for many minutes when it occurs and also suggested the following sequence of events: inspiratory obstruction, decrease in lung volume, and finally volume increase in shunt related to collapse of alveoli. Dr Phillipson suggested that the effect of negative thoracic pressure – the Müller maneuver – may persist beyond the episode of obstruction and may also participate in this process.

8
Effects of Oxygen Administration in Sleep-Induced Apneas

Jorge Motta and Christian Guilleminault

INTRODUCTION

Cyclical hypoxemia secondary to cessation of effective ventilation is one of the hallmarks of sleep-induced apnea [1]. The effect of reversal of hypoxemia by oxygen administration in sleep-induced apnea has received little attention from the investigators interested in this disorder. This study reports the effects of oxygen administration in patients with sleep-induced apnea.

METHOD

As part of the sleep apnea hemodynamic study protocol, four male patients underwent oxygen interventions during overnight monitoring. A detailed description of the techniques employed for overnight monitoring is presented in Chapter 11. Three patients had predominantly obstructive apneas (apnea per sleep-hour 51, 81, and 78), while the fourth had mostly central apneas (apnea per sleep-hour 53). The four patients' mean age was 52 years (range 39–73); none had symptoms of significant lung disease. Oxygen was administered intermittently via nasal prongs and/or mask at a rate of 5 to 10 liters/min during rapid eye movement (REM) and non-rapid eye movement (NREM) sleep. Oxygen tension was constantly monitored by an indwelling arterial oxygen electrode, and arterial blood gases were randomly drawn as close as possible to the end of the apneas in three patients. The duration of each apnea was calculated by measuring the time elapsed between cessation of ventilatory air flow, as determined by the nasal thermistor deflection, and the first major onset of air flow, also determined from the thermistor deflection. Four consecutive apneas were then measured during

Sleep Apnea Syndromes, pages 137–144

NREM and REM sleep with and without oxygen administration. Statistical analysis was done by the paired t test.

RESULTS

Hyperoxia During NREM Sleep

All patients achieved pO_2 levels of > 120 mm Hg during oxygen administration. The mean duration of apneas during NREM sleep for the four patients increased from 28 ± 1 (mean ± SEM), 31 ± 2, 27 ± 2, and 21 ± 2 seconds to 41 ± 2, 62 ± 10, 35 ± 2, and 46 ± 3 seconds, respectively, after the administration of oxygen. In three patients the increase was found to be statistically significant ($P < 0.05$, Table I). Arterial blood gases obtained in three patients during oxygen administration revealed increases in carbon dioxide (pCO_2) tension and acidosis as compared to blood gases obtained on room air (Table II).

Hyperoxia During REM Sleep

In two of the patients significant increases in the mean duration of apneas from 37 ± 2 to 85 ± 8 seconds ($P < 0.01$) and 54 ± 6 to 106 ± 9 seconds ($P < 0.05$) were noted during oxygen administration (Table I). In the other two patients the mean duration of apneas also increased, from 42 ± 2 to 85 ± 18 seconds and from 32 ± 2 to 99 ± 25 seconds, but these failed to reach statistical signficance ($P < 0.10$).

In two patients arterial blood gases obtained during oxygen administration revealed further increases in carbon dioxide and acidosis compared to samples obtained on room air (Table II). The mean increase in the length of apneas with oxygen administration was noted to be greater during REM sleep, 52 ± 5 seconds, than during NREM sleep, 19 ± 5 seconds ($P < 0.01$).

DISCUSSION

Transient depression of ventilation during wakefulness with the inhalation of high concentrations of oxygen has been well documented [2, 3]. Less is known of the effects of hyperoxia on ventilation during the different stages of sleep and, particularly, of its effects on sleep-induced apneas. Bolton and Herman reported that breathing high concentrations of oxygen reduced minute volume ventilation during sleep in the newborn [4]. Phillipson and Sullivan (Chapter 4) have noted the prolongation of spontaneous REM apneas in dogs during oxygen administration.

TABLE I. Duration (seconds) of Apneas by Sleep Stage and Oxygen Administration*

Patient	NREM	NREM + O_2	REM	REM + O_2
1) Obstructive	28	38	38	105
	25	48	37	90
	30	38	39	82
	30	39	35	65
Mean ± SEM	28 ± 1	41 ± 2	37 ± 1	85 ± 8
Significance		$p < 0.05$		$p < 0.01$
2) Obstructive	22	30	67	107
	28	37	55	87
	32	35	38	130
	26	38	55	102
Mean ± SEM				
Significance	27 ± 2	35 ± 2	54 ± 6	106 ± 9
		$p < 0.025$		$p < 0.05$
3) Obstructive	26	38	45	60
	20	50	37	90
	24	47	47	135
	16	48	41	55
Mean ± SEM				
Significance	21 ± 2	46 ± 3	42 ± 2	85 ± 18
		$p < 0.025$		$p < 0.10$
4) Central	30	52	35	122
	35	40	29	50
	33	70	32	125
	25	85		
Mean ± SEM	31 ± 2	62 ± 10	32 ± 2	99 ± 25[a]
Significance		$p < 0.10$		$p < 0.10$

*Abbreviations: NREM, non-rapid eye movement sleep; NREM + O_2, oxygen given during NREM sleep; REM, rapid eye movement sleep; REM + O_2, oxygen given during REM sleep.
[a]Only three cycles obtained with REM + O_2

Our observations in the four studied patients indicate a consistent prolongation of NREM apneas during oxygen administration (Figs 1, 2, and 3). In one of the patients this prolongation was not statistically significant, probably because of the small sample of apneas obtained. According to Phillipson and Sullivan, ventilation during NREM sleep in dogs appears to be regulated by the automatic respiratory control system responding to chemical stimuli like hypoxia, hypercapnia, and acidosis (Chapter 4; see also [5]). Prolongation of apneas during

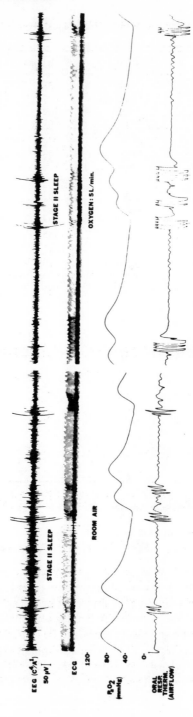

Fig 1. Demonstration of lengthening of apneas during NREM sleep by oxygen administration.

TABLE II. Arterial Blood Gases During Different Sleep Stages and Oxygen Administration*

Patient	Sleep stage	Oxygen administration	pO$_2$ (mm Hg)	pCO$_2$ (mm Hg)	pH
1	Awake	No	87	39	7.38
	NREM	No	55	45	7.35
	NREM	Yes	127	51	7.28
2	Awake	No	70	39	7.45
	NREM	No	41	43	7.35
	NREM	Yes	111	46	7.35
	REM	No	33	50	7.37
	REM	Yes	36	60	7.24
3	Awake	No	81	36	7.42
	NREM	No	63	39	7.41
	NREM	Yes	126	43	7.35
	REM	No	64	43	7.37
	REM	Yes	131	43	7.32

*Abbreviations: pCO$_2$, carbon dioxide tension; pO$_2$, oxygen tension; all other abbreviations as in Table I.

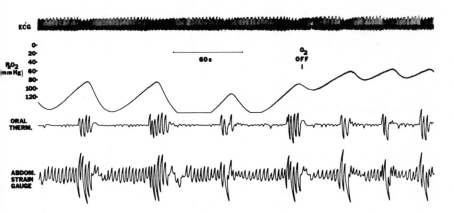

Fig 2. Demonstration of shortening of apneas with discontinuation of oxygen.

NREM sleep after oxygen administration can be explained by the removal of "hypoxic drive," leaving the other chemical stimuli to induce the initiation of breathing or arousal. It can be argued that a longer time will be required to achieve a critical level of these other chemical stimuli, and, in this fashion, the longer apneas are produced. The existence of this mechanism is also suggested by the arterial blood gases obtained with and without oxygen intervention at

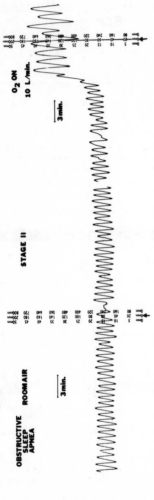

Fig 3. Continuous oxygen tension tracing demonstrating effects of oxygen administration. Note the increase in distance between the peaks of the tracing before and after oxygen administration, indicating apnea lengthening. Oxygen tension is demonstrated by the arrow. Note that apnea ends during oxygen administration at higher than normal levels.

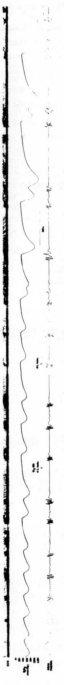

Fig 4. Demonstration of apnea lengthening during REM sleep by oxygen administration.

the end of NREM apneas. In three patients increases in carbon dioxide tension and acidosis were noted after oxygen administration.

During REM sleep hyperoxia also appeared to prolong the duration of apneas, suggesting some interaction between oxygen and the mechanism which controls the initiation of breathing or arousal (Fig 4). Nevertheless, during oxygen administration, we have noted that the onset of ventilation occurs during REM sleep, sometimes at normal and supernormal arterial oxygen tension. This suggests independence of the mechanism terminating REM apneas from arterial oxygen tension. We also observed an increase in arterial carbon dioxide tension and acidosis as compared to NREM sleep levels during oxygen administration (Table II). It appears that there is a difference between REM and NREM sleep in the response to these stimuli as related to the end of the apneas. In dogs, ventilation during REM sleep appears not to be related to the automatic respiratory control system, retaining responsiveness to hypoxic stimuli (Chapter 4). The other sources of control of ventilation remain poorly defined.

The clinical importance of the prolongation of sleep-induced apneas with oxygen administration resides in the marked deterioration in arterial blood gases noted during this intervention, particularly during REM sleep. The extreme levels of acidosis recorded in two patients represent a potential risk factor for cardiovascular catastrophies by lowering ventricular fibrillation thresholds and depressing myocardial contraactivity [6].

We conclude that administration of high levels of oxygen prolongs sleep-induced apneas occurring during REM and NREM sleep. These observations suggest that oxygen has an effect on the mechanism which controls the end of apneas during both REM and NREM sleep.

ACKNOWLEDGMENTS

This research was supported by National Institute of Neurological Diseases and Stroke grant NS 10727 and by INSERM to Dr Guilleminault.

REFERENCES

1. Guilleminault C, Tilkian A, Dement WC: The sleep apnea syndromes. Annu Rev Med 27: 465–484, 1976.
2. Lambertsen CJ: Effects of oxygen at high partial pressure. In Fenn W, Rahn H (eds): "Handbook of Physiology. Section III, Respiration," vol 2. Baltimore: Williams & Wilkins, 1965, pp 1027–1046.
3. Comroe JH: The response to oxygen and oxygen lack. In Comroe JH (ed): "Physiology of Respiration," 2nd Ed. Chicago: Year Book, 1974, pp 33–54.

4. Bolton DPG, Herman S: Ventilation and sleep state in the newborn. J Physiol (London) 240:67–77, 1974.
5. Cunningham DJC: The control system regulating breathing in man. Q Rev Biophys 6: 433–483, 1974.
6. Ng ML, Levy MN, Sieske HA: Effects of change of pH and of carbon dioxide tension on left ventricular performance. Am J Physiol 213:115–120, 1967.

DISCUSSION

Dr Weil asked if there was some critical point during apnea at which breathing always resumes. Dr Phillipson commented that in dogs there are very short apneas during REM sleep which terminate long before hypoxia develops; therefore, giving oxygen would not alter the response. He noted, however, that some very long apneic episodes may be programmed otherwise, and hypoxia may contribute to termination of this dangerous state in these instances. Dr Guilleminault agreed with Dr Phillipson, mentioning that when a patient is given oxygen and presents apnea, CO_2 and acidosis seem to be factors in the termination of NREM apneas, as they terminate fairly quickly. Of particular interest are the REM apneas of lengthy duration despite hypercapnia and acidosis, and the difference in the critical breathing points seen in REM and NREM sleep. These indicate that similar mechanisms exist in dogs and man.

Analysis of Apnea in Sleep Apnea

Daniel Kurtz and Jean Krieger

Polygraphic recordings of wakefulness and sleep during circadian periods [1–] have demonstrated in Pickwickian patients a sleep-related disturbance of respiration, characterized by transient respiratory arrests occurring as soon as the patient falls asleep or as soon as his sleep deepens. Three types of sleep apnea are usually distinguished [3]: central apnea, characterized by absence of respiratory airflow, with complete cessation of activity in both intercostal and diaphragmatic muscles; obstructive apnea, ie, absence of respiratory airflow despite the persistence of thoracoabdominal respiratory movements; and mixed apnea, a combination of central and obstructive respiratory arrests.

New techniques applied to respiratory recordings have allowed the semiology of these respiratory arrests to be specified. These techniques include determination of inspiratory and expiratory gasflow by pneumotachography, measurement of the percentage of CO_2 in the expired airflow, immediate determination of the partial pressures of O_2 and CO_2 by mass spectrometry, and analyses of thoracic and abdominal respiratory movements using either strain gauges or impedance plethysmography [5, 6]. Data obtained confirm the variability of percentages of central, obstructive, and mixed apneas, both in one patient recorded on several occasions and from one patient to another. Furthermore, several authors [9–] could not confirm the exclusive occurrence of obstructive apneas. Finally, our latest results suggest that the different types of respiratory arrests are based on a single physiopathological mechanism.

MATERIALS AND METHODS

Our study was based on polygraphic recordings made during wakefulness and sleep during the circadian period in 38 patients; 32 of these patients were classified as Pickwickian.

Sleep Apnea Syndromes, pages 145–159
1978 Alan R. Liss, Inc., 150 Fifth Avenue, New York, NY 10011

Recordings were always done in a quiet but not soundproof room. The following were studied: electroencephalogram (EEG) using eight channels (Reega Alvar XVI Tr), electrooculogram (EOG), body movements, direct and integrated electromyogram (EMG) of the chin muscles by means of flexible steel wire electrodes, and electrocardiogram (ECG) and instantaneous heart rate (NC). Analysis of respiration was based on the following four procedures.

1) The first was measurement of the respiratory gas flow ($\dot{V}_{air}$) and inspiratory (V_{air} insp.) and expiratory (V_{air} exp.) volumes by Goddart's pneumotachograph these measurements the patient breathes through a Fleish Flow Transducer head 2), thereby creating within the transducer head alternating differential pressures positive during inspiration and negative during expiration. The alternating differential pressure is then fed by thin-gauge polythene tubing to a capacitance-type pressure transducer where it is converted into electrical signals that are directly proportional to the respiratory gas flow. The signals (100 mV/mm H_2O) are then amplified (up to -5 V nominal for inspiratory flow) and transmitted to five separate integrators for processing. The time response of the pressure transducer is 15 milliseconds and its sensitivity about 6 mm + 2 mm H_2O.

2) The percentage of CO_2 in the expired air was measured by a capnograph (Cosma Rubis 3000) which continuously analyzes the CO_2 concentration in a small air volume taken at bucconasal level. The resulting curve is linear from 0 to 6% CO_2.

3) The third procedure was instantaneous mass spectrometrical analysis of CO_2 and O_2 partial pressures in expired air.

4) Thoracic movements were studied by measuring the variation in impedance of the chest and abdominal movements by a strain gauge. The variation at the abdominal transducer is proportional to the volume of mobilized air and is linear up to 6 liters.

The polygraphic records are always analyzed second by second. In this chapter we report only the results related to sleep apnea.

RESULTS

Central Apnea With Open Glottis (Fig 1)

During the two to three respiratory cycles preceding apnea, respiratory airflow is reduced. But as soon as the patient falls asleep, breathing stops; the last respiratory movement is expiratory. After 10–30 seconds, respiration starts again, with an inspiration. In the interval, no air output is recorded.

During this type of apnea the glottis remains open; this is demonstrated by the persistence of a high level of CO_2, resulting from free diffusion of CO_2 through the upper airways. This diffusion is facilitated by the pump of the capnograph, which continuously takes air samples at the bucconasal level.

The open position of the glottis during the apnea contrasts with the arrest of intercostal and diaphragmatic muscular activity. Absence of thoracic and abdominal movements results not from a tonic contraction of those muscles but from inhibition of their activity, and is shown by disappearance of EMG activity in the inferior intercostal muscles during apnea. When the patient awakens or his sleep lightens, breathing starts again, and thoracic and/or diaphragmatic EMG activity reappears.

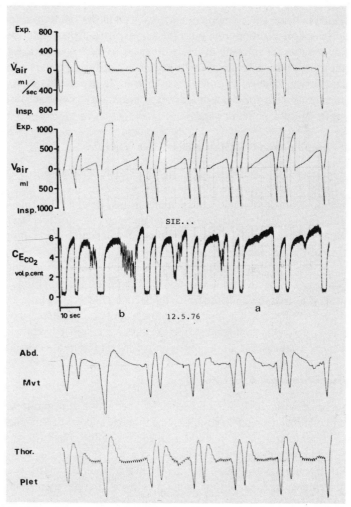

Fig 1. Central apnea a) with open glottis, b) with secondary closing of the glottis. Abbreviations: $\dot{V}_{air}$, respiratory gas flow; V_{air} insp, inspiratory volume; V_{air} exp, expiratory volume; C_{ECO_2}, Concentration of CO_2 in expired air; Abd. Mvt, abdominal movements measured by a strain gauge; Thor. Plet, thoracic impedance plethysmography.

The recovery of respiration is followed by a fall in CO_2 concentration in the upper airways, and the capnographic curve reaches the zero level. Sometimes the respiratory arrest is followed by a period of hyperventilation.

Central Apnea With Secondary Closing of the Glottis

The initial stages in this event are similar to those previously described. However, in this type of respiratory arrest, there is a secondary closing of the glottis after a variable time. The consequence is a decrease in CO_2 concentration in the supraglottic space, resulting from both the action of the capnographic pump and passive penetration of ambient air inside the mask to the supraglottic level. Closing of the glottis does not coincide with recurrence of thoracic and abdominal muscular activity, which starts a few seconds later. As previously noted, the first respiratory movement following the apnea is inspiratory; simultaneously, the glottis opens and the patient awakens.

Central Apnea Followed by Obstructive Apnea (Fig 2)

There is no difference between the semiology of an isolated central apnea and that of a central respiratory arrest followed by an obstructive one. Both start after an expiration, and, in both, the glottis remains open and the capnographic curve shows a high level of CO_2. After a certain point, the glottis closes; this is followed by a fall, at a constant slope, of the CO_2 concentration in the supraglottic space. Unlike central apneas with secondary closing of the glottis, however, in this case the occlusion of the glottis is more or less simultaneous with the beginning of thoracic and/or abdominal movements. The amplitude of these movements is at first low, but progressively becomes higher. Regardless of the intensity of intercostal or diaphragmatic muscle contraction, there is no airflow, either expiratory or inspiratory, because the glottis is completely closed. As soon as the patient awakens, the glottis opens and effectual respiration resumes.

Immediate Obstructive Apnea (Fig 3)

The respiratory arrest is often preceded by a reduction in respiratory airflow and a proportional decrease in amplitude of thoracic and/or diaphragmatic movements. The apnea starts after an expiration and is simultaneous with closing of the glottis and the subsequent decrease, at a constant slope, of the CO_2 concentration in the supraglottic space and persistence of thoracic and/or diaphragmatic movements, at an amplitude sometimes low at first but increasing after a few seconds. These movements, however, whatever their amplitude, remain ineffectual since no respiratory gas flow is recorded.

The patient's awakening is always accompanied by opening of the glottis; respiration resumes with an inspiratory movement, and the amplitude of the thoracic and/or abdominal movements increases.

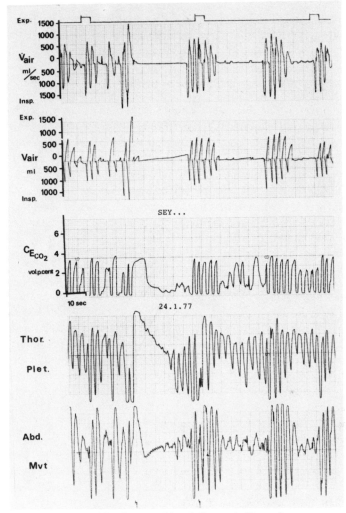

Fig 2. Mixed apnea; abbreviations as in Figure 1.

Obstructive Apnea With a Valve Phenomenon (Fig 4)

The major characteristics of this type of respiratory arrest are similar to those in an immediate obstructive apnea. However, the closing of the glottis is presumably incomplete since low expiratory outputs without subsequent inspiration are recorded. These low expiratory gas flows (< 50 ml/sec for 1–2 seconds) are never accompanied by increase in amplitude of thoracic and/or abdominal movements; they may occur at any moment during the respiratory arrest, and some variations in amplitude of the expiratory airflow are noticed. Recovery of respiration is again marked by inspiration.

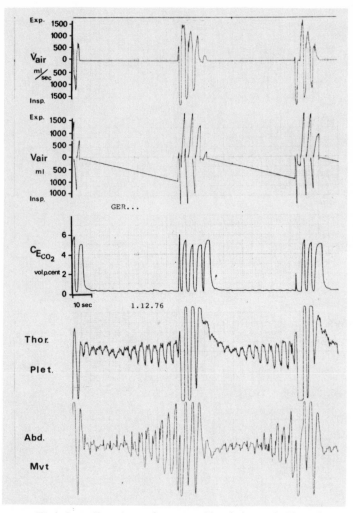

Fig 3. Immediate obstructive apnea; abbreviations as in Figure 1.

Detection and Significance of Hypopneas

Hypopneas, ie, decrease in respiratory airflow, were first noticed in 1965 by Jung and Kuhlo [4] during preapneic periods. In 1971, Kurtz et al [7] described hypopneas characterized by both a decrease in respiratory airflow to one-third of its basal value and a parallel reduction in amplitude of thoracic and abdominal movements (see Fig 5).

We consider hypopnea equivalent to minor central apnea, the only difference between the two being intensity. These central hypopneas contrast with the

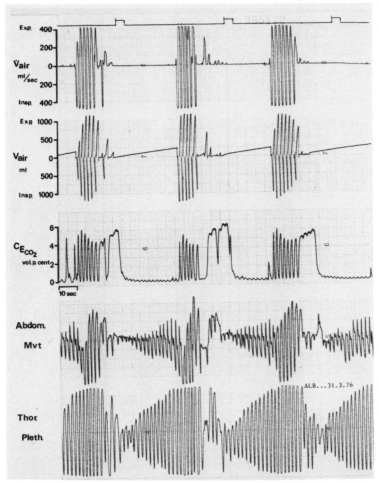

Fig 4. Obstructive apnea with the valve phenomenon. Abbreviations as in Figure 1.

"obstructive" hypopneas reported by Lugaresi et al [12] and Schwartz and Granelet-Eprinchard [13] and characterized as "semieffectual" periodic respiration. In the latter case, respiratory airflow was lowered despite stability of, or increase in, the amplitude of thoracic and abdominal movements.

Although respiratory airflow can be measured, it is not yet possible to measure the amplitude of thoracic and/or abdominal movements. In fact, the variation of the thoracic wall impedance is correlated to variation in size, but this relationship varies from one subject to another as well as with the patient's position. However, the indications given by an abdominal strain gauge transducer are proportional to the respiratory gas flow and linear up to a 6-liter tidal volume. This relationship also varies with the position of the sleeping patient and the tension

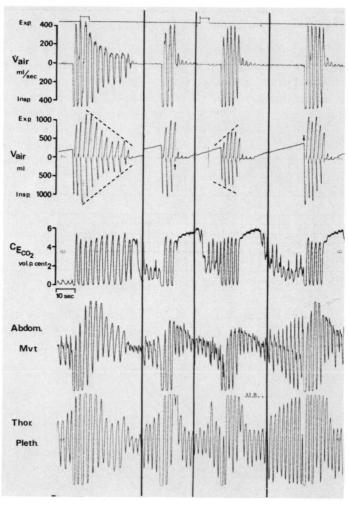

Fig 5. Respiratory pattern after an apnea. Abbreviations as in Figure 1.

applied to the transducer. Thus, a close correlation between the response of the abdominal transducer and the air output presupposes an absence of any body movement during sleep. Therefore, we could not accurately distinguish between "central" and "obstructive" hypopneas. This is regrettable considering the frequency of hypopneas during sleep: Among 2,616 respiratory events in six patients, Krieger [6] reported 1,410 hypopneas, 948 of which were associated with apneas.

Pattern of Postapneic Respiration

The first respiration after apnea is an inspiration, regardless of whether the apnea started after an expiration [14] or an inspiration. The postapneic respiratory pattern often varies. Sometimes respiratory airflow increases progressively and the final values are far beyond the basal values; at times hyperventilation starts immediately after the respiratory arrest. In both instances, hyperventilation is maintained for several respiratory cycles, and breathing then falls to the basal level. The next apnea may start during a period of hyperventilation, hypoventilation, or normal respiration. Thus, it appears that the onset of respiratory arrest does not depend on the pattern of ventilation.

Snoring and Respiratory Arrests

Duron [15] reported in 1972 the importance of snoring in patients with sleep-related obstructive apneas; he considered snoring essentially an expiratory nasal dyspnea. The importance of snoring, either inspiratory or expiratory and especially during deep slow-wave sleep, is emphasized by Tassinari et al [16]. These data are confirmed by Lugaresi et al [17], but according to these authors snoring usually takes place during inspiration, is related to partial obstruction of the upper airways, and occurs even in light slow-wave sleep. Our own findings were in agreement with the results of Lugaresi et al [17], but it appears that snoring does not necessarily precede apnea.

Groups and Trains of Apneas

Isolated apneas are rare. Kurtz et al [18], studying the night sleep of 12 Pickwickians, found only 78 respiratory arrests preceded and followed by at least one minute of sleep or wakefulness without respiratory disturbance. Similarly, respiratory events of a single type, ie, only central or only obstructive apnea, are less frequent than groups of more than one type of apnea or hypopnea. In 2,616 respiratory events analyzed by Krieger [6], 118 isolated central apneas and 18 obstructive apneas were found. In contrast, groups of more than one type of apnea and sometimes including hypopnea represent more than 50% of respiratory disturbances during sleep. Analysis of these groups shows that in the case of mixed apnea, ie, a group of central and obstructive apneas possibly associated with hypopneas, the central apnea almost always precedes the obstructive one. The contrary is rarely observed [6, 16]. In such mixed groups, hypopneas are followed by either central or obstructive apneas; therefore, low airflow does not determine the type of the subsequent respiratory arrest. In such groups, hypopneas may be bordered by apneas of the same type or of two different types; if they are different, the central apnea precedes the obstructive one.

Several groups of apneas can constitute trains of apneas; these may occur at various times during the circadian period but always during sleep [6]. For a given patient, the structure of such trains does not depend on the time of day or night, but may vary from one circadian period to another [6, 7]. Finally, in fully decompensated Pickwickians, hypopneas and apneas occur without interruption as soon as the patient falls asleep, and there is no period of either slow-wave or REM sleep without respiratory disturbances.

DISCUSSION

Characteristics of Respiratory Arrests During Sleep

Our polygraphic recordings of sleep-related respiratory disturbances (previously described by Gastaut [4, 19], Duron and Tassinari [20], Kuhlo [21], and Coccagna et al [21]) confirmed the existence of central, obstructive, and mixed apneas and specified some aspects of these respiratory arrests. Furthermore, two new patterns of apnea were described: central apnea with secondary closing of the glottis, and obstructive apnea with the valve phenomenon.

What are the significance and importance of these various respiratory patterns? According to Boonstra et al [23], Smirne et al [24], Lugaresi et al [25–27], Kuhlo and Doll [26], Hishikawa et al [27], and Tambling et al [28], the sleep-related obstructive apneas are of major importance. Their opinion is based on results obtained by tracheal intubation or tracheostomy, after which the obstructive apneas are suppressed, daytime sleepiness disappears, and nocturnal sleep becomes normal. Nevertheless, there is no suppression of either central apneas [16, 29] or what Coccagna et al [29] call "periodic respiration," which, occurring particularly during stage 2 slow-wave sleep and rapid eye movement (REM) sleep, may correspond to groups of hypopneas. But Kuhlo and Doll [26] suggest that these persisting respiratory events are only an exaggeration of what happens under normal conditions during falling asleep, ie, slow and irregular breathing.

Taking into account the results published by Nevsimal et al [30], Guilleminault et al [31], and Krieger [6], central and obstructive events may be equally important and may have the same significance: In some patients with daytime sleepiness and disorganized nighttime sleep, the respiratory arrests are always or predominantly of the central type. Furthermore, in mixed apnea, the central event always precedes the obstructive one. Finally, in most cases, central and obstructive apneas coexist and only the percentage of the two types of respiratory patterns varies. Therefore, it seems useless to differentiate patients with predominantly obstructive sleep-related apneas from those in whom central respiratory arrests are predominant.

Inspiratory and Expiratory Apneas

For a given patient, the respiratory arrest, whatever its type, always arises in the same respiratory phase. Frequently, the last respiratory movement is expiratory, but onset of apnea after an inspiration has been described [32]. In either case, as soon as the patient awakes, respiration resumes with an inspiration. These data are very important considering the physiopathology of obstructive apnea: Closing of the glottis certainly is increased by the inspiratory depression that develops at the onset of apnea, regardless of the phase of respiration.

Accordingly, we first discuss the role of the laryngeal and perilaryngeal muscles in normal breathing and in cases of respiratory arrest, and second, the possible dissociation of the activity of the three muscle groups — the laryngeal, intercostal, and diaphragmatic muscles — that take part in respiration.

Respiratory functions of the laryngeal and perilaryngeal muscles. According to Andrew [33] and Burgat-Cadilhac [34], the hyoglossal, omohyoid, and sternohyoid muscles are not activated during respiration. But the sternothyroid [33–35], genioglossal, sternoglossal, stylopharyngeal [33], and posterior cricoarytenoidian [36, 37] are used during inspiration. During expiration, activity is recorded in the lateral cricoarytenoidian, interarytenoidian [36, 37], thyrohyoidian, and thyroarytenoidian muscles [34, 35]. Andrew [33] and Nakamura et al [37] could not record any respiratory activity in the thyrohyoidian and thyroarytenoidian muscles in anesthetized dogs and rats, respectively.

The predominant action of the cricothyroidian muscle is inspiratory according to Andrew [33], Buchthal and Faaborg-Andersen [38], Hiroto et al [39], Faaborg-Andersen [40], Konrad and Rattenborg [41], and Burgat-Cadilhac [34], and is expiratory according to Murtagh [42], Fink et al [35], Nakamura et al [37], and Rudomin [43]. Arnold [44] and Suzuki et al [45] consider that the cricothyroidian muscle has a double function, inspiratory and expiratory. Part of this disagreement could be explained by the recent results published by Sherrey and Megirian [46] who suggested that the inspiratory or expiratory function of the cricothyroidian muscle depends on factors such as level of vigilance and blood gases. In awake animals, that muscle acts during expiration, but it becomes inspiratory in animals under barbiturate anesthesia; during hypoxia with hypercapnia, its activity is both inspiratory and expiratory. This functional plasticity of the laryngeal muscles may explain previously noticed discrepancies.

Dissociated activity of the muscles used in respiration. The activities of the intercostal muscles and the diaphragm are dissociated in sleeping healthy subjects [Duron, personal communication] and in adults with sleep-related apneas [7]. Recently, Curzi-Dascalova and Plassart [47] demonstrated the same fact in newborns. Therefore, a respiratory movement results either from combined action of the intercostal muscles and the diaphragm or from predominant activity of one of these two groups of muscles.

Our results suggest a somewhat similar dissociation between the function of the laryngeal muscles and that of the thoracic and/or diaphragmatic muscles. Thus, central apneas would be characterized by activation of the posterior crico-arytenoidian (which opens the glottis) associated with inhibition of the thoracic and diaphragmatic muscles. In contrast, obstructive apnea would be correlated with an inhibition of laryngeal muscles (with subsequent closing of the glottis) and persistent activation of the thoracic and/or diaphragmatic muscles. In the latter case, the inspiratory depression would reinforce the closing of the glottic barrier (obstructive apnea with the valve phenomenon).

This hypothesis is reinforced by direct fibroscopic examination of the vocal cords during obstructive respiratory arrests [48]. The obstruction is produced by progressive closing of the vocal cords and remains complete despite an increase in amplitude of thoracic and/or abdominal movements. But as soon as the patient awakes, there is sudden abduction of the vocal cords, allowing respiratory movements to become effectual again. One must also keep in mind a particular form of dissociated laryngeal paralysis due to a supranuclear lesion, described by Gerhardt (in [49]). This syndrome is characterized by dysfunction of the laryngeal muscles responsible for abduction of the vocal cords during inspiration. What happens during an obstructive apnea is perhaps similar to what was described by Gerhardt. If that hypothesis is correct, closing of the glottis, with subsequent obstruction of the upper airways, would be determined by a central mechanism, whereas factors such as adenopathy, goiter, hypertrophic amygdala, and micrognathia [8, 15, 27, 50] would play only a secondary role.

SUMMARY

Whatever the type of apnea, all are based on the same physiopathological mechanism: an impaired coupling of sleep and respiration. Dissociation of the activities of the three major muscle groups that take part in respiration may explain the different types of respiratory arrests and the variability of relative percentages of central and obstructive apneas during sleep.

REFERENCES

1. Gerardy W, Herberg D, Kuhn HM: Vergleichende Untersuchungen der Lungenfunction und des Electroencephalogramms bei zwei Patienten mit Pickwickian-Syndrom. Z Klin Med 156:362–380, 1960.
2. Drachmann DB, Gumnit RJ: Periodic alteration of consciousness in the Pickwickian syndrome. Arch Neurol 6:471–477, 1962.
3. Gastaut H, Tassinari CA, Duron B: Etude polygraphique des manifestations épisodiques (hypniques et respiratoires) du syndrome de Pickwick. Rev Neurol 112:568–579, 1965.

4. Jung R, Kuhlo W: Neurophysiological studies of abnormal night sleep and the Pickwickian syndrome. In Akert K, Bally C, Schadé (eds): "Progress in Brain Research," vol 18. Amsterdam: Elsevier, 1965, pp 140–159.

5. Kurtz D, Lonsdorfer J, Meunier-Carus J, Micheletti G, Lampert-Benignus E: Contribution à l'étude du type et de la répartition des apnées au cours du syndrome de Pickwick. Rev Electroencephalogr Neurophysiol Clin 2:367–378, 1972.

6. Krieger J: Les séquences hypno-apnéiques chez les sujets Pickwickiens. Leur séméiologie et leur répartition. Thèse Méd, Strasbourg, 1975.

7. Kurtz D, Meunier-Carus J, Bapst-Reiter J, Lonsdorfer J, Micheletti G, Benignus E, Rohmer F: Problèmes nosologiques posés par certaines formes d'hypersomnie. Rev Electroencephalogr Neurophysiol Clin 1:227–230, 1971.

8. Lugaresi E, Coccagna G, Mantovani M, Brignani F: Effects of tracheostomy in two cases of hypersomnia with periodic breathing. J Neurol 36:15–26, 1973.

9. Guilleminault C, Eldridge FL, Dement WC: Insomnia with sleep apnea: A new syndrome. Science 181:856–858, 1973.

10. Kurtz D, Bapst-Reiter J, Fletto R, Micheletti G, Meunier-Carus J, Lonsdorfer J, Lampert-Benignus E: Les formes de transition du syndrome Pickwickien (séméiologie et distribution des apnées). Bull Physiopathol Respir 8:1115–1125, 1972.

11. Autret A, Lafont F, Minz M, Beillevaire T, Cathala HP, Castaigne P: Étude de la relation entre les troubles du rythme respiratoire et hypersomnie. Rev Neurol (in press).

12. Lugaresi E, Coccagna G, Mantovani M: Pathophysiological, clinical and nosographic considerations regarding hypersomnia with periodic breathing. Bull Physiopathol Respir 8:1249–1256, 1972.

13. Schwartz BA, Granelet-Eprinchard MF: Traitement et surveillance des Pickwickiens: trois modes évolutifs typiques. Rev Electroencephalogr Neurophysiol Clin 4:79–88, 1974.

14. Kurtz D, Krieger J, Lonsdorfer J: Etude pneumotachographique des apnées au cours du sommeil. In Koella WP, Levin P (eds): "Sleep, 1976." Basel: Karger (in press).

15. Duron B: La fonction respiratoire pendant le sommeil physiologique. Bull Physiopathol Respir 8:1031–1037, 1972.

16. Tassinari CA, Dalla-Bernardina B, Cirignotta F, Ambrosetto G: Apneic periods and the respiratory related arousal patterns during sleep in the Pickwickian syndrome: A polygraphic study. Bull Physiopathol Respir 8:1087–1102, 1972.

17. Lugaresi E, Coccagna G, Fanetti P, Mantovani M, Cirignotta F: Snoring. Electroencephalogr Clin Neurophysiol 39:59–64, 1975.

18. Kurtz D, Micheletti G, Lonsdorfer J, Trapp C, Krieger J: Le sommeil pré and post apnéique du Pickwickien. Rev Electroencephalogr Neurophysiol Clin 5:278–282, 1975.

19. Gastaut H, Duron B, Papy JJ, Tassinari CA, Waltregny J: Etude polygraphique comparative du cycle nychthémérique chez les narcoleptiques, les Pickwickiens, les obèses et les insuffisants respiratoires. Rev Neurol 115:456–462, 1966.

20. Duron B, Tassinari A: Syndrome de Pickwick et syndrome cardiorespiratoire de l'obésité. A propos d'une observation. J Fr Med Chir Thorac 20:207–222, 1966.

21. Kuhlo W: Neurophysiologische und Klinische Untersuchungen beim Pickwick-Syndrom. Arch Psychiatr Nervenkr 211:170–192, 1968.

22. Coccagna G, Petrella A, Berti-Ceroni G, Lugaresi E, Pazzaglia P: Polygraphic contribution to hypersomnia and respiratory troubles in the Pickwickian syndrome. In Gastaut H, Lugaresi E, Berti-Ceroni G, Coccagna G (eds): "Abnormalities of Sleep in Man." Bologna: Gaggi, 1968, pp 215–221.

23. Boonstra S, Blokzijl EJ: Diagnosis and dramatic cure in two patients suffering from severe diurnal hypersomnia. Electroencephalogr Clin Neurophysiol 28:428–429, 1970.

24. Smirne S, Castellotti V, Graziani G: Aspetti patogenetici in un caso respirazione periodica e ipersonnia. Riv Neurol 41:342–349, 1971.

25. Lugaresi E, Coccagna G, Mantovani M, Brignani F: Effets de la trachéotomie dans les hypersomnies avec respiration périodique. Rev Neurol 123:267–268, 1970.

26. Kuhlo W, Doll E: Pulmonary hypertension and the effect of tracheotomy in a case of Pickwickian syndrome. Bull Physiopathol Respir 8:1209–1216, 1972.

27. Hisikawa Y, Furuya E, Wakamatsu H, Yamamoto J: A polygraphic study of hypersomnia with periodic breathing and primary alveolar hypoventilation. Bull Physiopathol Respir 8:1139–1151, 1972.

28. Tammeling GJ, Blokzijl EJ, Boonstra S, Sluiter HJ: Micrognathia, hypersomnia and periodic breathing. Bull Physiopathol Respir 8:1229–1238, 1972.

29. Coccagna C, Mantovani M, Brignani F, Parchi C, Lugaresi E: Tracheostomy in hypersomnia with periodic breathing. Bull Physiopathol Respir 8:1217–1227, 1972.

30. Nevsimal O, Nevsimalova S, Ourednik A: Different forms of sleep and breathing disorder in obese patients: Deep sleep stages deprivation in patients with alveolar hypoventilation. Bull Physiopathol Respir 8:1154–1155, 1972.

31. Guilleminault C, Eldridge F, Dement WC: Insomnia, narcolepsy and sleep apneas. Bull Physiopathol Respir 8:1127–1138, 1972.

32. Lonsdorfer J, Meunier-Carus J, Lampert-Benignus E, Kurtz D, Bapst-Reiter J, Fletto R, Micheletti G: Aspects hémodynamiques et respiratoires du syndrome Pickwickien. Bull Physiopathol Respir 8:1181–1192, 1972.

33. Andrew BL: The respiratory displacement of the larynx: A study of the innervation of accessory respiratory muscles. J Physiol 130:474–487, 1955.

34. Burgat-Cadilhac J, Dapres G, Botella JP, Cadilhac J: Les fonctions des muscles prélaryngés. Etude électromyographique. Rev Electroencephalogr Neurophysiol Clin 2: 344–351, 1972.

35. Fink BR, Basek M, Epanchin V: The mechanism of opening of the human larynx. Laryngoscope 66:410–425, 1956.

36. Green JM, Neil E: The respiratory function of the laryngeal muscles. J Physiol 129: 134–141, 1955.

37. Nakamura F, Uyeda Y, Sonoda Y: Electromyographic study on respiratory movements of the intrinsic laryngeal muscles. Laryngoscope 68:109–119, 1958.

38. Buchthal F, Faaborg-Andersen K: Electromyography of laryngeal and respiratory muscles. Ann Otol Rhinol Laryngol 73:118–123, 1964.

39. Hiroto H, Hirano M, Toyozumi Y: Function of laryngeal muscles. Otol Rhinol Laryngol Clin 57:1–9, 1964.

40. Faaborg-Andersen K: "Current Problems in Phoniatrics and Logopedics," suppl. Folia Phoniatrica, vol 3. Karger: New York, 1965, pp 1–70.

41. Konrad HR, Rattenborg LL: Combined action of laryngeal muscles. Acta Otolaryngol 67:646–649, 1969.

42. Murtagh JA: The respiratory function of the larynx. Ann Otol Rhinol Laryngol 54: 307–321, 1945.

43. Rudomin P: Some aspects of the control of cricothyroid muscle activity. Arch Int Physiol Biochim 74:154–168, 1966.

44. Arnold E: Physiology and pathology of the cricothyroid muscle. Laryngoscope 71: 687–753, 1961.

45. Suzuki M, Kirchner JA, Murakami Y: The cricothyroid as a respiratory muscle. Its characteristics in bilateral recurrent laryngeal nerve paralysis. Ann Otol Rhinol Laryngol 79:976–984, 1970.

46. Sherrey JH, Megirian D: State dependence of upper airway respiratory motoneuron: Functions of the cricothyroid and nasolabial muscles of the un-anesthezied rat. Electroencephalogr Clin Neurophysiol (in press).

47. Curzi-Dascalova L, Plassart E: Mouvements respiratoires au cours du sommeil du nouveau-né à terme: Comparaison des enregistrements thoraciques et abdominaux. Rev Electroencephalogr Neurophysiol Clin 6:97–104, 1976.

48. Krieger J, Kurtz D, Roeslin N: Observation fibroscopique directe au cours des apnées hypniques chez un sujet Pickwickien. Nouv Presse Méd 5:2890, 1976.

49. Alajouanine T, Bouchet M, Pialoux P, Lhermitte F: La paralysie des dilateurs de la glotte dans la sclérose latérale amyotrophique. Rev Neurol 89:157–158, 1953.

50. Coccagna G, Di Donato G, Verucchi P, Cirignotta F, Mantovani M, Lugaresi E: Hypersomnia with periodic apneas in acquired micrognathia (a bird-like face syndrome). Arch Neurol 33:769–776, 1976.

10
EEG Changes Before and After Apnea

Jean Krieger and Daniel Kurtz

This chapter presents results obtained by analyzing polygraphic recordings made during sleep or circadian periods* in patients with hypopneic or apneic episodes. The patients were of the following types: a) those with the typical Pickwickian syndrome, presenting all the symptoms of obesity, daytime drowsiness, alveolar hypoventilation and/or pulmonary arterial hypertension, and right or total cardiac decompensation [1−3]; b) those with atypical Pickwickian syndromes [4, 5], combining obesity, sometimes moderate, with at least one other element of the Pickwickian syndrome; c) subjects who, whether obese or non-obese, drowsy or not, had isolated alveolar hypoventilation not of bronchopulmonary origin; d) subjects with an apparently primary polycythemia reflecting alveolar hypoventilation which could have taken place only during sleep [6]; and e) dyssomniacs with disturbed sleep − either irregular breathing at night noted by a family member or sleep interrupted by distressed arousals. Thus, the population included the three major classes of subjects with respiratory arrests during sleep: Pickwickians, subjects with Ondine syndrome [7−10], and subjects with insomnia accompanied by periodic respiration [11, 12]. The similarity of the polygraphic data collected in such syndromes justifies their classification as a single group [11, 13, 14].

We analyzed EEG changes before and after sleep apneas according to the type of respiratory disturbance (hypopnea, central or obstructive apnea) and the level of vigilance when the apnea began.

---

* For methods see D Kurtz and J Krieger, Analysis of apneas in sleep apnea, pp 145−159 of this volume.

Sleep Apnea Syndromes, pages 161−176
© **1978 Alan R. Liss, Inc., 150 Fifth Avenue, New York, NY 10011**

APNEA IN THE WAKING STATE

In addition to apneas during sleep, some subjects had occasional apneas while awake, ie, in a state characterized by the persistence of abundant alpha activity predominant in the posterior EEG derivations. The apneas we observed in such cases were always of the central type (characterized by arrest or resumption of respiratory airflow simultaneous with thoracic and abdominal movements). The persistence of a state of wakefulness is subject to some reservations, however. In some cases, despite EEG activity characteristic of wakefulness, there were some behavioral changes suggesting drowsiness, ie, disappearance of small movements of the eyelids and a sudden drop in the amplitude of the chin EMG. In one case, direct observations showed that apneas, when they occurred with the eyes open, were accompanied by a change in the quality of the gaze, which became empty, and by a general loss of contact with the surroundings.

Thus, central apneas can occur during physiological states that combine EEG activity characteristic of wakefulness and behavioral changes suggesting sleep. Such features have not been previously reported, and they emphasize the problem of polygraphically defining levels of wakefulness [14, 16] and stages of sleep.

APNEAS DURING LIGHT SLOW-WAVE SLEEP (KLEITMAN'S STAGES 1A, 1B, AND 2) (FIGS 1 AND 2)

The majority (90%) of sleep apneas appeared during light slow-wave sleep. Their course was consistent with respiratory changes paralleling somnolence; the decrease in amplitude of thoracoabdominal movements which often precedes apnea occurred shortly after movements of the eyes and eyelids ceased. In 75% of the cases, the apnea itself was concomitant with fragmentation or disappearance of alpha waves and an increase in theta waves (stages 1A or 1B). In 15%, apnea began later, during stage 2 sleep. Electromyogram (EMG) activity of the chin decreased or disappeared at the beginning of an apneic episode. The EEG changes preceding apnea were identical in hypopneas, central apneas, obstructive apneas (cessation of airflow with persistence of thoracoabdominal movements), and mixed apneas (a central apnea succeeded by an obstructive one).

The sleep pattern during apnea depended upon the length and type of the apnea; when the apnea was short, only stage 1B sleep was reached (30%). When apnea was prolonged, stage 2 sleep was reached before the end of the episode (60%). When apnea began during stage 2 sleep, it usually was not accompanied by further deepening of sleep. K Complexes sometimes occurred during apnea, but they did not influence its course.

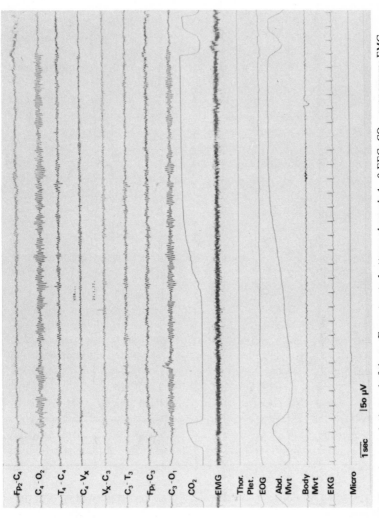

Fig 1. Central apnea during wakefulness. From top to bottom: channels 1–8 EEG; CO_2, capnogram; EMG, electromyogram of the chin muscles; Thor. Plet., thoracic impedance plethysmography; EOG, eye movements; Abd. Mvt, abdominal strain gauge, body movements; EKG, electrocardiogram; Micro, microphone.

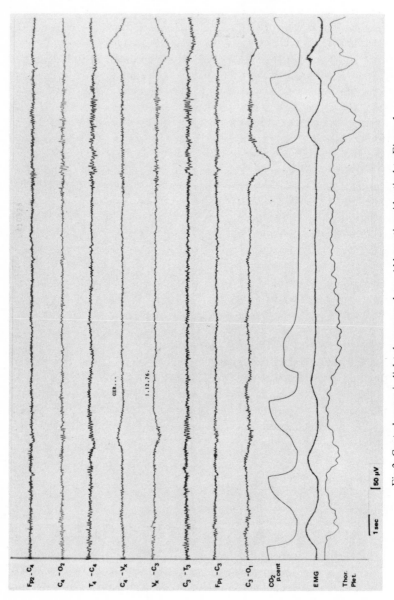

Fig 2. Central apnea in light slow-wave sleep. Abbrevations identical to Figure 1.

The parallel course of falling asleep and onset of apnea has been reported by all authors who have studied the polygraphy of sleep-related apneas [17–26].

The EEG pattern occasionally became more diversified towards the end of apnea. The episode could end with simple awakening, characterized by acceleration of the pattern, with reappearance of alpha waves, or with desynchronization of electrical activity (see Fig 3). The resumption of respiratory activity, usually inspiration, was generally preceded by two or three seconds of EEG signs of arousal, and was accompanied by reappearance or accentuation of EMG tonicity of the chin muscles, acceleration of heart rate, and often overall movement. Tassinari et al [27] advanced the hypothesis offered by Gastaut et al [19] that these repeated "respiration-related arousals" in the night produced daytime sleepiness.

Other aspects of EEG changes upon resumption of respiration have been described [15, 28, 29]. In some cases, a burst of slow delta activity appeared, with a high amplitude, frontotemporal predominance, and a morphology differing from that of K complexes (Fig 4). This burst of slow activity began a few seconds before respiration resumed and was at first superimposed by theta waves and sometimes by sleep spindles. When respiration resumed, the slow activity decreased in amplitude, became fragmented, and was associated with alpha waves which progressively increased and replaced it. The three- to ten-second burst of slow activity thus accompanied transition from a sleeping to a waking state and was generally associated with movement and increased heart rate. It was followed at times by a transitory desynchronization of electrical activity and, in this respect, resembled phases of transitory activation [30, 31].

Such bursts of slow activity appeared only following apneas occurring in sleep that reached at least stage 1B (31%) and more often stage 2 (63%). They were more frequent at the end of hypopneas (25%) and obstructive (24%) or mixed apneas (40%) than at the end of central apnea (11%). However, they were not directly related to the ineffectual respiratory movements of obstructive apneas, since during mixed apneas bursts of slow activity and the subsequent arousal occurred within 5 to 100 seconds of the resumption of these movements.

APNEAS DURING DEEP SLOW-WAVE SLEEP (KLEITMAN'S STAGES 3 AND 4) (SEE FIG 5)

In our experience, apneas during slow-wave sleep were very rare (5%). We did, however, sometimes observe apneas in stage 3 deep slow-wave sleep; there was no change in electroencephalographic activity, either before the onset of apnea, usually of the central type, or when breathing resumed. In the rare examples we saw, chin EMG activity reappeared briefly several seconds before the apnea began, accompanied by general movement. No behavioral change accompanied resumption of breathing.

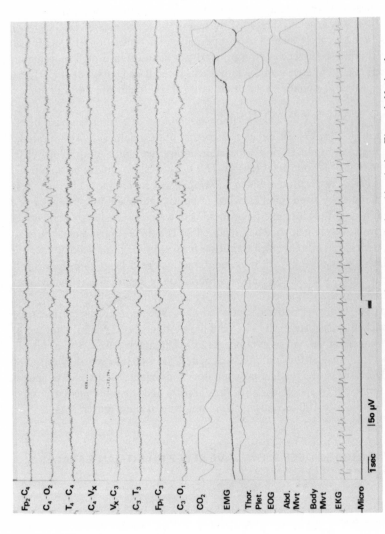

Fig 3. Mixed apnea in light slow-wave sleep. Abbreviations identical to Figure 1. Notice the occurrence of K complexes without subsequent modification of respiration.

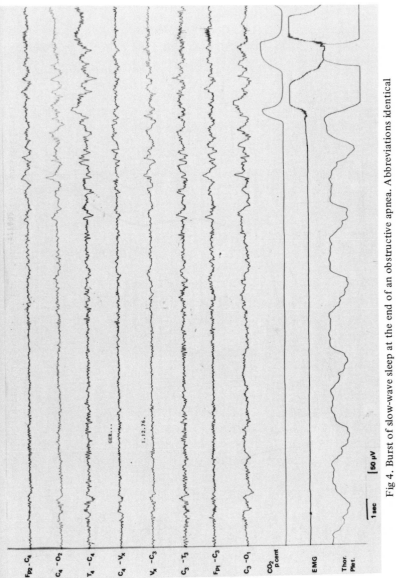

Fig 4. Burst of slow-wave sleep at the end of an obstructive apnea. Abbreviations identical to Figure 1.

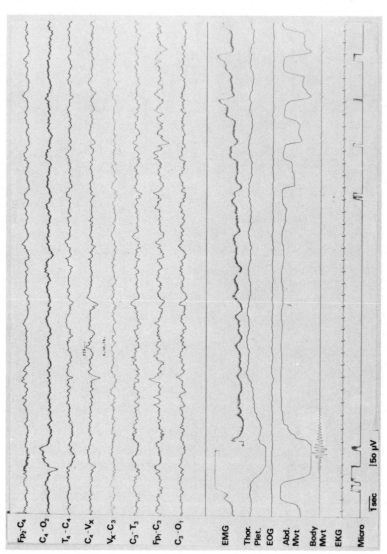

Fig 5. Central apnea in deep slow-wave sleep. Abbreviations identical to Figure 1.

Many authors agree that apneas during deep slow wave sleep are rare, and that this type of sleep is unusual in patients with hypnic apneas [15, 18, 19, 32—36]. However, Mantovani et al [37] reported a normal amount of deep slow-wave sleep in such patients. This quasipermanent absence of deep slow-wave sleep identifies these often drowsy patients as insomniacs.

APNEAS IN REM SLEEP (FIGS 6 AND 7)

The occurrence of REM sleep in subjects with sleep-related apneas has been variously evaluated, as normal by Lugaresi et al [39], rare by Schwartz et al [38] and Tammeling et al [39], and absent by Gastaut et al [19], Jung and Kuhlo [18], and Terzian [40]. We found the same variations in rapid eye movement (REM) sleep not only from patient to patient, but also in the same patient from one recording to another [15]. Although Gastaut et al [29] and Lugaresi et al [41] reported longer and proportionally more apneas in REM sleep, we found the frequency of apnea in REM sleep to be highly variable among subjects. Sometimes apneas were absent, other times the irregularities of amplitude and frequency were comparable to those in the respiration of normal subjects in REM sleep, and on other occasions, genuine apneas, which reached their maximal length and frequency in REM sleep, did occur.

Obstructive or mixed apneas were much more frequent in REM sleep than were central apneas, but the EEG patterns during each type of apnea were identical. With or without eye movement, REM sleep was established rapidly after an arousal; apnea began five to ten seconds following transition into REM sleep, and the EEG pattern remained unchanged throughout the episode. The end of the apneic episode was characterized by a transition to wakefulness or to stage 1A sleep, with the simultaneous reappearance of typical alpha activity and chin muscle activity (Fig 7). A burst of slow activity upon resumption of breathing was an exception. There was no correlation between bursts of eye movement and the beginning or end of apnea. Repeated apneas resulted in REM sleep interrupted by continuous shifts from wakefulness to REM sleep, in rhythmicity with the apneas.

DISCUSSION

Relationship Between Sleep and Respiration

A relationship became apparent between falling asleep and the onset of apnea, and between the end of apnea and arousal: A transition from wakefulness or stage 1A to stage 1B or 2 sleep was associated with an apnea and a sudden return

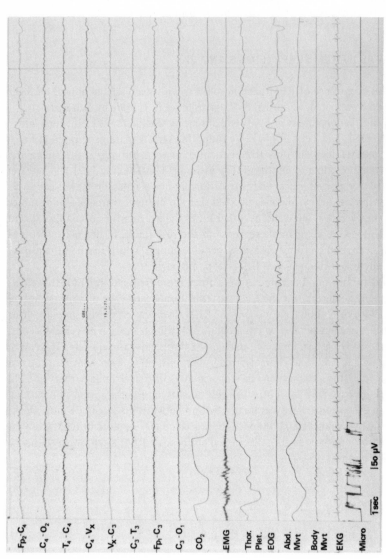

Fig 6. Central apnea starting in REM sleep. Abbreviations identical to Figure 1.

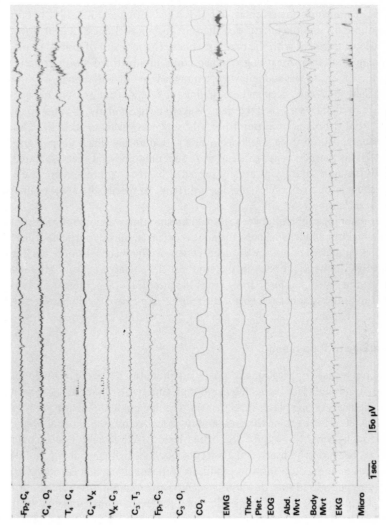

Fig 7. Obstructive apnea during REM sleep. Abbreviations identical to Figure 1.

to wakefulness or to stage 1A sleep just prior to the resumption of breathing. Apneas during REM sleep were characterized by a shift from one state of sleep to another, ie, from light slow-wave to REM sleep just before apnea began, and a return to light slow-wave sleep before resumption of breathing. This pattern resulted in REM sleep of broken quality. However, dividing sleep into stages and assigning a nomenclature (such as that of Rechtschaffen and Kales [42]) masks the continuous, unbroken nature of the shift from wakefulness to light slow-wave sleep coincident with the onset of apnea. The moment of arousal or of lightening of sleep as breathing resumed could be identified more precisely when the transition was sudden; we often saw a burst of slow activity beginning during light slow-wave sleep and continuing for several seconds after the reappearance of alpha waves, characterizing wakefulness. Similarly, in cases of apneas during REM sleep, the transition from light slow-wave sleep to REM sleep was not instantaneous, but was extended over a period during which the polygraphic characters of the two types of sleep were superimposed and then separated. Finally, the apnea itself was usually preceded by two or three progressively diminishing respiratory cycles, making it difficult to specify the exact beginning of the respiratory event.

This pathological link between sleep and respiration was not uniform throughout the night in all Pickwickians; the apneas occurred only at particular times during sleep and were usually grouped in series. The mechanism of this link constitutes the basic problem in the study of sleep-related apneas. Although most authors agree that respiratory arrest has a central origin, there is no satisfactory hypothesis as yet to explain the relationship between falling asleep and the onset of apnea.

Resumption of Respiration

The resumption of breathing is usually attributed to the preceding lightening of sleep or arousal. This lightening of sleep, in turn, is attributed to gas concentration changes taking place during apnea. Drachmann and Gumnit [17] and Semerano et al [43] (citing the mechanisms described by Hugelin et al [44]), considered hypoxia to be the cause, while Kuhlo [23] favored hypercapnia. However, because we observed that sleep sometimes lightened at the end of hypopneas or apneas too short to produce significant changes in gas concentration, we hypothesized that the arousal encouraging resumption of breathing can take place independently of changes in blood gas levels. Tammeling et al [39] suggested that increased intrapulmonary pressures play a role in the lightening of sleep. In obstructive apneas, the ineffectual respiratory movements constitute proprioceptive stimulations that probably contribute to lightening of sleep; however, the duration of such movements (30 to 120 seconds) suggests that they alone are not sufficient to stimulate arousal.

EEG and Changes in Respiration During Sleep in the Normal Subject

Relatively few studies have been made of the normal subject's breathing during sleep. Reed and Kleitman [45], Haab et al [46], Robin et al [47], Bulow and Ingvar [48, 49], Bulow [50], and Gillam [51] reported respiratory arrests of 10 to 40 seconds during somnolence in normal subjects; however, these authors did not analyze EEG changes before, during, and after apneas. Duron et al [52, 54] and Duron [55] pointed out the central nature of these apneas, but did not analyze their polygraphic concomitants either.

Regarding REM sleep of normal subjects, Snyder et al [56], Batini et al [57], Rohmer et al [58] as well as Duron and his colleagues have noted irregular breathing with pauses; in Duron's subjects, such apneas were of the central type. But again, although EEG recordings confirmed the REM sleep, pre- and post-apneic EEG changes were not analyzed. Aserinsky et al [59] and Duron et al [52, 54] merely stated that periods of irregular breathing were concomitant with bursts of eye movement.

We have not undertaken a systematic study of respiratory changes in the sleeping normal subject since the introduction of polygraphic methods of measuring respiration. Nevertheless, we have observed hypopneas and apneas in normal subjects during somnolence and light slow-wave sleep. Such episodes were rare (10 to 20 per night), lasted 10 to 20 seconds, and were always central in type. During REM sleep (with or without eye movement) of normal subjects, we have observed a very distinctive breathing pattern, irregular in both amplitude and frequency, and with central or obstructive apneas not necessarily associated with the bursts of eye movement. The termination of such apneas was usually followed by a transitory acceleration of the EEG trace associated with a brief burst of chin EMG activity.

CONCLUSION

We found some similarity between the sleep of normal subjects and that of Pickwickians; the sleep of Pickwickians differed definitively only in the number and duration of apneas and the different sleep pattern (deep slow-wave sleep was unstable and rare or absent). Thus, we question the nature of the link between sleep and pathological respiration observed in our patients. Is there a primary disturbance of the sleep-deepening process that maintains the patient in light slow-wave sleep, which is associated with apneas? If so, the presence of apneas in this phase would be physiological. (The absence of obstructive apneas in the normal subject, although not yet verified, would militate against this hypothesis.) Alternatively, does the primary trouble lie in the occurrence during light slow-wave sleep of abnormally frequent and prolonged apneas, which induce repeated arousals and subsequently prolong the state of unstable, light slow-wave sleep? These are the basic questions to be resolved in the study of sleep-related apneas.

REFERENCES

1. Auchincloss JH, Cook E, Renzetti AD: Clinical and physiological aspects of a case of obesity, polycythemia and alveolar hypoventilation. J Clin Invest 34:1537–1545, 1955.
2. Sieker HO, Estes EH, Kelser GA, MacIntosh HD: A cardiopulmonary syndrome associated with obesity. J Clin Invest 34:916, 1955.
3. Burwell CS, Robin ED, Whaley RD, Bikelmann AG: Extreme obesity associated with alveolar hypoventilation: A Pickwickian syndrome. Am J Med 21:811–818, 1956.
4. Kretschly A, Muhar F: Formes frustes bzw. Frühfälle vom Pickwick-syndrom. Wein Klin Wochenschr 76:389–393, 1964.
5. Kurtz D, Bapst-Reiter J, Fletto R, Micheletti G, Meunier-Carus J, Lonsdorfer J, Lampert-Benignus E: Les formes de transition du syndrome Pickwickien. (Seminologie et distribution des apnées.) Bull Physiopathol Respir 8:1115–1125, 1972.
6. Kurtz D, Meunier-Carus J, Bapst-Reiter J, Lonsdorfer J, Micheletti G, Benignus E, Rohmer F: Problèmes nosologiques posés par certaines formes d'hypersomnie. Rev Electroencephalogr Neurophysiol Clin 1:227–230, 1971.
7. Atlan G, Hatzeld C, Brille D: Hypoventilation alvéolaire primitive ou d'origine centrale chez le non-obèse. Presse Méd 75:2650–2654, 1967.
8. Lugaresi E: La "maledizione di Ondine" il disturbo del respiro e del sonno nell" ipoventilazione alveolare primaria. Sist Nerv 20:27–37, 1968.
9. Kuhlo W: Sleep attacks with apnea. In Gastaut H, Lugaresi E, Berti-Ceroni G, Coccagna G (eds): "Abnormalities of Sleep in Man." Bologna: Gaggi, 1968, pp 205–207.
10. Fruhmann G; Hypersomnia with primary hypoventilation syndrome and following corpulmonale (Ondine's Curse Syndrome). Bull Physiopathol Respir 8:1173–1179, 1972.
11. Guilleminault C, Eldridge F, Dement WC: Insomnia, narcolepsy, and sleep apnea. Bull Physiopathol Respir 8:1127–1138, 1972.
12. Guilleminault C, Eldridge FL, Dement WC: Insomnia with sleep apnea: A new syndrome. Science 181:856–858, 1973.
13. Lugaresi E, Coccagna G, Mantovani M: Pathophysiological, clinical and nosographic considerations regarding hypersomnia with periodic breathing. Bull Physiopathol Respir 8:1249–1256, 1972.
14. Tassinari CA: Nosologie et frontières des syndromes avec respiration périodique au cours du sommeil (syndrome de Pickwick, syndrome d'Ondine, obstruction des voies aériennes supérieures, syndrome avec microsommeil, insomnie et narcolepsie). Rev Electroencephalogr Neurophysiol Clin 5:53–61, 1976.
15. Krieger J: Les séquences hypno-apnéiques chez les sujets Pickwickiens: leur séméiologie et leur répartition. Thèse Méd, Strasbourg, 1975.
16. Simon O, Schultz H, Rassmann W: The definition of waking stages on the basis of continuous polygraphic recording in normal subjects. Electroencephalogr Clin Neurophysiol 42:48–56, 1977.
17. Drachmann DB, Gumnit RJ: Periodic alteration of consciousness in the Pickwickian syndrome. Arch Neurol 6:471–477, 1962.
18. Jung R, Kuhlo W: Neurophysiological studies of abnormal night sleep and the Pickwickian syndrome. Prog Brain Res 18:140–159, 1965.

19. Gastaut H, Tassinari CA, Duron B: Etude polygraphique des manifestations épisodiques (hypniques et respiratoires) du syndrome de Pickwick. Rev Neurol 112:568–579, 1965.

20. Gastaut H, Duron B, Papy JJ, Tassinari CA, Waltregny J: Etude polygraphique comparative du cycle nycthémérique chez les narcoleptiques, les Pickwickiens, les obèses et les insuffisants respiratoires. Rev Neurol 115:456–462, 1966.

21. Duron B, Tassinari A: Syndrome de Pickwick et syndrome cardiorespiratoire de l'obésité: à propos d'une observation. J Fr Méd Chir Thorac 20:207–222, 1966.

22. Escande JP, Schwartz BA, Gentilini M, Hazard J, Choubrac P, Domart A: Les syndromes Pickwickiens. Evolution des idées. Conceptions actuelles. (A propos de 3 observations.) Bull Mem Soc Méd Hop Paris 118:273–294, 1967.

23. Kuhlo W: Neurophysiologische und klinische Untersuchungen beim Pickwick Syndrom. Arch Psychiatr Nervenkr 211:170–192, 1968.

24. Hishikawa Y, Furuya E, Wakamatsu H, Yamamoto J: A polygraphic study of hypersomnia with periodic breathing and primary alveolar hypoventilation. Bull Physiopathol Respir 8:1139–1151, 1972.

25. Kurtz D, Lonsdorfer J, Meunier-Carus J, Micheletti G, Lampert-Benignus E: Contribution à l'étude du type et de la répartition des apnées au cours du syndrome de Pickwick. Rev Electroencephalogr Neurophysiol Clin 2:367–378, 1972.

26. Kurtz D, Micheletti G, Lonsdorfer J, Trapp C, Krieger J: Le sommeil pré et post apnéique du Pickwickien. Rev Electroencephalogr Neurophysiol Clin 5:278–282, 1975.

27. Tassinari CA, Dalla Bernardina B, Cirignotta F, Ambrosetto G: Apneic periods and the respiratory related arousal patterns during sleep in the Pickwickian syndrome: A polygraphic study. Bull Physiopathol Respir 8:1087–1102, 1972.

28. Schwartz BA, Granelet-Eprinchard MF: Traitement et surveillance des Pickwickiens: Trois modes évolutifs typiques. Rev Electroencephalogr Neurophysiol Clin 4:79–88, 1974.

29. Kurtz D, Krieger J, Lonsdorfer J: Séquences hypno-apnéiques chez les sujets Pickwickiens: Groupements apnéiques et trains d'apnées. Rev Electroencephalogr Neurophysiol Clin 6:62–69, 1976.

30. Schieber JP, Muzet A, Ferriere PJR: Les phases d'activation transitoire spontanées au cours du sommeil normal chez l'homme. Arch Sci Physiol 25:443–465, 1971.

31. Muzet A, Schieber JP, Ehrart J, Lienhard JP: Les phases d'activation transitoire et les changements de stades électroencéphalographiques de sommeil. Rev Electroencephalogr Neurophysiol Clin 3:219–222, 1973.

32. Roth B, Bruhova S, Lehovsky M: On the problem of pathophysiological mechanisms of narcolepsy, hypersomnia and dissociated sleep disturbances. In Gastaut H, Lugaresi E, Berti-Ceroni G, Coccagna G (eds): "Abnormalities of Sleep in Man." Bologna: Gaggi, 1968, pp 191–203.

33. Lugaresi E, Coccagna G, Berti-Ceroni G: Syndrome de Pickwick et syndrome d'hypoventilation alvéolaire primaire. Rev Neurol 116:678–679, 1967.

34. Coccagna G, Petrella A, Berti-Ceroni G, Lugaresi E, Pazzaglia P: Polygraphic contribution to hypersomnia and respiratory troubles in the Pickwickian syndrome. In Gastaut H, Lugaresi E, Berti-Ceroni G, Coccagna G (eds): "Abnormalities of Sleep in Man." Bologna: Gaggi, 1968, pp 215–221.

35. Bapst-Reiter J: Contribution à l'étude du nycthémère des hypersomnies paroxystiques (syndromes de Gélineau et de Pickwick). Thèse Med, Strasbourg, No. 175, 1970.

36. Gunella G: Interprétation pathogénique des troubles du sommeil et de la respiration dans le syndrome de Pickwick et dans l'hypoventilation alvéolaire primaire. Bull Physiopathol Respir 8:1257–1276, 1972.

37. Mantovani M, Cirignotta F, Vela Bueno A, Lugaresi E: Sleep organization in Pick-wickian syndrome and in primary alveolar hypoventilation. Bull Physiopathol Respir 8:1154, 1972.

38. Schwartz BA, Escande JP: Respiration hypnique Pickwickienne. In Gastaut H, Lugaresi E, Berti-Ceroni G, Coccagna G (eds): "Abnormalities of Sleep in Man." Bologna: Gaggi, 1968, pp 209–214.

39. Tammerling GJ, Blokzijl EJ, Boonstra S, Sluiter HJ: Micrognathia, hypersomnia and periodic breathing. Bull Physiopathol Respir 8:1229–1238, 1972.

40. Terzian H: Syndrome de Pickwick et narcolepsie. Rev Neurol 115:184–188, 1966.

41. Lugaresi E, Coccagna G, Mantovani M, Cirignotta F, Ambrosetto G, Baturic P: Hyper-somnia with periodic breathing: Periodic apneas and alveolar hypoventilation during sleep. Bull Physiopathol Respir 8:1103–1113, 1972.

42. Rechtschaffen A, Kales A: "A Manual of Standardized Terminology, Techniques and Scoring System for Sleep Stages of Human Subjects. Los Angeles: BIS, UCLA, 1968.

43. Semerano A, Bevilacqua M, Battistin L: Blood gas analysis and polygraphic observa-tions in the Pickwickian syndrome. Bull Physiopathol Respir 8:1193–1201, 1972.

44. Hugelin A, Bonvallet M, Dell P: Activation réticulaire et corticale d'origine chémoceptive au cours de l'hypoxie. Electroencephalogr Clin Neurophysiol 11:325–340, 1959.

45. Reed L, Kleitmann N: Studies on the physiology of sleep: The effect of sleep on respiration. Am J Physiol 75:600–608, 1926.

46. Haab P, Ramel F, Fleisch A: La respiration périodique lors de l'assoupissement. J Physiol 49:190–194, 1957.

47. Robin ED, Whaley RD, Crump LL, Travis DM: Alveolar gas tensions, pulmonary venti-lation and blood pH during physiological sleep in normal subjects. J Clin Invest 37: 981–989, 1958.

48. Bulow K, Ingvar D: Respiration and state of wakefulness in normals, studied by spirography capnography and EEG. Acta Physiol Scand 51:230–238, 1961.

49. Bulow K, Ingvar DH: Respiration and electroencephalography in narcolepsy. Neuro-logy 13:321–326, 1963.

50. Bulow K: Respiration during sleep. Electroencephalogr Clin Neurophysiol 17:441, 1964.

51. Gillam PMS: Patterns of respiration in human beings at rest and during sleep. Bull Phy-siopathol Respir 8:1059–1070, 1972.

52. Duron B, Tassinari CA, Gastaut H: Analyse spirographique et électromyographique de la respiration au cours du sommeil contrôlé par l'EEG chez l'homme normal. Rev Neurol 115:562–574, 1966.

53. Duron B, Tassinari CA, Laval P, Gastaut H: Les pauses respiratoires survenant au cours du sommeil chez l'homme. C R Soc Biol 161:634–639, 1967.

54. Duron B, Andrag C, Laval P: Ventilation pulmonaire globale, Coz alvéolaire et consom mation d'ozygène au cours du sommeil normal. C R Soc Biol 162:139–145, 1968.

55. Duron B: La fonction respiratoire pendant le sommeil physiologique. Bull Physio-pathol Respir 8:1031–1037, 1972.

56. Hobson JA, Morrison DF, Goldfrank F: Changes in respiration, heart rate and systolic blood pressure in human sleep. J Appl Physiol 19:417–422, 1964.

57. Batini C, Fressy J, Coquery JM: Critères polygraphiques du sommeil lent et du sommeil rapide. In "Le Sommeil de Nuit Normal et Pathologique," Paris: Masson, 1965, pp 156–183.

58. Rohmer F, Schaff G, Collard M, Kurtz D: La motilité spontanée, la fréquence cardiaque et la fréquence respiratoire au cours du sommeil chez l'homme normal. In "Le Sommeil de Nuit Normal et Pathologique," Paris: Masson, 1965, pp 192–205.

59. Aserinsky E: Periodic respiratory pattern occuring in conjunction with eye movements during sleep. Science 150:763–766, 1965.

1
Hemodynamic Studies in Sleep Apnea

John S Schroeder, Jorge Motta, and Christian Guilleminault

INTRODUCTION

The Pickwickian syndrome consisting of obesity, periodic breathing with hyperventilation, somnolence, and progressive cor pulmonale was described in 1956 [1]. In the 1960s a syndrome, sleep-induced obstructive apnea, characterized by daytime hypersomnolence but multiple apnea episodes only during sleep, secondary to transient upper airway obstruction, was described [2]. Multiple cardiovascular abnormalities have been reported in these patients [3, 4]. This study will describe the hemodynamic changes observed during wakefulness and sleep in a group of patients with documented sleep apnea who have undergone overnight hemodynamic and polygraphic monitoring. The therapeutic effect of tracheostomy on these hemodynamic abnormalities will be presented. These findings and pharmacologic intervention results will be used to develop proposed mechanisms for the cardiovascular abnormalities observed.

MATERIALS AND METHODS

Patients were selected from adult patients referred to the Stanford Sleep Disorders Clinic because of a suspected sleep disorder. Patients who had documented sleep-induced apnea on routine diagnostic polygraphic and Holter ECG monitoring studies gave informed consent for overnight hemodynamic monitoring. All patients had complete physical examinations, detailed neurologic and otolaryngologic examinations, routine chemistries and hematologic studies, pulmonary function studies, chest x rays, and resting electrocardiograms (ECG).

Sleep Apnea Syndromes, pages 177–196
© 1978 Alan R. Liss, Inc., 150 Fifth Avenue, New York, NY 10011

The predominant type of sleep-induced apnea had been determined by polygraphic monitoring of thoracic and abdominal respiratory movements, oral and nasal airflow, continuous recording of endoesophageal pressures with an endoesophageal pressure tip transducer (Bio-Tec BT5F), and ear oximetry prior to the hemodynamic investigation. All patients presented a disabling sleep apnea syndrome (see Chapter 1). The predominantly obstructive sleep apneic patients had Apnea Indices (number of apneas per sleep-hour, see Chapter 1) over 40, and the predominantly central sleep apneic patients over 30.

After one night of polygraphic EEG monitoring in the Clinical Research Center, a standard right heart catheterization was performed in all patients. Cardiac outputs were measured by the thermodilution method and confirmed by the Fick method. A No. 7.0 French Swan-Ganz catheter (Edwards Laboratory, Santa Ana, California) and a polyethylene arterial catheter were left in the femoral and pulmonary arteries, respectively, for the following 14 to 16 hours which included overnight pressure monitoring. Overnight sleep monitoring included continuous Holter ECG recording, a separate ECG (lead II) simultaneously recorded on paper with an electroencephalogram (C_3/A_2), electrooculogram, digastric electromyogram, oral and nasal thermistors, thoracic and abdominal movements, as well as pulmonary and femoral arterial pressures. A continuous record of arterial pO_2 was obtained with an intraarterial oxygen electrode (International Biophysics Corporation, Model #625-001, Irvine, California) in 18 patients. Arterial blood samples were obtained during wakefulness and at least three times during sleep for blood gas movements in all cases. All medicines were stopped one week before the studies. Statistical analysis of this study was done by the paired t test.

RESULTS

Patients With Predominant Obstructive Sleep Apnea

Twenty-two patients with predominantly obstructive apnea completed the study. Their ages ranged from 30 to 63 years (mean 47 years). All of them had typical clinical symptoms (see Chapter 1) with disabling excessive daytime sleepiness and loud snoring at night. The majority were overweight with a mean weight of 104 kg (range 78 to 143 kg) and a mean height of 189 cm (range 175 to 203 cm). In all patients the symptom of heavy snoring preceded obesity by a mean of ten years. Six of the 22 patients had systemic hypertension. Electrocardiographic abnormalities during wakefulness included left ventricular hypertrophy (three patients), left anterior hemiblock (one patient), and ST-T wave abnormalities (three patients). Borderline cardiomegaly was noted in two patients on x rays. The mean Apnea Index in this group of patients was 79 range 48 to 160), a mean of 88% of sleep apneic episodes was obstructive, and patients spent a mean of 45% of total sleep time without air exchange (range 28 to 78%). Partial results of the right heart cardiac catheterization are presented in Table I. There were few abnormalities present during wakefulness and at rest.

Studies during sleep. Table I shows the number of apneic episodes per sleep-hour, arterial oxygen tension, and pulmonary and systemic arterial pressures during sleep. Pressures reported during sleep are the highest sustained values observed for each patient during the entire sleep period. Cardiac output values during sleep with a mean of three measurements (thermodilution) were performed in rapid succession during one episode of sleep apnea and did not necessarily correspond in time to recorded pressures. Blood gas values during sleep reflect the extremes of recorded values. Twenty patients developed significant rises in systemic arterial pressure during sleep, six exceeding 200 mm Hg (systolic), and seven reaching or exceeding 120 mm Hg (diastolic). These pressure elevations were generally transient and occurred cyclically with each episode of apnea (Fig 1). When episodes of apnea occurred in rapid succession, systemic arterial pressures did not return to control values but showed a stepwise increase as shown in Figure 2.

Twenty-one patients developed moderate rises in pulmonary arterial pressure. The degree of pulmonary hypertension increased gradually with each apneic episode and returned towards control levels at resumption of ventilation. Upon awakening, with unobstructed respiration, both systemic and pulmonary artery pressures rapidly returned to control levels. There was no definite trend in cardiac outputs in the seven patients in whom this was measured during sleep.

Marked degrees of hypoxemia occurring transiently with each episode of apnea were documented, with arterial pO_2 values falling below 50 mm Hg in 17 of the 22 patients. These episodes of hypoxemia were accompanied by moderate elevations in arterial pCO_2 (mean 48.5 mm Hg; range 42–65 mm Hg) and respiratory acidosis.

Hemodynamic Studies in Predominantly Central Apneic Patients

Four patients with predominantly central apnea (over 55% of the total number of apnea of "central type") were studied under a protocol similar to that for the predominantly obstructive sleep apneic patients. Their ages ranged from 40 to 73 years (mean 56). Their mean weight was 72.75 kg (range 65–97 kg). One patient had systemic hypertension, and one had ST-T wave abnormalities during wakefulness. Their mean Apnea Index was 59 (range 30–104), and they spent a mean of 56% of their total sleep time without air exchange. Right heart catheterization demonstrated normal resting hemodynamics during wakefulness in three patients; one patient had moderately severe hypertension. During exercise, mild pulmonary hypertension with elevation of pulmonary arterial wedge pressure was seen in one case.

TABLE I. Obstructive Sleep Apneic Patients

Patient	Apnea index	Femoral arterial pressure (mm Hg)		Pulmonary arterial pressure (mm Hg)		Lowest PaO$_2$ (mm Hg)	
		Awake supine (S/D)[a]	Asleep (S/D)	Awake supine (S/D)	Asleep (S/D)	Awake supine	Asleep
1	60	130/80	200/145	28/18	70/50	87	38
2	80	150/90	170/110	32/26	38/32	76	43
3	65	145/80	190/110	20/10	64/36	73	48
4	50	120/80	120/80	20/10	22/12	73	—
5	74	115/65	140/80	36/16	55/30	74	42
6	78	140/90	150/100	35/20	80/50	60	25
7	48	140/80	140/80	22/18	40/25	83	53
8	59	120/75	180/110	28/14	60/25	80	26
9	81	105/70	140/80	35/20	50/30	70	36
10	65	160/90	190/100	32/20	48/24	69	30
11	90	160/94	280/170	34/20	68/40	80	30
12	63	160/110	194/124	28/12	60/48	85	30
13	78	130/80	200/120	30/20	80/54	83	35
14	64	120/70	168/100	17/7	38/24	84	34
15	81	120/74	160/100	28/14	60/40	98	50
16	70	110/80	240/130	23/12	54/30	76	33
17	51	120/64	178/100	34/22	52/30	87	52
18	90	130/70	180/104	24/16	42/20	90	47
19	120	180/110	230/130	35/18	60/38	87	41
20	140	130/80	160/90	30/18	64/32	80	33
21	78	170/96	220/120	50/30	80/34	68	40
22	57	140/88	180/96	32/18	50/32	89	40
Mean	75	136/83	182/108	30/17	56/33	80	38

aHere and in Tables II–IV, S/D refers to systolic/diastolic.

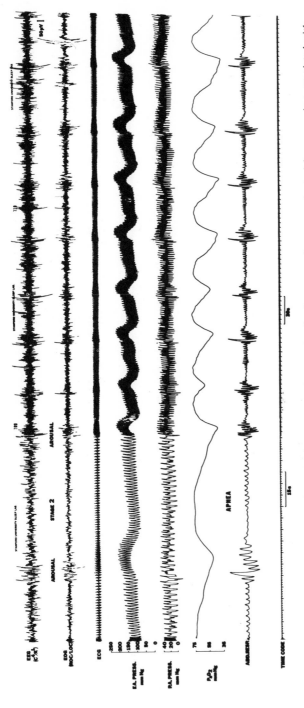

Fig 1. Polygraphic recording in obstructive sleep apnea patient showing the simultaneous pulmonary and arterial pressure rises associated with transient falls in PaO₂.

Studies during sleep. Table II shows the Apnea Index, arterial oxygen tension, and pulmonary and systemic arterial pressures during sleep. The pressures are the highest values recorded during the entire sleep period for each patient and occurred primarily during rapid eye movement (REM) sleep. Blood gas values during sleep reflect the lowest values recorded, which were generally not as extreme as in the obstructive group.

Patients' cyclical systemic and pulmonary hypertension during sleep was similar to that in predominantly obstructive patients. The transient increases in pressures were moderate compared to those seen in obstructive patients. The systemic pressure tracing showed a gradual rise during progressive hypoxemia and a further brief rise at the onset of respiration and arousal similar to the obstructive patients. Mean pulmonary arterial pressure rose progressively with development of hypoxemia. During central apnea, pulmonary arterial pressure was easy to measure as respiratory movements did not interfere (Fig 1).

Intervention Studies

The similarity of the cyclic arterial and pulmonary arterial pressure changes in the obstructive and central apnea patients suggests that the hypoxemia with the associated mild hypercapnia and acidosis plays a central role in these hemodynamic abnormalities. We therefore undertook several intervention studies to identify the reflex pathways involved in the pathophysiologic response to sleep apnea.

Parasympathetic blockade. Five patients (four obstructive, one central type) were given 1 mg of atropine sulfate intravenously twice, three minutes apart, during non-rapid eye movement (NREM) sleep. Arterial pO_2, state of sleep, cardiac rhythm, and pressures were determined to be stable before the injection. No change in the number or duration of apneas or arterial pO_2 changes could be observed after the injections. The patients remained in NREM sleep, and the typical cyclical pattern of apnea respiration was observed on the polygraph.

The atropine administration resulted in sustained sinus tachycardia with abolition of the sinus arrhythmia and marked cyclical sinus bradycardia (Fig 3). The hemodynamic responses to atropine are shown in Table III. With the onset of tachycardia, there was a slight fall in both systemic and pulmonary pressures. The transient rise in systemic pressure at the onset of respiration was still evident but blunted.

Shy-Drager patients (see Chapter 21). Two patients with sleep apnea were also identified as having Shy-Drager syndrome, a unique combination of autonomic insufficiency and extrapyramidal derangement [5]. Both of these patients presented with progressive symptoms of autonomic insufficiency as well as sleep apnea. The patients were observed to have marked periodic respiration during sleep with multiple periods of apnea characterized by increased respiratory effort and loud snoring. Holter monitoring recording revealed minimal variation in

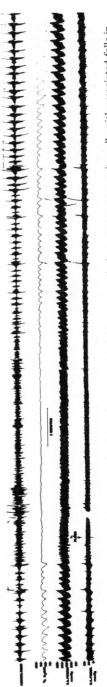

Fig 2. Polygraphic recording showing progressive femoral pressure rise during progressively more severe apneic spells with associated falls in arterial oxygen saturation.

TABLE II. Central Apnea Patients

Patient	Apnea index	Femoral arterial pressure (mm Hg)		Pulmonary arterial pressure (mm Hg)		PaO$_2$ (mm Hg)	
		Awake supine (S/D)	Asleep (S/D)	Awake supine (S/D)	Asleep (S/D)	Awake supine	Asleep
1	53	120/68	180/120	25/16	34/18	92	50
2	104	150/90	160/100	20/10	54/38	90	33
3	48	140/67	170/89	40/22	50/30	97	62
4	30	210/110	240/160	20/16	26/19	86	63
Mean	59	155/84	188/117	56/16	41/26	91	52

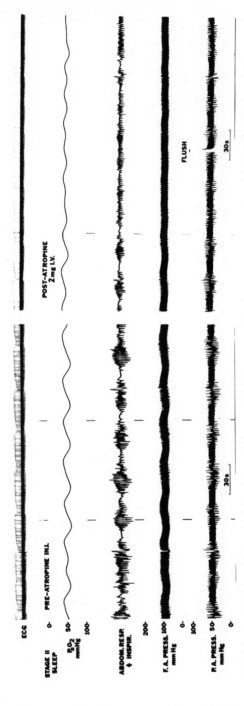

Fig 3. Vagal blockade with atropine during sleep apnea. Note the blunting of transient femoral pressure rises with little alteration in the pulmonary pressure or O_2 saturation after atropine.

TABLE III. Parasympathetic Blockade During Sleep Apnea

| | Pre-atropine | | Post-atropine[a] (two minutes) | |
| | Femoral arterial pressure (mm Hg) (S/D) | Pulmonary arterial pressure (mm Hg) (S/D) | Femoral arterial pressure (mm Hg) (S/D) | Pulmonary arterial pressure (mm Hg) (S/D) |
Patient				
12	184/116	47/25	180/110	44/26
14	140/80	22/14	140/80	18/8
17	160/98	52/30	150/98	34/20
22	168/108	58/36	150/80	40/24
2	160/100	55/28	160/100	50/25
(central) Mean	162/100	47/27	156/94	37/21

[a] Atropine, 2 mg, IV.

heart rate during awake and asleep periods, reflecting autonomic denervation. The patients underwent right heart catheterization and overnight hemodynamic monitoring in an effort to evaluate the integrity of the reflex pathways and responses to hypoxia. Both patients had an increase in the resting heart rate of approximately 30 beats per minute after intravenous (IV) administration of 2 mg of atropine, suggesting residual vagal nerve function and influence on the vagus nerve.

During overnight hemodynamic monitoring, wide swings of the pulmonary arterial pressure occurred in response to marked increases in respiratory effort during obstruction with transient rises in pulmonary artery systolic pressure to 70 mm Hg without changes in systemic arterial pressure. These episodes were associated with marked falls in PaO_2 to as low as 32 mm Hg and rises in $PaCO_2$ to 55 mm Hg.

The lack of systemic pressure rise in these two cases confirms the involvement of the autonomic nervous system in the progressive rise in systemic arterial pressure. However, the persistence of cyclical pulmonary hypertension in these patients, and its persistence after treatment with atropine sulfate in obstructive and central apnea patients, indicates a greater direct role of hypoxia in pulmonary pressure changes. In order to further define the role of hypoxemia in the cyclic hemodynamic changes, the effect of oxygen administration was studied.

Effect of oxygen. Four patients, three with predominantly obstructive and one with predominantly central type apnea, received oxygen during sleep by means of a nasal cannula and/or mask which was held in front of the patient's face without touching him. Five to 10 liters of oxygen per minute in room air were administered in an acute, intermittent procedure, during NREM sleep. Arterial pO_2, state of sleep, and pressures were continuously monitored: blood gases were measured during control and oxygen administration. In two cases, atropine sulfate, 1 mg IV, was administered while the patient was receiving oxygen. The results are presented in Table IV. All patients' PaO_2 values rose to > 120 mm Hg. Within two minutes after oxygen administration, the cyclic systemic and pulmonary arterial pressure rises during apnea were blunted despite the fact that the length of apnea greatly increased (see Chapter 8). When atropine sulfate was injected intravenously in combination with oxygen, pressure changes were further blunted.

Effect of Tracheostomy

Six patients underwent repeat hemodynamic monitoring after tracheostomy. Except for systemic hypertension in two patients, few abnormalities were noted at rest. After tracheostomy no significant differences were observed in pO_2 or pulmonary systemic pressure during wakefulness. After tracheostomy, however, the mean number of apneic episodes per hour decreased from 73 ± 5 to 6 ± 2 ($P < 0.001$). All posttracheostomy apneas were of the central type. The

TABLE IV. Effect of Oxygen*

| Patient | Room air | | | Oxygen[a] | | Oxygen + atropine sulfate | |
	FA (S/D)	PA (S/D)	PaO$_2$	FA (S/D)	PA (S/D)	FA	PA
16	150/92	50/30	65	130/80	34/18	—	—
17	160/98	52/30	58	140/90	45/28	140/90	34/20
22	168/108	58/36	57	140/64	40/28	120/64	34/18
1 (central)	180/120	54/38	63	160/100	50/34	—	—
Mean	165/105	54/34	61	143/84	42/27	—	—

*All measures given in mm Hg. FA, femoral arterial pressure; PA, pulmonary arterial pressure.
[a]Mean oxygen administration 8 liters/min. All PaO$_2$ > 120 mm Hg.

lowest mean arterial pO_2 during apnea increased from 38 ± 3 to 71 ± 2 mm Hg ($P < 0.001$). Significant reductions were noted in the mean femoral and pulmonary arterial pressures after tracheostomy. For the group, pulmonary artery mean pressure decreased from 35 ± 6 to 22 ± 2 mm Hg ($P < 0.05$) and the femoral arterial mean pressure decreased from 137 ± 6 to 97 ± 3 mm Hg ($P < 0.005$). Episodes of obstructive apnea were essentially totally abolished and there were no typical cyclic elevations of pressure rise.

DISCUSSION

Since Gastaut's report that periods of apnea are associated with sleep, multiple reports have appeared describing patients with sleep-induced apnea [2]. It appears that the syndrome need not occur in obese patients. Complete pulmonary function studies have been reported to be entirely normal in many patients, with normal CO_2 responsiveness and without obvious anatomic abnormalities of the hypopharynx during wakefulness. We have found overnight Holter monitoring to be extremely helpful in diagnosis of patients with sleep-induced obstructive apnea, the pathognomic finding being a characteristic and marked variation in sinus heart rate in phase with respiration and apnea as reported by Tilkian et al [6].

It appears that in the early stages of this syndrome there are few abnormalities during wakefulness, as confirmed by normal hemodynamics in our patients. Six patients did have mild to moderate systemic hypertension but no pulmonary hypertension. During exercise there was a rise in pulmonary artery wedge pressure in five patients, which may reflect mild abnormalities of left ventricular function [7].

Normal sleep is generally characterized by reduction in systemic arterial pressure, the lowest values being reported in stages 3 and 4 of sleep. Episodes of acute elevation of blood pressure in sinus rhythm can occur during REM sleep [4, 8, 9]. These changes rapidly resolve on arousal, as does the blood pressure return to normal. The hemodynamic changes during sleep are quite different in our patients. In none was there a progressive fall in arterial pressure. In fact, 21 of the 22 patients had characteristic rises of a cyclic nature of their arterial pressure which was initiated at a time of ventilation after a period of apnea. This cyclic systemic pressure rise was associated with sinus tachycardia and appeared to occur at the time of EEG arousal and inspiration. As seen in Figure 1, it appears that there are actually two phases to the systemic arterial pressure rise. There is a progressive slow rise in pressure associated with a progressive fall in PaO_2 during the apneic episodes. However, at the onset of EEG arousal, tachycardia and ventilation occur as the apneic episode is broken, and there is a rapid bump or rise in the arterial pressure associated with the sinus tachycardia. This further arterial pressure rise appears to be initiated by the first breath and lasts only 10 to 15 seconds as the arterial oxygen tension rapidly rises back to normal. This cycle then recurs as apnea recurs, and the PaO_2 progressively falls.

The hemodynamic findings in the two patients with Shy-Drager syndrome suggest that autonomic vasomotor reflexes are important factors responsible for cardiovascular abnormalities observed in patients with sleep apnea syndrome. In the absence of these reflexes, apnea during sleep was not associated with cyclic changes in systemic blood pressure, suggesting that reflex changes in sympathetic tone due to hypoxia are the predominant mechanisms for the changes rather than a direct vasoconstrictive effect of the hypoxia. The fact, however, that pulmonary hypertension did occur with apneic episodes suggests that other factors such as local and central hypoxia or local pulmonary vascular reflexes are important to the generation of these pressures.

Vagal blockade with atropine blunted the sinus bradycardia and tachycardia associated with the cyclic apneic episodes. However, there continued to be transient cyclical rises in pulmonary, as well as arterial, pressure, which suggest a mechanical or nonparasympathetically mediated response to the hypoxia.

The presence of cyclic pulmonary hypertension in our two Shy-Drager patients during sleep apnea and the blunting of the pressure changes during oxygen administration suggest a direct effect of the hypoxemia and acidosis on the pulmonary vasculature. The systemic pressure rises, however, appear to be multifactorial. Since the cyclic systems and pressure rises were absent in the Shy-Drager patients, this indicates the involvement of the autonomic nervous system. Since this cyclical response is blunted by oxygen administration, the response is presumably initiated by the chemoreceptor reflex. Further intervention studies will be required to further define the direct versus reflexly induced pressure changes.

Response to Tracheostomy

Tracheostomy has been utilized with success in the treatment of patients with sleep-induced apnea [10]. These studies have reported the prompt disappearance of daytime somnolence and return to normal sleep patterns after tracheostomy. Resolution of the hemodynamic abnormalities has been reported by Kuhlo and Doll [11], Lugaresi et al [12], and Motta et al [13]. Furthermore, children with chronic upper airway obstruction secondary to enlarged tonsillar and adenoid tissue who develop cor pulmonale and hypersomnolence have marked response to tonsillectomy and adenoidectomy [14, 15]. In these cases, falls in pulmonary artery pressure have been documented before and after cardiac catheterization [14]. Our results confirm that relief of upper airway obstruction by tracheostomy can produce marked symptomatic improvement and almost complete return to normal of hemodynamic and cardiac rhythm abnormalities. After tracheostomy, the overnight hemodynamic monitoring documented almost complete resolution of the cyclical changes in pulmonary and femoral artery pressures. Although there were small falls in PaO_2 in response to periods of central apnea in patients after tracheostomy, these changes tended to be small and characterized by only slight increases in pulmonary artery and systemic pressures. Therefore, it appears that normalization of arterial blood gases and pH by tracheostomy is the most important contributor to the resolution of these abnormalities. Furthermore, with closure of the tracheostomy, in several patients we can document rapid return of the obstructive apneic episodes accompanied by the same pretracheostomy hemodynamic and rhythm abnormalities. In view of these findings, airway obstruction appears to play the primary role in inducing cardiovascular reflexes resulting in hemodynamic and rhythm abnormalities.

Proposed Mechanisms of Cyclic Hemodynamic Changes (Figs 4 and 6)

The mechanisms responsible for the cyclic changes in pressures and sinus rhythm are not completely understood. The marked relief of these abnormalities by tracheostomy, however, would suggest that hypoxia which causes stimulation of arterial chemoreceptors must play an important role in the production of these cardiovascular abnormalities.

The striking abnormality during sleep apnea is the profound degree of hypoxemia in these patients which cannot be attributed solely to hypoventilation. This abnormality suggests that a widening of the alveolar arterial oxygen gradient occurs, for which the mechanism is not known. It is suspected that there is a cyclic ventilation perfusion mismatch during obstructive respiration [3]. Pulmonary edema due to negative intrapulmonary pressure generated by the Müller maneuver or due to left ventricular dysfunction has also been proposed as a mechanism, but is unlikely to be an important factor [16]. Continuous arterial pO_2 measurements by intraarterial electrode have allowed us to document marked falls in PaO_2 to as low as 25 mm Hg at the end of prolonged apneic episodes. These extreme degrees of transient hypoxemia might put the patient at higher risk for ischemic events or arrhythmias. It is likely that, during periods of undisturbed sleep, patients achieve even more prolonged periods of apnea and hypoxemia.

Heart rate slowing induced by breath-holding has been well described in man [17]. In canine preparations, Daly and Scott have demonstrated that stimulation of carotid chemoreceptors by hypoxic blood produced marked sinus bradycardia at a time when ventilation was controlled at low lung volumes [18]. However, a change in respiration, sometimes with even a single breath, caused accelerations of heart rate. Daly and Scott concluded that chemoreceptor stimulation by hypoxic blood caused the vagally mediated sinus bradycardia, and this was over-come or reversed by reflex-activated pulmonary stretch receptors. It appeared that the magnitude of rate increase was related to the amount of lung volume increase and could be abolished by lung denervation. It appears that a similar mechanism is present in sleep-induced apnea patients. This vagal response explains the marked sinus bradycardia resulting from the progressive hypoxia and limitation of lung expansion produced by upper airway obstruction. The heart rate changes are thoroughly discussed in Chapter 12 and will not be repeated here.

It can be seen that sinus tachycardia occurs at the onset of respiration and EEG arousal despite a further fall for several more seconds of arterial pO_2 until reversed by the hyperventilation. Thus, the pulmonary stretch reflexes appear to dominate as far as control over heart rate, despite the falling PaO_2. It is of

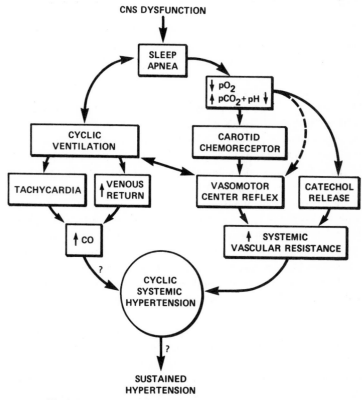

Fig 4. Proposed mechanism for cyclic systemic hypertension.

interest that there is also a further rise in arterial pressure at the onset of ventilation, presumably reflecting further sympathetic influences or release of vagal tone at the onset of ventilation. This hypothesis is further strengthened by the recording in a patient with central apnea of transient tachycardia and rise in blood pressure initiated by a sigh just prior to onset of sleep apnea (Fig 5). Additionally, we hypothesize that initiation of ventilation, frequently with an initial large breath, increases central venous return and stroke volume via the Frank-Starling mechanism. The transient rise in cardiac output for five to ten beats most likely contributed to the further rise in blood pressure at the onset of ventilation. Since ventilation, sinus tachycardia, and systemic pressure rise all occur during EEG arousal, it is possible that these changes may have a centrally mediated component as well.

Thus, the transient rises in systemic blood pressure have at least these components: a) a slow rise during progressive fall in PaO_2 that reflects primarily a reflex-induced rise in systemic vascular resistance via carotid chemoreceptors; and b) a further bump or rise in pressure at the onset of effective ventilation probably secondary to release of vagal tone, heightened sympathetic tone, and increased cardiac output due to pulmonary stretch reflex-induced tachycardia, as well as the increase in central venous return. The cyclic increases in systemic pressure are probably partly explained in the chemoreceptor stimulation by hypoxia and acidosis, leading to vasomotor center-mediated arteriolar constriction. Thus, there is a progressive rise in systemic pressures associated with progressive falls in PaO_2 and rising $PaCO_2$ levels.

The cyclic changes in pulmonary artery pressure are most likely multifactoral (Fig 6). As can be seen during vigorous respiratory efforts, there are mild rises in systolic and falls in diastolic pulmonary pressure characteristic of marked changes in intrathoracic pressures. However, during this marked respiratory effort there is little change in mean pulmonary artery pressures, reflecting varying combinations of the Müller and Valsalva maneuvers. However, there are progressive rises in mean pulmonary artery pressure during the night in response to progressive falls in PaO_2 and $PaCO_2$ as apneic episodes continue. These elevations in pulmonary artery pressure are most likely secondary to the combined effects of acidosis and hypoxemia, both directly on the pulmonary vasculature as well as reflex induced. The transient rise in cardiac output at the onset of effective ventilation, causing a rise in systemic pressure, probably also accounts for the rise in pulmonary arterial pressure. Upon awakening, these changes rapidly return to normal, as does the systemic arterial pressure.

In conclusion, cyclical hypoxemia occurring during both obstructive and central apnea is the predominant initiating event which precipitates a series of direct and chemoreceptor-induced changes in observed pulmonary and arterial pressures. These changes are nearly completely reversed by tracheostomy.

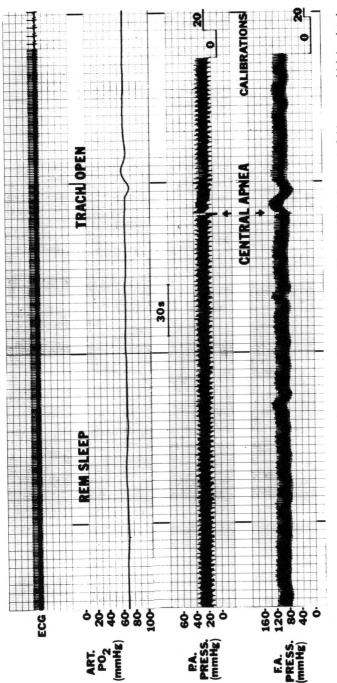

Fig 5. Isolated central apnea during REM sleep recorded in a posttracheostomy patient. Note the biphasic aspect of this apnea, which is related to physiological compensatory mechanisms: hyperoxia followed by apnea.

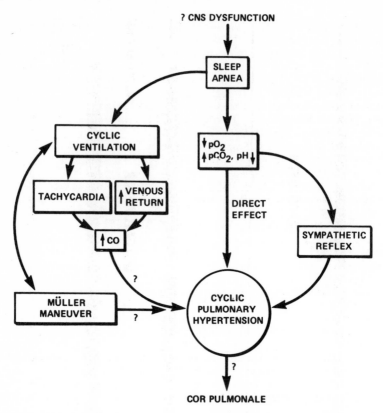

Fig 6. Proposed mechanism for cyclic pulmonary hypertension.

ACKNOWLEDGMENTS

This research was supported by National Institute of Neurological Diseases and Stroke grant NS 10727, Public Health Service Research Grant RR-70 from the General Clinical Research Centers, Division of Research Resources, and by INSERM to Dr Guilleminault.

REFERENCES

1. Burwell CS, Robin ED, Whaley RD, Bikelman A: Extreme obesity associated with alveolar hypoventilation: A Pickwickian syndrome. Am J Med 21:811–818, 1956.
2. Gastaut H, Tassinari CA, Duron B: Étude polygraphique des manifestations épisodiques (hypniques et respiratoires), diurnes et nocturnes, du syndrome de Pickwick. Rev Neurol 112:568–579, 1965.

3. Guilleminault C, Eldridge FL, Simmons FB, Dement WC: Sleep apnea syndrome: Can it induce hemodynamic changes? West J Med 123:7–16, 1975.
4. Khatri IM, Freis ED: Hemodynamic changes during sleep. J Appl Physiol 22:867–873, 1967.
5. Shy GM, Drager GA: A neurologic syndrome associated with orthostatic hypotension. Arch Neurol 2:511, 1960.
6. Tilkian AG, Guilleminault C, Schroeder JS, Lehrman KL, Simmons FB, Dement WC: Sleep induced apnea syndrome: Prevalence of cardiac arrhythmias and their reversal after tracheostomy. Am J Med 63:348–358, 1977.
7. Tilkian AG, Guilleminault C, Schroeder JS, Lehrman KL, Simmons FB, Dement WC: Hemodynamics in sleep-induced apnea. Studies during wakefulness and sleep. Ann Intern Med 85:714–719, 1976.
8. Bristow JD, Honour AJ, Pickering TG, Sleight P: Cardiovascular and respiratory changes during sleep in normal and hypertensive subjects. Cardiovasc Res 3:476–485, 1969.
9. Coccagna G, Mantovani M, Brignani F, Manzini A, Lugaresi E: Arterial pressure changes during spontaneous sleep in man. Electroencephalogr Clin Neurophysiol 31:277–281, 1972.
10. Guilleminault C, Tilkian A, Dement WC: The sleep apnea syndromes. Annu Rev Med 27:465–484, 1976.
11. Kuhlo W, Doll W: Pulmonary hypertension and the effect of tracheostomy in a case of Pickwickian syndrome. Bull Physiopathol Respir 8:1205–1216, 1972.
12. Lugaresi E, Coccagna G, Mantovani M, Brignani F: Effects of tracheostomy in two cases of hypersomnia with periodic breathing. J Neurol Neurosurg Psychiatry 36:15–26, 1973.
13. Motta J, Guilleminault C, Schroeder JS, Dement WC: Changes in hemodynamics after tracheostomy in sleep induced obstructive apnea. Ann Intern Med, in press.
14. Bland JW Jr, Edwards KF, Brinsfield D: Pulmonary hypertension and congestive heart failure in children with chronic upper airway obstruction. Am J Cardiol 22:830–837, 1969.
15. Guilleminault C, Eldridge FL, Simmons FB, Dement WC: Sleep apnea in eight children. Pediatrics 58:23–31, 1976.
16. Luke MJ, Mehrizi A, Folger GM Jr, Rowe R: Chronic nasopharyngeal obstruction as a cause of cardiomegaly, cor pulmonale, and pulmonary edema. Pediatrics 37:762–768, 1966.
17. Moore TO, Elsner R, Lin YC, Lally DA, Hong SK: Effects of alveolar PO_2 and PCO_2 on apneic bradycardia in men. J Appl Physiol 34:795–798, 1973.
18. Daly M de B, Scott MJ: The effects of stimulation of the carotid body chemoreceptors on heart rate in the dog. J Physiol 144:148–166, 1958.

DISCUSSION

Questions about the mechanisms involved in pulmonary hypertension were raised by several investigators. Dr Schroeder and Dr Weil insisted on the major role of hypoxia. As stated in the text, two components apparently exist in pulmonary hypertension: a slow rise in pulmonary artery (PA) pressure related to hypoxia, and a more rapid component related to increased stroke volume and cardiac output during inspiration. During exercise, cardiac output may rise two- to threefold with only minimal increase in PAP. But as Dr Severinghaus noted, when a subject is hypoxic, doubling the cardiac output greatly increases PA pressure, whereas very little effect on PA pressure is seen in a normoxic individual. Dr Weil stated that the Müller maneuver must also be taken into consideration as it produces changes in afterload. It should also be remembered that the lung is very poor at diverting blood away from underventilated areas when pressure is high in the left ventricle. Dr Phillipson and Dr Severinghaus stressed that the severe pulmonary hypertension which develops during the hypoxic episodes in sleep apnea may be sufficient in itself to produce pulmonary edema and may also contribute to pathogenic PAP, particularly in older patients who progressively develop hypertension, obesity, and in some cases, pulmonary arterial disease.

Dr Coccagna referred to the fact that two separate groups of patients could be delineated — one group with normal ventilation during wakefulness and in whom PAP drops nearly instantaneously to normal levels when the patient awakens, and the second group of patients who gradually develop alveolar hypoventilation which persists during wakefulness. These two groups, however, may be representative of a continuum.

Dr Hill was struck by the fact that in the different patient populations reported here by multiple investigators, about 50% are hypertensive during daytime wakefulness; he raised a question as to the mechanisms responsible for persistence of daytime hypertension. Dr Weil suggested studying the renin-angiotensin system in sleep apneic patients, using Saralasin (an angiotensin II inhibitor) infusion after sodium depletion to demonstrate whether angiotensin is inhibited during sleep-related hypertensive episodes. Dr Coccagna reported that his patients with daytime hypertension became normotensive after tracheostomy. Dr Guilleminault reported differing findings and mentioned that again two groups could be observed, one in whom daytime hypertension disappeared after tracheostomy and a second group which improved (decreased medication as index of improvement) but retained elevated readings during the daytime. He felt it possible that sleep apnea (and its implications of hypoxia, etc) may contribute to the appearance of daytime hypertension and that if this condition is neglected for many years, the patient may develop secondary lesions (eg, kidney) which will maintain hypertension after tracheostomy.

12
Cardiac Arrhythmias in Sleep Apnea

Ara G Tilkian, Jorge Motta, and Christian Guilleminault

Cardiovascular manifestations of the sleep apnea syndrome have received recent attention. The hemodynamic changes observed in patients with sleep apnea were the first to be investigated. The development of pulmonary and systemic hypertension in this syndrome is now well recognized and their reversal after tracheostomy has been repeatedly confirmed [1, 2]. These findings are summarized in Chapter 11. The present discussion will be limited to the cardiac arrhythmias associated with sleep apnea and their response to various interventions.

MATERIALS AND METHODS

Patients were selected from 450 adults referred to the Stanford Sleep Disorders Clinic during a 30-month period. Twenty-five patients were documented to have sleep-induced apnea on routine diagnostic polygraphic studies. All gave written informed consent for the present study and approval of the Stanford University School of Medicine Committee on the Use of Human Subjects in Research was obtained.

The following studies were performed in all patients: medical history, physical examination, detailed neurological and otolaryngologic evaluation, routine laboratory studies, chest X ray, and electrocardiogram. All patients underwent 24 hours of continuous electrocardiographic recording (Holter recording) using a single channel Avionics ECG tape recorder. A second 24 hours of ECG recording was obtained in nine of the patients, during atropine administration. In five, 1.2 mg of atropine was given orally just prior to sleep and repeated in four hours if the patient was awake. In four, atropine was given intravenously (1.0–2.0 mg)

Sleep Apnea Syndromes, pages 197–210

during sleep. In 17 patients in whom a therapeutic tracheostomy was performed, an additional 24-hour ECG recording was obtained six to eight weeks following the operation. In nine patients, ECG recordings were repeated with the tracheostomy plugged during part of the sleep. In addition to the Holter ECG recordings, a separate ECG lead (lead II) was also continuously recorded on paper simultaneously with recordings of the electroencephalogram (C_3/A_2), electrooculogram, digastric electromyogram, thoracic and abdominal movements, oral and nasal temperatures and ear oximetry. All ECG tapes were processed by computer methods described previously [3]. This technique permits visual inspection of every R-R interval, QRS duration and vector for the entire 24-hour period allowing accurate determination and quantification of all arrhythmias (Fig 1). Once detected, arrhythmias were recorded in conventional form (Fig 2).

Marked sinus arrhythmia was considered present when rhythmic alteration in heart rate during sleep exceeded 40 beats per minute *and* recurred cyclically, in phase with apnea and respiration.

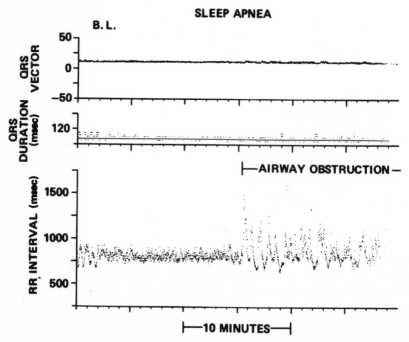

Fig 1. Computer printout of 30 minutes of ECG recording during sleep. Each QRS complex is characterized by three dots indicating the R-R interval, QRS duration, and QRS vector. Periodic obstructive apnea (second half of recording) is accompanied by marked variation in the R-R interval, occurring cyclically with each apnea (sinus bradycardia) and ventilation (sinus tachycardia).

APNEA DURING SLEEP

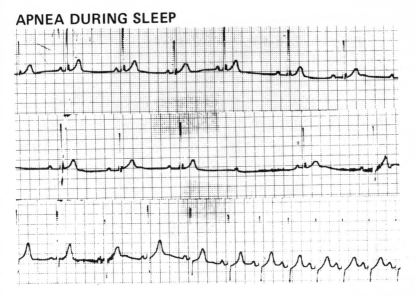

Fig 2. Twenty-five seconds of continuous ECG recording during sleep. Sinus bradycardia during apnea is accompanied by transient type I second-degree AV block. Sinus tachycardia accompanies onset of ventilation.

One patient with an advanced case of Shy-Drager syndrome and sleep apnea had additional hemodynamic studies to evaluate the integrity of his autonomic reflex pathways. Almost complete autonomic denervation was documented on various provocative tests and later confirmed on postmortem examination [4].

RESULTS

Pertinent clinical findings are summarized in Table I. All patients were men and all presented with disabling daytime sleepiness. Unusually loud snoring was present in all but one for many years. Most were overweight and half had systemic hypertension during wakefulness. One patient also suffered from autonomic nervous system dysfunction (Shy-Drager syndrome) and another had spinobulbar poliomyelitis at age 17.

Diagnostic polygraphic recordings during sleep revealed the pattern of predominantly obstructive (upper airway obstruction) type of apnea in all but one. The exception was the patient with poliomyelitis who had mild nocturnal snoring and in whom the majority of apneas were central (nonobstructive) with no detectable intercostal or diaphragmatic muscular effort.

TABLE I. Clinical Data

Number of patients	25
Age (years)	30–63 (mean 44)
Sex	All males
Weight (kg)	76–165 (mean 115)
Disabling daytime sleepiness	25
Loud, severe snoring	24
Systemic hypertension	12
Other diagnoses	Shy-Drager syndrome – 1
	Spinobulbar poliomyelitis – 1

Arrythmias recorded during wakefulness and sleep are summarized in Table II. Normal sinus rhythm was present during wakefulness in all, while a cyclic pattern of marked sinus arrhythmia appeared in all except one during sleep and apnea (Fig 1). This rhythm pattern was characterized by progressive sinus bradycardia during apnea (heart rate < 30/min in seven) with abrupt reversal and sinus acceleration at the onset of ventilation (heart rate 85–120/min) with recurrent cycles of 1 to 1.5 minutes each. The exception was the patient with autonomic dysfunction (Shy-Drager syndrome) who had a qualitatively similar response during sleep; ie, cyclic sinus slowing and speeding in phase with apnea and ventilation cycles were noted, but sinus rate variation was minimal and ranged from 70 to 90/min. Second degree Atrio-Ventricular (AV) block was noted in four patients (Fig 2) and prolonged sinus pauses ranging from 2.5 to 13 seconds accompanied the apnea and the bradycardia in seven patients (Fig 3). Premature ventricular contractions (PVCs) were seen more frequently during sleep, and in two patients self-limited runs of ventricular tachycardia accompanied the sinus bradycardia during sleep (Fig 4). Paroxysmal atrial tachycardia was recorded only once during sleep.

The effect of atropine on these arrhythmias was tested in nine patients. Marked sinus arrhythmia was present in all before atropine. Following oral administration of 1.2 to 2.4 mg of atropine in five patients, there was abolition of sinus bradycardia in all. The cyclical pattern of sinus arrhythmia continued but the marked sinus rate variation was abolished. When atropine was administered intravenously (1–2 mg) in four patients, a sustained sinus tachycardia resulted with complete suppression of all sinus arrhythmia (Fig 5). Oral administration of atropine successfully prevented extreme sinus bradycardia in three, second degree AV block in one, and sinus pauses of up to 6.3 seconds in three patients. Atropine had no apparent effect on the disturbed sleep pattern or the cyclic upper airway obstruction. Edrophonium hydrochloride (Tensilon, 10 mg, intravenous) was given to one patient while the effect of atropine was still present. Marked cyclic sinus arrhythmia in phase with the respiration-apnea cycles resumed promptly (Fig 5).

TABLE II. Arrhythmias During Wakefulness and Sleep

	Awake	Sleep
Number of patients	25	25
Normal sinus rhythm	25	0
Marked sinus arrhythmia	0	24
Extreme sinus bradycardia (HR $<$30/min)	0	9
Asystole (2.5–13 seconds)	0	9
Second-degree AV block	0	4
Ventricular tachycardia	0	2
Atrial tachycardia	0	1

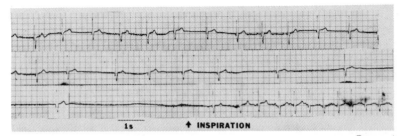

Fig 3. Forty-two seconds of continuous ECG recording during sleep and apnea. Progressive sinus bradycardia and junctional escape rhythm are interrupted by a 5.8-second asystole. Inspiration initiated sinus tachycardia.

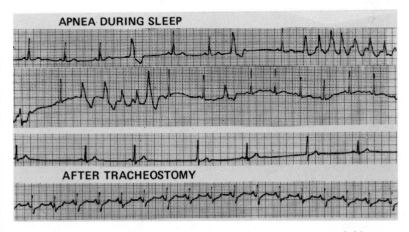

Fig 4. ECG recording during sleep and apnea. Sinus bradycardia is accompanied by premature ventricular beats and a brief run of ventricular tachycardia. Following tracheostomy, ventricular arrhythmias are not seen.

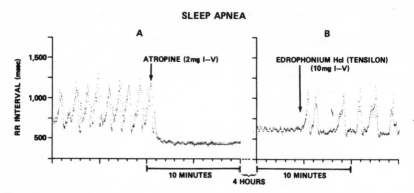

Fig 5. Computer printout of 30 minutes of ECG recording during sleep. Each QRS complex is characterized by one dot, indicating the R-R interval. A) The first ten minutes reveal marked sinus arrhythmia with sinus rate varying from 120/min to 50/min every minute. Intravenous administration of atropine (2 mg) abolishes the cyclic sinus arrhythmia and results in sinus tachycardia while sleep with intermittent apnea continues. B) Four hours later, following intravenous administration of edrophonium (Tensilon), cyclic sinus arrhythmia recurs.

Seventeen patients underwent tracheostomy as treatment for their disorder. Marked sinus arrhythmia, present in all prior to surgery, was completely abolished in all patients immediately after tracheostomy (Fig 6). This coincided with the normalization of their sleep pattern and abolition of obstructive apnea during sleep. Extreme sinus bradycardia, second degree AV block, and ventricular tachycardia were not detected after tracheostomy, while complex premature ventricular contractions were less frequent. Asystole was abolished in seven patients. Although obstructive apnea was prevented by tracheostomy in all patients, brief episodes of central apnea accompanied by 2.5–3.5 and 6.5 seconds of asystole occurred in two patients after tracheostomy (Fig 7).

Tracheostomy site was temporarily occluded in nine patients during sleep, while the cuff balloon was left deflated, permitting a respiratory pattern similar to the pretracheostomy state. In all six, the pretracheostomy pattern of arrhythmias (marked sinus arrhythmia and extreme sinus bradycardia) recurred promptly and was abolished on unplugging the tracheostomy (Fig 6). During tracheostomy occlusion, sleep was not interrupted and the abnormal sleep pattern characterized by intermittent obstructive apnea appeared in all patients.

DISCUSSION

Cardiac rhythm in normal sleep has been previously studied. A progressive decrease in sinus rate occurring during sleep, with slight increases in the average

SLEEP APNEA

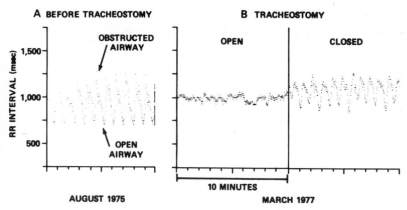

Fig 6. Computer printout of 30 minutes of ECG recording during sleep. QRS complexes are characterized by dots indicating the R-R interval. A) Ten minutes of marked sinus arrhythmia during cyclic apnea. B) Twenty minutes of recording following tracheostomy. With the tracheostomy open, normal sinus rhythm is present. Temporary plugging of the tracheostomy with the balloon deflated brings out the characteristic pattern of sinus arrhythmia and obstructive apnea.

rate and wider variability during rapid eye movement (REM) sleep, has been described [5]. Tzivoni reported that the lowest sinus rate during normal sleep was 76 to 78% of the average awake heart rate in both normals and patients with ischemic heart disease [6]. Sinus arrhythmia with slight variation of sinus rate is present during wakefulness and during most stages of sleep in normal controls. This rhythmic alteration in heart rate ranged from a minimum of one to as high as 28 beats per minute [7]. Animal experiments have suggested that sinus arrhythmia during wakefulness and sleep is dependent on phasic inhibition of vagal and sympathetic activity [8].

The incidence and type of arrhythmias occurring during sleep have received recent attention because of their suspected relationship to sudden death. Although Smith reported that 18 acutely ill cardiac patients showed no change in premature atrial contraction (PAC) or premature ventrical contraction (PVC) frequency during sleep [9], REM sleep has been reported to be associated with increased frequency of premature ventricular contractions [10]. During non-EEG-monitored sleep of 54 ambulatory patients, the majority with stable cardiac disease, 78% showed decreased frequency of PVCs during sleep. In many cases sleep was more effective in controlling ventricular arrhythmias than antiarrhythmic medications [11]. A single case has been reported where ventricular tachycardia consistently was abolished by sleep [12]. Another recent case report

CENTRAL SLEEP APNEA IN STAGE 3 NREM SLEEP

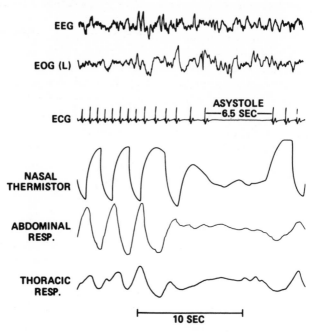

Fig 7. Twenty seconds of polygraphic recording during sleep. Ten seconds of central apnea is characterized by absence of abdominal or respiratory effort and no nasal airflow; 6.5 seconds of asystole is present. EEG) Electroencephalogram; EOG) electrooculogram; ECG) electrocardiogram.

describes increased frequency of PVCs during REM sleep in one patient with an episode of ventricular fibrillation during the early morning hours. The author suggested that emotionally charged dreams trigger a central nervous system mechanism, provoking the ventricular ectopic beats and the ventricular fibrillation [13]. Thus, normal sleep is characterized by sinus slowing with episodes of sinus arrhythmia and, in general, suppression of any preexisting premature ventricular contractions. Rapid eye movement sleep may be associated with faster sinus rates, more frequent PVCs, and, rarely, major ventricular arrhythmias.

A recent study of 50 clinically normal male medical students by 24 hours of Holter ECG recording adds valuable information on arrhythmias during sleep [14]. Sinus bradycardia was frequently present, with the longest R-R interval being 2.06 seconds. Sinus arrhythmia with changes in adjacent cycle length of 100% or more was noted in half the subjects, but it was episodic and not reported as recurring cyclically, in a continuous pattern. Three subjects had type I

Wenckebach AV block, one of whom had this arrhythmia also during wakefulness and another had first-degree AV block during wakefulness. Sleep in these presumably normal subjects was not monitored and their respiratory pattern was not observed. History of snoring, if any, was not reported.

Information on arrhythmias in the sleep apnea syndrome is scanty and limited to case reports. A well-documented case of obstructive sleep apnea was shown to have sinus bradycardia during apnea as well as paroxysms of atrial fibrillation with a high degree of AV block (up to ten seconds of ventricular asystole) [15]. Atropine was effective in controlling these bradyarrhythmias, and no arrhythmias were observed after tracheostomy. Figures of hemodynamic monitoring in this syndrome published by Coccagna et al clearly show phasic sinus slowing and speeding, suggesting the presence of marked sinus arrhythmia, although no mention was made of rhythm disorders [1]. "Bradycardia and EKG changes — QRS widening and T inversion" during apnea have been mentioned without further details by others [16]. Sinus bradycardia, first- and second-degree AV block (Wenckebach) were reported in a 56-year-old man with congestive heart failure during REM sleep [17]. The patient was described as "sleep deprived" and having "frequent arousals," but no apnea was mentioned. Apneic spells in low-birthweight infants are frequent and are commonly associated with bradycardia [18, 19]. Prolonged apnea and Sudden Infant Death syndrome have been closely associated [20], and the occurrence of bradycardia with apnea has been noted [21]. It has been suggested that sinus bradycardia in such infants is secondary to the effect of hypoxia [22]. It is still controversial whether the immediate cause of Sudden Infant Death syndrome is respiratory (apnea) or cardiac.

Our prospective study of sleep apnea-associated arrhythmias in adults suggests that the arrhythmias observed in these patients are not random events unrelated to the sleep disorder, but that they are a *direct* result of the altered and abnormal sleep state. The ECG hallmark of the syndrome seems to be abnormal and exaggerated sinus arrhythmia (Fig 1). This abnormality was present in all patients except in one with autonomic dysfunction. Although sinus arrhythmia is a normal physiological event, the type and degree of phasic sinus rate change in our patients appears to be grossly exaggerated and abnormal. During normal respiration with a frequency of 10 to 14 per minute, the accompanying sinus arrhythmia will go through 10 to 14 cycles per minute. In the absence of hypoxemia and apnea, severe bradycardia is not seen. In sleep apnea, where one episode of apnea and subsequent ventilation usually occupy 50 to 100 seconds, there is only one cycle of sinus acceleration and deceleration within this period, and this pattern recurs until apnea is relieved. Also, the apnea with marked hypoxemia causes severe bradycardia, thus producing the extreme degree of sinus arrhythmia. Such a pattern has not been reported in otherwise normal subjects and appears to be quite specific for sleep apnea. We suggest that a sleep ECG recording may be the easiest method of screening for this syndrome. More serious arrhythmias accompanied the characteristic marked sinus arrhythmia. Apparent sinus arrest or sinoatrial block with 2.5 to 13 seconds of ventricular asystole was observed in nine patients during periods of apnea and sinus brady-cardia. All such arrhythmias occurred during sleep, in supine posture, and rarely were associated with symptoms — urinary incontinence in one patient with 13 seconds of asystole. Wenckebach's second-degree AV block accompanied the bradycardia in four patients. Atropine was effective in preventing both the pro-longed periods of asystole and AV block, suggesting that the underlying mecha-nism was one of increased parasympathetic tone triggered by the apnea and the progressive hypoxia. The reversal of atropine effect by Tensilon with unmasking of the sinus arrhythmia further strengthens this concept. The absence of marked sinus arrhythmia in the patient with a Shy-Drager syndrome and severe obstruc-tive apnea is also consistent with this view.

Tracheostomy bypasses the sleep-induced upper airway obstruction and nor-malizes the sleep pattern as well as the hemodynamic changes during sleep [23; see also Chapter 11]. Our data indicate that the majority of arrhythmias are also abolished. The complete disappearance of marked sinus arrhythmia and extreme sinus bradycardia as well as AV block after tracheostomy, and their reappear-ance during sleep when the tracheostomy site was occluded, indicate that this characteristic rhythm disorder is directly related to the upper airway occlusion during sleep. In patients with mixed (central and obstructive) apnea, episodes of central apnea can continue after tracheostomy and may be accompanied by bradyarrhythmias. Sinus arrest with ventricular asystole of 2.5–3.5 and 6.5 seconds were documented during brief episodes of central apnea in two patients. We suspect that a central mechanism simultaneously causes the respiratory pause and the cardiac standstill.

Figure 8 outlines proposed mechanisms for arrhythmia production. The pri-mary dysfunction seems to reside in the central nervous system. Even in the cases of predominantly obstructive apnea, the central nervous system is impli-cated since abnormal degrees of genioglossus and other oropharyngeal muscle atonia during obstructed sleep apnea has been demonstrated [24; see also Chapter 16]. Direct observation of the tongue during sleep has also confirmed that this organ collapses into the hypopharynx and can completely occlude the airway [25, 26]. The subsequent airway obstruction produces alveolar hypo-ventilation with hypoxia and respiratory acidosis. The degree of hypoxemia can-not be accounted for only on the basis of hypoventilation and is probably re-lated to intrapulmonary shunts and the Müller maneuver. The marked and pro-gressive hypoxemia (PaO_2 30–45 mm Hg) stimulates carotid body chemorecep-tors producing primary reflex bradycardia of vagal origin. Associated with this increased vagal tone are periods of sinus arrest, ventricular asystole and Wencke-

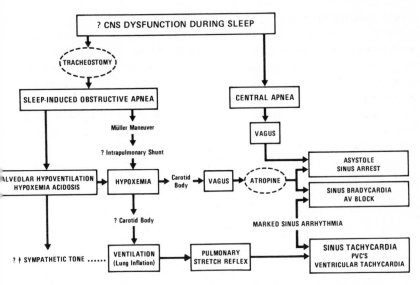

Fig 8. Proposed mechanism of arrhythmia production in sleep apnea. See text.

ach's type AV block. After 10 to 100 seconds of total upper airway occlusion with progressive hypoxemia and bradycardia, there is an arousal pattern on the electroencephalogram, the airway occlusion is relieved, and ventilation resumes. This event is easily recognized at the bedside by a loud snore. At this moment, the Müller maneuver abruptly ceases, effective inspiration with inflation of the lungs is accomplished triggering a reflex cardioacceleration — the pulmonary stretch reflex — again via vagal mechanisms [27]. Heightened sympathetic tone previously obscured by the vagus and triggered by the hypoxemia and acidosis may contribute to this sinus acceleration as well as to the production of ventricular ectopic beats and ventricular tachycardia. Since the apnea respiration cycle typically repeats itself every one to two minutes, this produces the marked sinus arrhythmia which seems to be the hallmark of patients with obstructive apnea (Fig 1). Tracheostomy, by bypassing the airway occlusion during sleep, prevents the hypoxemia and the reflex bradycardia and the subsequent cardioacceleration at the moment of ventilation. Atropine has no effect on airway obstruction and does not prevent the hypoxemia. It is effective in blocking the bradyarrhythmias by its effect on vagally mediated reflexes. The mechanism(s) of arrhythmia production in central apnea where upper airway occlusion cannot be demonstrated is not well understood but a centrally mediated parasympathetic discharge is most likely.

CONCLUSIONS AND CLINICAL APPLICATIONS

The data presented here have several areas of clinical application. The marked sinus arrhythmia present only during sleep seems to be highly characteristic of patients with sleep apnea syndrome. Thus, nocturnal ECG monitoring (Holter type ECG) promises to be both a sensitive and specific diagnostic tool in evaluation of patients suspected to have sleep apnea syndrome. If such arrhythmias are detected in otherwise healthy subjects, evaluation for possible occult sleep apnea seems indicated. Although in these series no arrhythmias were *documented* to be directly responsible for serious morbidity or mortality, their potential danger cannot be denied. One patient in this series with 13-second asystole also gave a history of urinary incontinence. A ten-second asystole was accompanied by seizure and urinary incontinence in another patient reported elsewhere [15]. Two of our patients with severe obstructive apnea died prior to tracheostomy. In one, the history suggested progressive airway occlusion and asphyxiation while the second patient died, during sleep, unobserved.

The possible contribution of sleep-associated arrhythmias to sudden death in the Pickwickian syndrome seems likely but remains to be proven. Presently, we offer tracheostomy only to patients disabled by symptoms (daytime somnolence). However, if further experience confirms the therapeutic role of tracheostomy for arrhythmias of obstructive apnea, it will be considered for patients with potentially lethal arrhythmias. Alternate modes of therapy — atropine and pacemakers — may also be effective but have had no long-term trials.

The role of sleep apnea in Sudden Infant Death syndrome has gained increasing attention [28]. Prolonged apnea (central or obstructive) in a susceptible infant may lead to sudden death through the production of brady- or tachyarrhythmias similar to those reported here.

Our data establish the presence of a characteristic rhythm disorder and frequent occurrence of potentially life-threatening arrhythmias in the sleep apnea syndrome. The mechanism of production, the long-term significance of these arrhythmias, and their possible role in Sudden Infant Death syndrome are currently under further study.

ACKNOWLEDGMENTS

Ms Pat Bell and Wendy Watkins helped in the technical analysis of Holter electrocardiograms. The technical assistance of Ms Gerry Derby was greatly appreciated.

Lola M Griggs helped in the preparation of the manuscript.

This research was supported in part by National Institute of Neurological Diseases and Stroke grant NS 10727, Public Health Service Research Grant

R-70 from the General Clinical Research Centers, Division of Research Re-
urces, and by INSERM to Dr Guilleminault.

EFERENCES

. Coccagna G, Mantovani M, Brignani F, Parchi C, Lugaresi E: Continuous recording of the pulmonary and systemic arterial pressure during sleep in syndromes of hyper-somnia with periodic breathing. Bull Physiopathol Respir 8:1159–1169, 1972.
2. Tilkian AG, Guilleminault C, Schroeder JS, Lehrman KL, Simmons FB, Dement WC: Sleep induced apnea syndrome; hemodynamic studies during wakefulness and sleep. Ann Intern Med 85:714–719, 1976.
3. Fitzgerald JW, Clappier RR, Harrison DC: Small computer processing of ambulatory arrhythmias. In "Computers in Cardiology." Bethesda, Maryland: IEEE Biomedical Proceedings, 1974, p 31.
4. Lehrman KL, Guilleminault C, Schroeder JS, Tilkian A, Forno LN: Sleep apnea syndrome in a patient with Shy-Drager syndrome. Arch Intern Med 138:206–209, 1978.
5. Snyder F, Hobson JA, Morrison DF, Goldfrank F: Changes in respiration, heart rate, and systolic blood pressure in human sleep. J Appl Physiol 19:417–421, 1964.
6. Tzivoni D, Stern S: Electrocardiographic pattern during sleep in healthy subjects and in patients with ischemic heart disease. J Electrocardiol 6(3):225–229, 1973.
7. Bond WC, Bohs C, Ebey J, Wolf S: Rhythmic heart rate variability (sinus arrhythmia) related to stages of sleep. Cond Reflex 8:98–107, 1973.
8. Baust W, Bohnert B: The regulation of heart rate during sleep. Exp Brain Res 7:169–180, 1969.
9. Smith R, Johnson L, Rothfeld D, Zir L, Tharp B: Sleep and cardiac arrhythmias. Arch Intern Med 130:721–753, 1972.
10. Rosenblatt G, Hartmann E, Zwilling G: Cardiac irritability during sleep and dreaming. J Psychosom Res 17:129–134, 1973.
11. Lown B, Tykocinski M, Garfein A, Brooks P: Sleep and ventricular premature beats. Circulation 48:691–701, 1973.
12. Shahaway M: Arrhythmias and the varieties of sleep. N Engl J Med 282:815–816, 1970.
13. Lown B, Temte J, Reich P, Gaughan C, Regestein Q, Hai H: Basis for recurring ventricular fibrillation in the absence of coronary heart disease and its management. N Engl J Med 294:623–629, 1976.
14. Brodsky M, Wu D, Denes P, Kanakis C, Rosen K: Arrhythmias documented by 24 hour continuous electrocardiographic monitoring in 50 male medical students without apparent heart disease. Am J Cardiol 39:390–395, 1977.
15. Kryger M, Quesney LF, Holder D, Gloor P, MacLeod P: The sleep deprivation syndrome of the obese patient. Am J Med 56:531–539, 1974.
16. Popoviciu L, Corfariu O, Pop I, Popa D, Gondos M, Pop R: Clinical, biochemical, functional-respiratory, electroencephalographic and polygraphic investigations of wakefulness-sleep in Pickwickian syndromes. Rev Roum Neurol Psychiatr 11(2):93–110, 1974.
17. Nevins DB: First- and second-degree A-V heart block with rapid eye movement sleep. Ann Intern Med 76:981–983, 1972.
18. Daily WJR, Klaus M, Meyer HBP: Apnea in premature infants: monitoring incidence, heart rate changes, and an effect of environmental temperature. Pediatrics 43:510–517, 1969.

19. Shannon DC, Gotay F, Stein SM, Rogers MC, Todres D, Moylan FMB: Prevention of apnea and bradycardia in low birthweight infants. Pediatrics 55:589–594, 1975.

20. Steinschneider A: Prolonged apnea and the SIDS: Clinical and laboratory observations. Pediatrics 50:646–654, 1972.

21. Bachman DS: Prolonged apnea, vagal overactivity, and sudden infant death. Pediatrics 51:755–756, 1973.

22. Girling DJ: Changes in heart rate, blood pressure and pulse pressure during apneic attacks in newborn babies. Arch Dis Child 47:405–410, 1972.

23. Coccagna C, Mantovani M, Brignani F, Parchi C, Lugaresi E: Tracheostomy in hypersomnia with periodic breathing. Bull Physiopathol Respir 8:1217–1227, 1972.

24. Sauerland EKG, Harper RM: The human tongue during sleep: Electromyographic activity of the genioglossus muscle. Exp Neurol 51:160–170, 1976.

25. Hishikawa Y, Furuya E, Wakamatsu H: Hypersomnia and periodic respiration – presentation of two cases and comment on the physiopathogenesis of the Pickwickian syndrome. Folia Psychiatr Neurol Jpn 24:163–173, 1970.

26. Walsh R, Michaelson E, Harkleroad L, Zighelboim A, Sackner M: Upper airway obstruction in obese patients with sleep disturbance and somnolence. Ann Intern Med 76: 185–192, 1972.

27. Daily MS: The effects of stimulation of the carotid body chemoreceptors on heart rate in the dog. J Physiol 144:148–166, 1958.

28. Guntheroth WG: Sudden infant death syndrome (Crib Death). Am Heart J 93:784–793, 1977.

DISCUSSION

In order to sort out the mechanisms involved in arrhythmias, it was suggested that an attempt be made to assess the role of the baroreceptors by plotting instantaneous pressures in relation to instantaneous heart rate. If an inverse relationship was found to exist, was this a function of pO_2? Dr Tilkian stated that when arterial pressure is rising and all other variables are constant, one would expect sinus slowing, but that is the time when sinus tachycardia occurs. He therefore considered it unlikely that there was a significant contribution to sinus slowing from the baroreceptor mechanism. It was his feeling that there was no inverse relationship and what is observed is an exaggeration of physiologic events with overriding of the baroreceptors.

Dr Phillipson mentioned that in the awake dog when the classic Hering-Breuer is elicited, progressive cardiac slowing is observed during the prolonged apnea but, concomitant with the first inspiration, profound tachycardia is seen. He stated that it would be helpful to be able to correlate heart rate with the pO_2 as there are reflexes in animals that will produce identical apnea and bradycardia unrelated to carotid bodies or pO_2. The J reflex, characterized by apnea and bradycardia, is an example of such a reflex wherein pO_2 and the carotid bodies play no known role.

13
Neural and Mechanical Factors Controlling Pharyngeal Occlusion During Sleep

John E Remmers, William J DeGroot, Eberhardt K Sauerland, and A Michael Anch

The precise pathogenesis of periodic upper airway occlusion (AO) during sleep is uncertain. We have recently reported results obtained during nocturnal sleep in ten obese, hypersomnolent patients [1]. While all displayed periodic breathing, significant nonocclusive (central) apnea appeared in one case only. Our analysis seeks to identify the physical and neural factors determining the state of the upper airways during the occluded and ventilatory phases of the periodic breathing cycle. We refer to occlusion rather than obstruction because the latter does not specifically denote total blockage of airflow. Mechanically, AO consists of unidirectional (inspiratory) occlusion, inasmuch as expiratory flow typically accompanies expiratory efforts during the occluded phase [1–3]. In other words, during the occluded phase the patient sustains inspiratory occlusion and expiratory obstruction. Patients with nonocclusive upper airway obstruction may sustain respiratory decompensation during sleep consequent to the mechanical loading of the respiratory muscles by elevated upper airway resistance, even though they do not display periodic breathing [1, 4].

Reports of radiographic studies indicate the presence of pharyngeal closure during AO [5, 6], and other reports describe amelioration of periodic AO with pharyngeal intubation. We have confirmed this latter finding in four patients in whom nasopharyngeal intubation eliminated the characteristic cyclic ventilation and reestablished regular breathing. Strong, confirmatory evidence of pharyngeal occlusion was derived from recordings of supraglottic pressure in the other six patients with periodic AO. A pressure transducer was positioned at the level of the tip of the epiglottis as shown in Figure 1. During occluded inspiratory efforts,

Sleep Apnea Syndromes, pages 211–217

pharyngeal (supraglottic) pressure (P_{ph}) closely approximated esophageal pressure (P_{es}), indicating a patent larynx and lower airway. This equivalence was generally maintained throughout the occluded phase, and divergence of the two pressures occurred coincident with the onset of inspiratory flow. In many cases this divergence occurred abruptly part way through the respiratory effort, as shown in Figure 2. Supraglottic pressure is plotted against esophageal pressure for four efforts. Each begins as an occluded inspiratory effort (last effort of the occluded phase) and ends as an unoccluded inspiration (first breath of the ventilatory phase). The initial portion of each occluded effort lies near the identity line (dashed line), and as the effort progresses P_{ph} and P_{es} rise equally, inscribing a 45° line (occluded/pharynx). The onset of inspiratory flow (release of occlusion) is marked by a precipitious drop in P_{ph} at a constant P_{es}. This "explosive" release of pharyngeal occlusion was followed by the unoccluded portion of the effort, where P_{es} either declines transiently or continues to rise as air flows through the pharyngeal lumen.

The foregoing findings demonstrate that pharyngeal inspiratory occlusion was of primary importance in our patients. The characteristics of this occlusion, its unidirectionality and its "explosive" release, suggest that the action of pharyngeal transmural pressure to constrict the pharyngeal lumen may be important. On the other hand, for a variety of reasons, we anticipate that the dilating action of muscles attached to the pharyngeal walls may be of importance. The principal muscle in this regard seems to be the genioglossus (GG) whose fibers

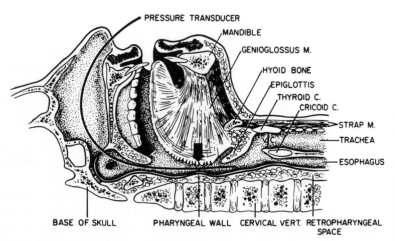

Fig 1. Drawing of a saggital section of the pharynx showing the position of the transducer-tipped catheter. VC) Vocal cords. The vertical arrow represents the constricting action of negative pharyngeal pressure which is opposed by genioglossal contraction.

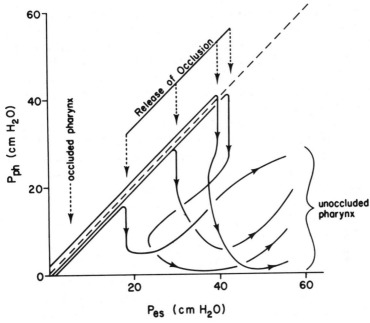

Fig 2. Pharyngeal (supraglottic) pressure (P_{ph}) is plotted against esophageal pressure (P_{es}) for four inspiratory efforts. During each effort pharyngeal occlusion was released, marking the end of the occluded phase and the beginning of the ventilatory phase. During the initial part of the effort (occluded pharynx) the two pressures are equal and values move up along the identity line (dashed line) until "explosive" release of occlusion occurs, and P_{ph} drops precipitously at a constant P_{es}. Thereafter, inspiratory flow occurs through the unoccluded pharynx.

course normally to the ventral pharyngeal wall. The important work of Sauer-land and co-workers [7, 8; see also Chapter 14] reveal respiratory motor regulation of the muscle during wakefulness and sleep, suggesting that genioglossal force (GGF) is important in controlling the size of the pharyngeal lumen.

The results of our studies are compatible with the notion that genioglossal activity influences the state of the pharynx in periodic upper AO; in all ten patients we observed periodicity in genioglossal electromyogram (GGEMG) in relation to the occluded/ventilatory cycle (Fig 3). Onset of occlusion was always associated with a relatively low level of discharge, and release consistently occurred when genioglossal discharge was the most intense. In one case, occlusion was uniquely correlated with electromyogram (EMG) activity; the lowest levels of discharge were recorded throughout the occluded phase and release of occlusion coincided with a sudden burst of genioglossal activity. However, in other cases, the correlation was nonunique; comparable GGEMG activity

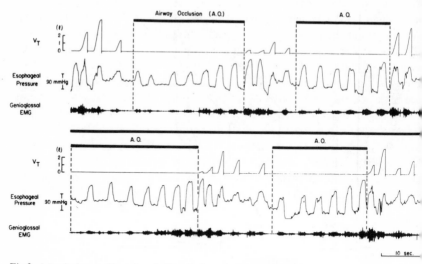

Fig 3. A typical recording of periodic AO showing periodicity of genioglossal activity. Note the low level of activity at the onset of occlusion and high level at the beginning of the ventilatory phase.

could be observed during selected portions of the occluded and ventilatory phases. Specifically, peak GGEMG during the terminal portion of the ventilatory phase was comparable to that recorded during most of the occluded phase. Interestingly, the one patient displaying a unique correlation had only minimal disease so that the occluded phase was brief and the fluctuations in P_{es} and P_{ph} were small (10 cm H_2O). This suggests that when the constricting effects of transmural pharyngeal pressure are negligible, genioglossal activity principally determines the state of the pharynx. However, in most cases occluded inspiratory efforts produce large values of P_{ph} (40–60 cm H_2O).

To discern the combined efforts of GGF and pharyngeal transmural pressure, we have plotted P_{ph} against GGEMG as shown for the peak values in Figure 4. The dashed line segregates all occluded from unoccluded respiratory efforts in a series of occlusive/ventilatory cycles, and the arrows show the position and direction of movement of sequential points in the occluded and unoccluded phases. The vertical shaded area indicates the range of GGEMG where comparable EMG values were recorded for occluded and unoccluded efforts. Clearly, some combination of the two variables, eg, their difference or ratio, will suffice to predict whether the pharynx is occluded or patent.

We speculate that there is a "critical" value for the difference, P_{ph}–GGF. For efforts where the actual difference is less than the "critical" difference, the

harynx is patent, and when the difference exceeds the "critical" value the
harynx will occlude. Applying this concept to the plot shown in Figure 4, we
an account for the dynamics of the occlusive/ventilatory cycle. The ventilatory
hase begins at the lower right and is characterized by a steady decline in
GEMG. At sleep onset, there is a further drop in EMG and rise in P_{ph} such that
he difference, $P_{ph}-GGF$, exceeds the "critical" value. At this juncture, points
cross the segregating line, the pharynx occludes. During sleep, pharyngeal occlu-
ion is maintained because activation of inspiratory muscles relative to the genio-
lossus is such that P_{ph} increases more than GGF. The "automatic" control of
he relative activity in these two sets of muscles during sleep is reflected in the
lope of the regression shown for the occluded phase in Figure 4. Since during
his phase P_{ph} equals P_{es} and since the inspiratory muscles are contracting iso-
netrically, the ordinate manifests inspiratory muscle activation. Because the re-
ression for occluded efforts is steeper than the segregating line, we concluded

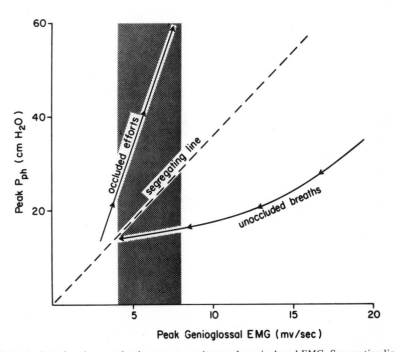

Fig 4. A plot of peak supraglottic pressure against peak genioglossal EMG. Segregating line
separates all points for occluded efforts and unoccluded breaths in a series of occlusive/
ventilatory cycles in one patient. Arrows represent mean values and show the sequence of
points during a cycle. Shaded area represents the overlap in range of EMG values for
occluded efforts and unoccluded breaths.

that the "automatic" control during sleep is such that the difference $P_{ph}-GGF$ increases, thereby maintaining occlusion even though GG activity increases.

Release of occlusion follows arousal and engagement of neural mechanisms which preferentially recruit the genioglossus, shifting points to the right in Figure 4. This decreases the difference, $P_{ph}-GGF$, below the critical value, and the pharynx opens. The dynamics of unocclusion are represented in Figure 5. The nearby vertical arrow represents the final inspiratory efforts in the occluded phase. The average for eight efforts during which occlusion was released is shown by the arrow displaced down and to the right of the segregation line. This indicates that release of occlusion is preceded by preferential activation of the genioglossus from the beginning of the effort.

In conclusion, we believe that the dynamic relationship of supraglottic pressure and genioglossal discharge adequately accounts for the onset, maintenance, and release of pharyngeal occlusion in our patients with periodic AO. Structural

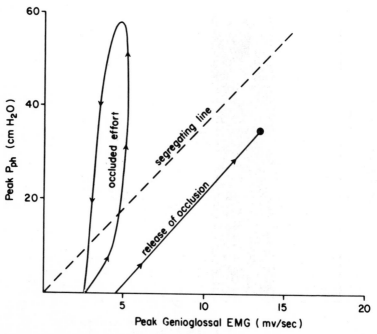

Fig 5. Supraglottic pressure is plotted against genioglossal EMG for the patient shown in Figure 4. The nearly vertical loop shows the average of occluded efforts just prior to termination of occluded phases. The line to the right of the segregating line shows the average relationship during eight efforts where occlusion was released during the occluded effort. The closed circle represents the average point of unocclusion.

encroachment on the pharyngeal lumen can be expected to decrease the "critical" value of the difference, $P_{ph}-GGF$, and increase P_{ph}. Such a dual action may explain the beneficial effects of moderate weight loss in obese patients with periodic upper airway obstruction. In two of our patients studied after weight reduction and relief of symptoms, AO was not present and GGEMG exhibited qualitatively normal behavior. This suggests that a disturbance in genioglossal motor control is not primary in the pathogenesis of periodic AO.

ACKNOWLEDGMENTS

The authors thank Ms Lucy Hairston for her assistance in carrying out experiments and preparation of the manuscript.

This research was supported by the National Heart, Lung and Blood Institute Research grant HL 18007 and by a Pulmonary Academic Award (HL 00131). Dr Anch is a NIH Postdoctoral Trainee (HL 07217).

REFERENCES

1. Remmers JE, deGroot W, Sauerland E, Anch M: Pathogenesis of upper airway occlusion during sleep. J Appl Physiol (in press).
2. Gastaut H, Tassinari CA, Duron B: Polygraphic study of the episodic diurnal and nocturnal (hypnic and respiratory) manifestations of the Pickwickian syndrome. Brain Res 2:167–186, 1966.
3. Walsh RE, Michaelson ED, Harkerload LE, Zighelboim A, Sackner MA: Upper airway obstruction in obese patients with sleep disturbance and somnolence. Ann Intern Med 76:185–192, 1972.
4. Simmons FB, Hill MW: Hypersomnia caused by upper airway obstructions. A new syndrome in otolaryngology. Ann Otol Rhinol Laryngol 83:670–673, 1974.
5. Schwartz BA, Escande JP: Respiration hypnique pickwickienne. In Gastaut H, Lugaresi E. Berti-Ceroni G, Coccagna G (eds): "The Abnormalities of Sleep in Man." Bologna: Gaggi, 1968, pp 209–214.
6. Smirne S, Comi G: The obstructive mechanism in Pickwickian syndrome: A serial x-ray study. Sleep Res 4:237, 1975.
7. Sauerland EK, Mitchell SP: Electromyographic activity of intrinsic and extrinsic muscles of the human tongue. Tex Rep Biol Med 33:444–455, 1975.
8. Sauerland EK, Harper RM: The human tongue during sleep: Electromyographic activity of the genioglossus muscle. Exp Neurol 51:160–170, 1976.

14
The Role of the Tongue in Sleep Apnea

Ronald M Harper and Eberhardt K Sauerland

INTRODUCTION

We have been describing the mechanisms of upper airway obstruction (UAO) in sleep apnea by studying the electromyographic activity of muscles involved in the maintenance of the upper airway. We have thus been concentrating on peripheral mechanisms of control of air flow; however, as shall be shown, these mechanisms are intimately related to central control of respiration.

There are several potential mechanisms for UAO resulting from increased muscle action or loss of muscle tone in the adult. The source of obstruction might be situated at the level of the larynx through loss of action of the posterior cricoarytenoid muscles, at the pharynx through constriction or atonia of the pharyngeal constrictor muscles, or at the level of the oropharynx by loss of tone of muscles which protrude the tongue.

The tongue is one source of obstruction which has long been familiar to clinicians. Relapse of the tongue, especially with the subject in the supine position, brings the tongue in apposition with the pharyngeal wall. This will cause occlusion of the airway with the attendant risk of suffocation.

Some of the pathological conditions under which relapse of the tongue can take place are well known. These conditions include bilateral lesion of the 12th cranial nerve (the motor supply to the tongue), destruction of motor nuclei of the 12th nerve in the midline of the brain stem, or deep general anesthesia. We will describe, however, a set of conditions under which relapse of the tongue can occur normally during sleep, and can combine with other structural pathologies to cause obstruction of the airway for long periods of time.

The tongue is a mass of striated muscle with a midline fibrous septum dividing the body into symmetrical halves. The main bulk of the tongue is made up

Sleep Apnea Syndromes, pages 219–234

of the genioglossus muscle together with some vertical, longitudinal, and transverse intrinsic fibers. The intrinsic muscle fibers principally alter the shape of the tongue. The paired genioglossi fibers arise from the genial tubercule of the mandible and radiate in a fan-shaped manner toward the mucosa of the tongue from tip to base (Fig 1). The principal action of the genioglossal muscle is to protrude the tongue. In doing so, it maintains an open airway between the pharyngeal wall and the body of the tongue.

There are other smaller extrinsic (ie, attached from mass of tongue to bone) muscles of the tongue in addition to the genioglossi; these include the palatoglossus, styloglossus, and hypoglossus attached to the palate, styloid process, and hyoid bone, respectively, and serve to position the tongue. The styloglossus retracts the tongue, while the hyoglossus draws the sides of the tongue downwards. The palatoglossus raises the tongue and narrows the transverse diameter of the oropharyngeal isthmus. Only the genioglossus, however, is capable of active protrusion [1, 2].

Our studies were oriented toward examining the electromyographic activity of this very large muscle during respiratory activities associated with sleep and wakefulness states in normal individuals and in individuals with UAO.

Recording Techniques

Detailed procedures of the recording methods have been described elsewhere [3]. For some of the electromyographic recording, bipolar fine wire electrodes of the type used by Basmajian and Stecko [4] were employed; a typical assembly is shown in Figure 1A. Two insulated wires were inserted into a hypodermic needle. The wires were bared 0.5 mm at each end and bent sharply. After autoclaving, the needle assembly was inserted 3 mm lateral from the midline and midway between the first mandibular incisor tooth and the sublingual fold to a depth of 22–25 mm (Fig 1B). The needle was then withdrawn, leaving the wires within the muscle because of their barbed wire configuration (Fig 1C). The electrodes were later removed with a gentle pull on the wires.

Since insertion of electrodes into the muscle substance is often inconvenient, undesirable, or not feasible, a noninvasive technique for recording genioglossal electromyogram (EMG) was developed [5]. The surface electrodes were placed midsagittally: 1) midway between the mental protuberance and the lower lip, and 2) midway between the inner aspect of the mandible and the hyoid bone. The validity of this recording technique was confirmed by comparison of EMG activity patterns simultaneously obtained from intramuscular and surface skin electrodes. The surface recording technique has the additional advantage of monitoring the entire bulk of the genioglossus, in contrast to only several motor units with small intramuscular electrodes. The disadvantage lies in the fact that other muscular activities (active opening of the mouth, lip movements during

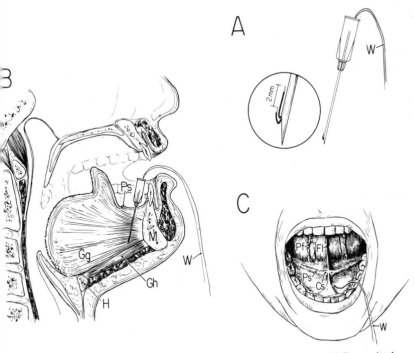

Fig 1. A) Bipolar recording electrode with disposable hypodermic needle. B) Parasagittal section through portion of head approximately 3 mm from midline. The tongue is actively reflected. Peroral and percutaneous needle insertion into the substance of the genioglossus muscle. C) Recording wires from left genioglossus muscle emerging from floor of mouth after withdrawal of needle. The inferior surface of the tongue is reflected. Abbreviations: Cs, caruncula sublingualis; Fl, Frenulum linguae; Gg, genioglossus muscle; Gh, geniohyoid muscle; H, hyoid bone; M, mandible; Ps, plica sublingualis with underlying submandibular duct; W, insulated wire of bipolar recording electrode. (Reprinted with permission from Sauerland and Mitchell: Bull LA Neurol Soc 35:69–73, 1970).

speaking) will obscure the genioglossal activity pattern. During sleep, however, excellent selective genioglossal activity patterns can be obtained. The new, convenient method was applied in 35 patients presenting UAO with the sleep apnea syndrome.

Cup electrodes for monitoring EEG (positions $C_3 - T_3$), mentalis musculature ("EMG of the chin"), and eye movements were placed on the subjects, while respiration was monitored with a bellows belt strapped to the chest (female subject) or to the anterior abdominal wall just below the rib cage (male subjects). Nasal and oral thermistors were also used to record respiratory activity. The ECG was monitored via cardiac disk electrodes attached to the right forearm and the left leg. All signals were displayed on a polygraph and stored on magnetic tape over an all-night (eight hours) recording period.

BASELINE MONITORING

Waking

Activity of the genioglossal muscles while awake in the supine position is characterized by high amplitude continuous background activity, together with transient bursts of discharge during inspiration (Fig 2A). This tonic activity is augmented with active protrusion of the tongue [6] or protrusion against the teeth, and served as a functional test for correct placement of the electrode.

The tonic activity, observed in the genioglossus while the subjects were in a supine position, indicates an active effort to maintain a tongue position away from the airway. The transient bursts of activity with inspiration suggest that to reduce airway resistance, the base of the tongue is actively moved forward from the pharyngeal wall to allow for a larger airway.

Quiet Sleep

Activity of the genioglossus in normal subjects during quiet sleep (QS) was very similar to that observed during waking. Tonic activity in the record was accompanied by strong inspiratory bursts of discharge, while only slight diminution in background tone was noted relative to the waking state (Fig 2B). Episodes

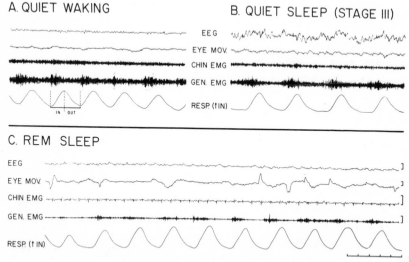

Fig 2. EEG, eye movements, mentalis ("chin") EMG, genioglossal EMG (GEN.), and respiration (RESP.) during waking and sleep states. Note continuous discharges with augmented inspiratory activity of the genioglossus muscle during quiet waking (A) and quiet sleep (B). In contrast, during REM sleep (C) the genioglossal activity almost ceases, except for small bursts during the inspiratory phase. Calibrations: time, one-second intervals; amplitudes, 50 μV. (Reprinted with permission from Sauerland and Harper: Exp Neurol, Vol 51, 1976).

of snoring were accompanied by extremely vigorous phasic genioglossal activity
[3].

Rapid Eye Movement (REM) Sleep

During REM sleep, tonic activity in the genioglossi was greatly diminished or
totally absent. Only small bursts of activity during the inspiratory phase of
respiration (Fig 2C) continued. Occasionally, the activity of a few muscle units
would totally cease for the duration of several respiratory cycles lasting from 15
to 90 seconds (Fig 3). These periods of silence were terminated by large inspiratory bursts. Tonic activity was resumed on waking from REM or after transition
to another sleep stage.

Relationship of Depth and Rate of Respiration to Tone

During the course of REM sleep, the tonic activity and the inspiratory bursts
occasionally reappeared. These reappearances of tonic and phasic EMG activity
were associated with increased depth of respiration and a slowing of respiratory

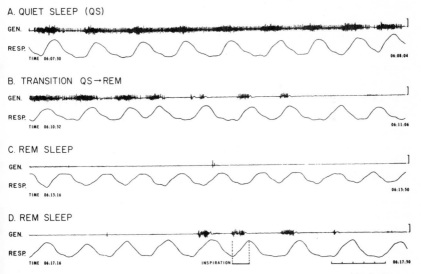

Fig 3. Activity of a small number of motor units in the right genioglossus muscle during
various sleep phases (subject D). Note the increased frequency of discharges during inspiration in quiet sleep (A). During transition from quiet sleep to REM sleep (B), the tonic discharges with expiration disappear and the inspiratory bursts become less pronounced. In
REM sleep, motor units may be totally silent for a number of respiratory cycles (C). However, this silence is regularly interrupted by a few inspiratory bursts (D). Calibrations: time,
one-second intervals; amplitudes, 50 μV. (Reprinted with permission from Sauerland and
Harper: Exp Neurol, Vol 51, 1976).

rate [7]. Figure 4 illustrates this relationship. In subject E, breaths 1 and 2, 8–16 and 22–26 are associated with increased EMG activity of inspiratory bursts and background activity. Breaths 3–7 and 17–21 are associated with reduced EMG activity in tonic and phasic bursts.

The relationship between these correlations is not fully understood. It is possible that the increased airway resistance caused by loss of tonic and phasic EMG activity results in increased rate as the respiratory mechanisms attempt to move air through a relative obstruction. The return of tone is accompanied by deeper and slower breaths. However, variability in respiratory rate is also observed after tracheostomy, with no upper airway resistance (see Orem, Chapter 5). It is more likely that the alterations in rate and depth of excursion are mediated by a common mechanism that regulates both genioglossal muscle tone and the primary respiratory musculature.

SCHEMATIC OUTLINE OF GENIOGLOSSAL ACTION

The implications of these findings in normal subjects can be schematically outlined in Figure 5. The importance of the tongue in maintaining an open airway is shown in Figure 5 which illustrates the role of the genioglossal muscles in tongue positioning in upright and supine positions. In the upright position the genioglossi muscles move the base of the tongue forward with each inspiration to allow for a large airway and decreased airway resistance. In the supine position (Fig 5) there is a tendency for the mobile tongue to relapse against the pharyngeal wall with the pull of gravity. For this reason, tonic activity of the genioglossi is necessary to maintain an open airway; this is indicated by the continuous background discharges upon which are superimposed bursts of activity with each inspiration to allow for decreased airway resistance. Loss of background activity, and decreased discharge during inspiration, as seen in REM sleep, will allow the tongue to relapse toward the posterior pharyngeal wall and thus restrict air flow (Fig 5). Of course, it is not essential that the

A. SUBJECT E IN REM SLEEP

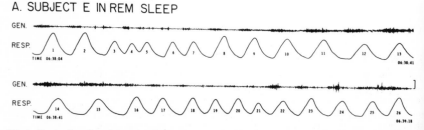

Fig 4. Genioglossal activity and respiration in REM sleep. There is an increased relationship between rate and depth of respiration and extent of background genioglossal EMG activity and inspiratory bursts.

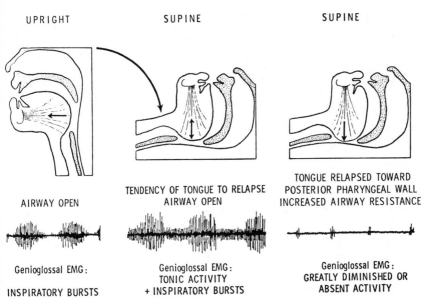

Fig 5. The relationship of the tongue to the pharyngeal wall during upright and supine positions, illustrating conditions of presence and absence of tonic activity. Strong inspiratory bursts of EMG activity in the genioglossi muscles, together with the help of gravity, maintain an open airway in the upright position. In the supine position, increased tonic activity, together with inspiratory bursts in the muscle maintain an open air passage against a natural relapse due to gravity. If this tone is diminished due to the suppression of muscle tone during REM sleep, or to pathological causes, the tongue is free to relapse towards the pharyngeal wall, thus producing increased airway resistance.

posterior base of the tongue physically come in contact with the pharyngeal wall to increase airway resistance. A narrowing of the airway itself would cause partial occlusion. One would predict from this schematic outline that an individual in a prone position would not suffer as great an increase in airway resistance during REM sleep, since the tongue would fall forward, away from the airway.

GENIOGLOSSAL ACTIVITY IN UAO

EMG — Relationships to Respiration

We have demonstrated that groups of genioglossal motor units may lose tone for periods of 90 seconds or more during sleep in normal subjects. These subjects did not exhibit sleep apnea, indicating that tongue relapse does not normally occlude the airway. However, the presence of a unique combination of structural or functional conditions, together with loss of genioglossal tone and a resulting relapsing tongue, may result in partial or total occlusion.

We have examined this possibility in patients with UAO. Figure 6 is part of a recording from an obese 52-year-old male. The genioglossal recordings were made using surface recording techniques described earlier. Multiple episodes of prolonged apnea occurred repeatedly throughout the night in this individual in both QS and REM, but were greatly prolonged in REM. Each apneic episode was accompanied by loss of tone in the genioglossal muscle and also in the mentalis musculature. The apnea shown lasted 45 seconds and was terminated by an arousal reaction (second arrow) with a return of muscle tone in the genioglossal recording. The sequence of loss of tone followed by apnea arousal with return of tone was repeated hundreds of times during the night.

Periods of apnea that occurred in QS were longer and more severe if the individual was in the supine position (Fig 7) rather than the semiprone position (Fig 8). In a semiprone position, of course, loss of tone in the genioglossus muscle would not cause relapse of the tongue since gravity would cause it to fall away from the pharyngeal wall.

In the semiprone position, occasional prolongations of a breath together with reduced genioglossal activity were occasionally seen, but no prolonged apnea episodes were observed.

This last finding is particularly relevant, since sleep apnea patients occasionally adopt bizarre sleeping positions such as kneeling at the bedside or sitting

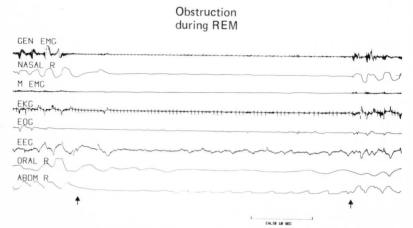

Obstruction
during REM

Fig 6. Loss of tone in the genioglossal and mentalis muscles occurs during this 45-second apnea experienced by an obese patient during REM (indicated by arrows). The apnea terminates in arousal, with a return of muscle tone. Note that although there is initial central apnea, abdominal excursions return shortly after cessation of air flow.

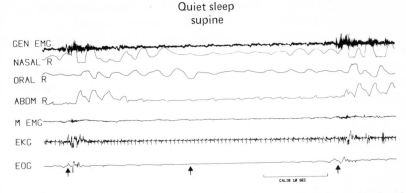

Fig 7. Partial occlusion during QS in an obese patient. The genioglossal tone is reduced during the obstruction, and tone in the mentalis muscle is lost. QS episodes of obstruction were not as severe as those during REM, but they were terminated by arousals as well (third arrow).

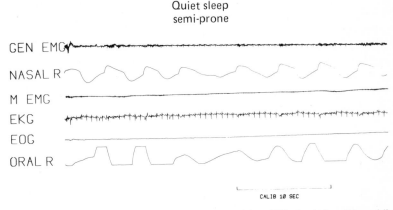

Fig 8. The same subject described in Figure 7 had much less difficulty in breathing while semiprone (almost completely face down, with head and body at $70°$ angle from the vertical). Occasionally, there were slight prolongations in respiration (fourth-breath), accompanied by a decreased phasic burst in the genioglossal recording. However, periods of prolonged apnea were not observed while in this position.

upright in a chair. Both of these positions facilitate recruitment of the accessory respiratory musculature, but, in addition, facilitate a posture which allows the tongue to fall forward.

Activity of the genioglossal muscles in UAO patients has also been examined using the indwelling electrode technique. Remmers et al used the fine wire procedure to examine the activity of the genioglossal muscles in four UAO patients during sleep [8]. A cyclic repetition of obstruction and release from obstruction was found across the recording period. The obstruction was supralaryngeal, since nasal intubation to the level of the larynx abolished the obstruction. There was a high correlation of decreased EMG activity in the genioglossal muscle during the obstructive periods and increased muscle tone during release of obstruction. Moreover, the increase in genioglossal activity slightly preceded the termination of occlusion.

Obesity Effects

One of Remmer's [8] patients subsequently improved symptomatically and clinically following a 27-kg weight loss, which agrees with a number of earlier reports [9, 10]. A recording of genioglossal activity during sleep following the weight loss showed no evidence of airway obstruction, and no evidence of the decreased genioglossal EMG activity followed by intense EMG activation seen earlier in obstructive episodes.

Relief of airway obstruction by weight loss should provide strong evidence that a constellation of conditions, both structural and functional, combine to cause obstruction. In particular, a tongue that is large due to infiltration of fat, and which relapses due to loss of tone in sleep, is a prime causative agent. Any hypothesis of airway obstruction must consider the improvement of conditions in some patients by weight loss. However, UAO is, of course, not confined to obese patients, and obese patients may obstruct for a variety of reasons.

Structural Defects Aiding UAO

It should be noted that distortion in the mandible to which the genioglossus is attached will have a large effect on airway maintenance. A recessed mandible (retrognathic facial syndrome with "Andy Gump" appearance), for example, would bring the tongue closer to the pharyngeal wall. Such cases with severe airway obstruction during sleep have been described [11, 12]. In these cases, relapse of the tongue during sleep may reduce the airway aperture sufficiently to lead to a sequence of passive obstruction.

Evidence that the tongue can play a role in UAO also comes from cases of obstruction that have been initiated by surgical reconstruction. Orr and co-workers [13] described the case of a young male child who developed severe sleep-related UAO immediately following surgical repair for a cleft palate. The child has a long and mobile frenulum linguae which facilitated a relapse of the tongue toward the posterior pharyngeal wall. Clinically, the symptoms of UAO during sleep were not apparent prior to surgery. During surgery, a flap of midline pharyngeal tissue was used to close the palate defect. Subsequently, the more lateral pharyngeal tissue edges were approximated, thus tensing the posterior ɔharyngeal wall and bringing it forward. With this newly established anatomy, ɔhe base of the relapsing tongue could reach the pharyngeal wall and effectively ɔbstruct the upper airway.

Termination of UAO by Stimulation

Recently, efforts were made to abort upper airway obstruction by artificial activation of the genioglossal musculature based on the hypothesis that tongue relapse is an essential element in UAO. Remmers and co-workers [personal communication] selected an obese male patient whose baseline recordings showed several hundred apneic episodes per night. Two stimulation wire electrodes were perorally inserted in such a manner that electric stimuli activated selectively the bilateral motor branches to the genioglossi muscles. On the other hand, stimulation of the lingual nerves, which carry sensory fibers from the tongue, was avoided. A volley of electrical stimuli produced moderate protrusion of the tongue. The patient stated that he was unaware of pain, tactile or taste sensations during stimulation. Throughout the night, the patient displayed the previously substantiated apneic episodes. However, when a volley of electrical stimuli (lasting approximately 1.5 seconds) was delivered to the genioglossi, an apneic episode could be instantly interrupted and free respiration was established for 10 to 15 seconds before the next apneic episode began. Upper airway obstruction could be arbitrarily terminated at any time. This procedure was repeated over 100 times. Although the patient stated that he was unaware of stimulus-induced sensations, there is still the possibility that the electrical stimulus led to a certain degree of arousal with subsequent termination of UAO. Work is now in progress to clarify this matter. During electrical genioglossal stimulation, EEG spectra will be analyzed to confirm or rule out any significant EEG changes [Remmers, Harper, and Sauerland, in preparation].

MECHANISMS OF UAO

If loss of motor control of the tongue is involved in UAO, then the question arises whether obstruction results from the tongue mass interfering with the normal flow of air, or whether a chain of events is triggered by loss of muscle tone during certain conditions which involve active constriction of the pharyngeal musculature.

Passive Constriction

Recently, Weitzman and co-workers [14] demonstrated that UAO is associated with a very substantial narrowing of the upper airway at the level of the base of the tongue. Fiberscopic examination during UAO showed a severe ring-shaped constriction. Considering the anatomy of this region, one can divide this ring into four regions: posteriorly, the posterior pharyngeal wall; bilaterally, the lateral pharyngeal walls; and anteriorly, the base of the tongue. Obviously, all these anatomical components must be involved in a ring-shaped constriction. It is of interest to note that Hill et al (Chapter 16) showed that pharyngeal constrictors lose their muscular tone during an apneic episode. The fiberscopic observations made by Weitzman et al [14] could be explained if one considers the recent work of Remmers et al [15]. The essential element of this explanation is that constriction is a passive process. The tongue relapses due to lack of tone, causing a certain degree of narrowing of the upper airway. At the same time, the lack of pharyngeal tone causes "floppiness" of the pharyngeal walls. When "floppiness" and narrowing have exceeded a critical point, a sudden and forceful inspiration will suck the structures (tongue; pharyngeal walls) together. An analogous process can be seen in the collapse of a straw upon sucking. The straw will only collapse and thus make further passage of fluid or air impossible if 1) it is soft (floppy) enough, 2) its inner diameter is sufficiently small, and 3) there is adequate negative pressure (suction). The small inner diameter of the straw, creating increased airway resistance, is analogous to the creation of a smaller airway by relapse of the tongue, aided perhaps by an additional functional or structural element (for example, enlarged adenoids, nasal congestion, or fat infiltration). The actual obstruction could occur at a number of vulnerable points including "collapse" of the pharyngeal wall or closure of the laryngeal aditus by the displaced epiglottis. There is, of course, an anatomical relationship between the tongue and epiglottis in that the epiglottis is positioned inferior to the base of the tongue. Thus, if the tongue moves posteriorly, this movement must be necessarily associated with some movement of the epiglottis.

Active Constriction

One must remember that a variety of local swallowing and gag reflexes are organized in the oropharyngeal region, and they are triggered by a number of proprioceptive and pressure receptors. Relapse of the tongue caused by loss of tone during sleep may not be differentiated from normal retraction of the tongue associated with the passage of a bolus of food during swallowing. Thus, a swallowing reflex might be initiated which would cause a sequence of constriction and relaxation of the pharyngeal walls; the negative pressure associated with inspiratory effort would maintain a collapse of these walls. The atonia observed in the pharyngeal musculature (Hill et al, Chapter 16) during the obstruction would argue against such a process. Moreover, a swallowing reflex would involve raising of the soft palate, and this is not observed during obstruction in fiberscopic observations (Weitzman et al, Chapter 15).

Paradoxical Atonia in QS

Since REM sleep is characterized by periods of atonia, the mechanisms of passive collapse just described would be totally adequate to describe UAO if obstruction occurred principally during REM sleep. However, although there are cases in which UAO is most severe in REM (see Fig 6), obstruction clearly is also prevalent in QS as well [16]. There is the possibility (depending on individual anatomical configuration) that even the slight loss of tone that normally occurs during QS is sufficient to cause a relaxation of the tongue musculature and a narrowing of the airway, which leads to a collapse of the pharyngeal walls from the negative inspiratory pressure. Thus we have a potential mechanism in the normal atonia of REM and the partial loss of tone in QS that would account for a number of cases of UAO, especially when combined with particular anatomical conditions.

In many patients with UAO, however, a large degree of atonia occurred in QS. This severe loss of tone in QS rather than in REM is a puzzle. The loss of facial and genioglossal tone is probably related to the loss of the first few diagraphragmatic movements that are observed in "mixed" apnea. During such an apnea, the return of diaphragmatic movement with a relapsed tongue leads to airway collapse from negative pressure, and prolongation of the apnea.

The mechanisms of EMG suppression in QS have yet to be described. This EMG suppression might, however, develop after a long period of airway obstruction and hypoxia through the mechanisms of increased airway resistance and occlusion that result from normal loss of tone in REM sleep (Lugaresi, Chapter 2).

IMPLICATIONS FOR UAO IN INFANTS

The significance of potential source of airway obstruction by the genioglossal muscles in adults should not be missed when considering the mechanisms of obstructive apnea in infants. The anatomy of the oropharyngeal region of infants is quite different from that of adults, however, and consequently, any extrapolation from this adult model should be considered with some care.

Infants are obligatory nose-breathers for the first few months of life; if nasal passages were partially occluded due to nasal discharge from a respiratory infection and air flow consequently restricted, collapse of the surrounding tissue might occur due to the large negative pressure in the same fashion as described for adults. It should be noted that the epiglottis in infants is considerably higher than in adults, being situated nearly at the level of the soft palate [17]. However, the tongue is also positioned more superiorly. Relapse of the tongue due to loss of genioglossal tone or relaxation of the mandible during sleep, and strong negative inspiratory pressure might lead to prolonged apnea of the obstructive variety, merely by passive movement of the tongue against the soft palate [18] or epiglottis.

The atonia of REM sleep might combine with congenital malformations to cause airway obstruction in the infant. Malformations of the first branchial arch result in hypoplasia of the mandible, together with a variety of other defects. The resulting micrognathia would bring the tongue more posterior, and hence more likely to occlude the airway when atonia occurs. If the palate is partially cleft, and the tongue unusually large (Pierre-Robin syndrome), the tongue may also relapse. If the infant is supine, further inspiration will suck the tongue into the cleft. These two syndromes could be treated by keeping the infant in a prone position to allow the tongue to fall forward, and by providing for a patent airway by insertion of an open-tipped rubber nipple into the infant's mouth until the infant is capable of spontaneous mouth breathing [19].

It should be noted that victims of the Sudden Infant Death Syndrome have an extraordinarily high incidence of mild respiratory infections [20] that might be expected to partially obstruct air passages and lead to increased airway resistance with the possibility of obstructive apnea. The mechanism of airway obstruction would be similar to that proposed for the soft-straw analogy; moving air through the clogged nasal passages would be similar to placing a finger on the end of the straw while simultaneously creating negative pressure on the opposite end. The result is collapse of the straw, or in this case, further relapse of the tongue against the palate and epiglottis, even more firmly sealing the airway.

SUMMARY

These studies demonstrate that a potential for airway obstruction exists with a relapsing tongue caused by normal processes that occur during sleep. The genioglossal muscle which protrudes the tongue undergoes loss of tone similar to that observed in most skeletal muscles in the body. The genioglossal muscles have a special importance in that they control the relative size of the oropharyngeal airway. In ordinary circumstances, such relapse is not sufficient to cause obstruction. However, if particular conditions exist, such as a large tongue resulting from fat infiltration, a tongue which is displaced posteriorly because of its attachment to a mandible that is in itself underdeveloped (as in the case of retrognathic facial syndrome), or a combination of circumstances that causes the mandible to fall back due to loss of tone, carrying the tongue back with it, then a potential for obstruction may result.

We are not suggesting that the mass of the tongue is the only obstructive element, but rather that this structure, on relapse, may increase airway resistance so much that the floppy pharyngeal walls will collapse with the negative pressure of inspiration, bringing the back of the tongue and the lateral walls together to ºomplete the occlusion. Increased airway resistance through the nasal cavities would aid in this collapse. It is perhaps significant that subjects suffering from :hronic nasal congestion would be at special risk for airway obstruction.

ACKNOWLEDGMENTS

This research was supported by the Veterans Administration. We would like to thank Mr Jerry Mason and Mr Steven Mandel for their help in these studies.

REFERENCES

1. Last RJ: "Anatomy Regional and Applied." Baltimore: Williams & Wilkins, 1954, p 638.
2. Sauerland EK, Mitchell SP: Electromyographic activity of instrinsic and extrinsic muscles of the human tongue. Tex Rep Biol Med 33:445–455, 1975.
3. Sauerland EK, Harper RM: The human tongue during sleep: Electromyographic activity of the genioglossus muscle. Exp Neurol 51:160–170, 1976.
4. Basmajian JV, Stecko G: A new bipolar electrode for electromyography. J Appl Physiol 17:849, 1962.
5. Yaksta-Sauerland BAT, Orr WC, Sauerland: EK: Non-invasive genioglossal EMG recording in normal subjects and patients with upper airway obstruction. AMSA-UTMB National Student Research Forum 63, 1977.
6. Sauerland EK, Mitchell SP: Electromyographic activity of the human genioglossus muscle in response to respiration and to positional changes of the head. Bull Los Angeles Neurol Soc 35:69–73, 1970.
7. Harper RM, Sauerland EK: The human tongue during sleep: Correlation of EMG activity with respiration. Sleep Res 5:44, 1976.
8. Remmers JE, deGroot WJ, Sauerland EK: Upper airway obstruction during sleep: role of the genioglossus. Clin Res 24:33A, 1976.
9. Coccagna C, Mantovani M, Brignani F, Parchi C, Lugaresi E: Continuous recording of the pulmonary and systemic arterial pressure during sleep in syndromes of hypersomnia with periodic breathing. Bull Physiopathol Respir 8:1217–1227, 1972.
10. Lugaresi E, Coccagna P, Farneti P, Mantovani M, Cirignotta F: Snoring. Electroencephalogr Clin Neurophysiol 39:59–64, 1975.
11. Imes NK, Orr WC, Smith RO, Rogers RM: Retrognathia and sleep apnea: A life threatening condition masquerading as narcolepsy. JAMA 237(15):1596–1597, 1977.
12. Coccagna G, Di Donato G, Verucchi P, Cirignotta F, Mantovani M, Lugaresi E: Hypersomnia with periodic apneas in acquired micrognathia (a bird-like face syndrome). Arch Neurol 33:769–776, 1976.
13. Orr WC, Imes NK, Sauerland EK, Kelly M: Upper airway obstruction following cleft palate surgery: A case report. (In preparation.)
14. Weitzman ED, Pollak C, Borowiecki B, Burack B, Shprintzen R, Rakoff S: The hypersomnia sleep-apnea syndrome (HSA): Site and mechanisms of upper airway obstruction. Sleep Res 6:182, 1977.

15. Remmers JE, deGroot WJ, Sauerland EK, Anch M: Pathogenesis of upper airway occlusion during sleep. (Submitted for publication.)
16. Guilleminault C, Tilkian A, Dement WC: The sleep apnea syndromes. Annu Rev Med 27:465–484, 1976.
17. Negus V: "The Comparative Anatomy and Physiology of the Nose and Paranasal Sinus." London: E and S Livingston, Ltd, 1958.
18. Tonkin S: Airway occlusion as a possible cause of SIDS. In Robinson RR (ed): "SIDS 1974." Toronto: Canadian Foundation for the Study of Infant Deaths, 1974, pp 73–75.
19. Ferguson CF: Treatment of airway problems in the newborn. Ann Otol 76:762–773, 1967.
20. Brandt C, Parrott R, Patrick J, Hyun Wha Kim, Arrobio J, Chandra R, Jeffries B, Chanock R: SIDS and viral respiratory disease in metropolitan Washington, DC. In Robinson RR (ed): "SIDS 1974." Toronto: Canadian Foundation for the Study of Infant Deaths, 1974, pp 117–141.

15
The Hypersomnia-Sleep Apnea Syndrome: Site and Mechanism of Upper Airway Obstruction

Elliot D Weitzman, Charles P Pollak, Bernard Borowiecki, Bernard Burack, Robert Shprintzen, and Saul Rakoff

It is now recognized that the syndrome of excessive daytime sleepiness (hypersomnia) and frequently recurring apnea associated with sleep forms an important clinical entity, called hypersomnia-sleep apnea syndrome (HSA) [1]. The syndrome can usually be easily recognized because of the major symptom of loud, intermittent snoring. The snoring results from partial obstruction of the upper air passages and terminates each apnea episode during which total functional airway obstruction has occurred [2]. In addition to the often serious emotional, social, and economic disability produced by the hypersomnia, the syndrome is also associated with systemic hypertension, cardiac arrhythmias, erythremia, pulmonary hypertension, cardiac hypertrophy and in some cases frank cerebral and myocardial infarcts. A number of previously separate clinical syndromes often share the essential features of HSA and may therefore be classified with it. These include Pickwickian syndrome [3], central alveolar hypoventilation and Ondine's curse syndrome [4]. In addition, many patients with daytime hypersomnolence but without the other symptoms of the narcolepsy-cataplexy syndrome have been increasingly recognized to have the HSA syndrome. Susceptible children with adenoidal and tonsillar enlargement [5, 6] and adults with micrognathia and temporomandibular joint disturbances [7] may also develop the HSA syndrome. It also has been suggested that the Sudden Infant Death syndrome (SIDS) and "near miss" may be disorders related to sleep apnea [8, for review].

It is clear that the functional airway obstruction takes place in the upper respiratory passages since treatment with a tracheotomy that is kept open during sleep dramatically reverses most of the symptoms and pathological findings [1,

Sleep Apnea Syndromes, pages 235–248

9] . Until now, however, the exact site and mechanism of the functional airway obstruction have remained obscure.

We have therefore studied the dynamic anatomical changes which take place in the oral and hypopharynx during sleep in several patients using the techniques of multiview video fluoroscopy and fiber-optic direct visual examination. Our findings indicate that the specific site of airway obstruction is in the oral pharynx at the velopharyngeal sphincter. The mechanism involves recurrent opposition of the superior lateral pharyngeal walls and posterior movement of the base of the tongue. A secondary downward displacement of the soft palate and hypopharynx subsequently occurs due to the negative pressure produced by vigorous respiratory efforts against a closed upper pharyngeal airway.

PATIENTS AND METHODS

During the past nine months, 33 patients with HSA were seen in the Sleep-Wake Disorders Unit at Montefiore Hospital and Medical Center (MHMC). Of these we have listed 25 who had repeated diagnostic polygraphic recordings of multiple physiological functions [polysomnograms (PSGs)] during the six-month period October 1, 1976 to March 31, 1977 (Table I).

All cases had either obstructive apnea or mixed (ie, diaphragmatic plus obstructive) apnea during sleep and in no case did fewer than 200 separate apneic episodes occur during one six- to eight-hour nocturnal recording. Only one patient (RY) was a female and only one patient (GE) did not have either systolic or diastolic hypertension when first examined. Most of the patients were at least moderately obese but 9 out of 25 were not.

Each patient was studied with several all night PSGs and the diagnosis of HSA with recurrent major airway obstruction was confirmed in each case. The technique for polysomnography includes the following physiological channels of information obtained on a Grass Model 78, 12-channel polygraphic machine: scalp electroencephalogram ($C_3 - A_1 + A_2$), lateral and vertical eye movements, mentalis electromyogram, right and left nasal and mouth thermistors, thoraco-abdominal pneumograph, electrocardiogram, continuous ear oximetry, and in some patients endoesophageal pressure (Fig 1). In addition, continuous video monitoring and recording of the patient were obtained to simultaneously visualize the pattern of breathing and movement patterns during sleep. Analysis of sleep stages was made according to standard criteria [10] , in 20-second or 10-second epochs. The episodes of apnea and hypopnea were counted and the duration of each was measured in relation to sleep stage in selected patients. These findings will be reported separately. Three of the patients were studied with the multidimensional video fluoroscopic (MDVF) technique and four with direct visualization by a fiber-optic endoscope during sleep.

Montefiore Hospital and Medical Center, October 1976 – April 1977

Patient	Presenting symptom	Sex	Age (years)	Weight (pounds)	Duration of illness (years)	Previous diagnosis	Blood pressure
NS	Hypersomnia	M	40	265	>10	Narcolepsy	190/120
NB	CVA	M	52	275	>10	CVD and hypertension	160/100
JV	Hypersomnia	M	37	300	>10	None	130/102
JJ	Hypersomnia	M	52	160	>10	Depression	165/90
HK	Hypersomnia	M	61	162	>10	Early dementia	160/96
TS	CVA	M	54	210	>10	Hypertension and CVA	215/140
CM	Hypersomnia	M	50	210	2	Hypertension	180/125
HV	Hypersomnia	M	45	200	>10	Hypertension	144/90
RG	Hypersomnia	M	59	207	8	None	130/95
JB	Hypersomnia	M	47	250	>10	Hypertension/obesity	150/110
RS	Hypersomnia	M	49	187	>10	Headaches/restless legs	165/115
RG	Hypersomnia	M	42	253	>10	Hypertension/obesity	165/110
AG	Insomnia/ Hypersomnia	M	41	280	5	Hypertension/obesity	160/115
TS	Hypersomnia	M	48	170	>10	None	125/95
WV	Hypersomnia	M	57	204	4	Narcolepsy	130/95
RK	Hypersomnia	M	52	290	7	Pickwickian syndrome	160/90
WL	Hypersomnia	M	56	175	6	Narcolepsy	180/120
TH	Hypersomnia	M	58	175	>10	None	175/115
FP	Hypersomnia/ Nocturnal cough	M	45	185	2	Hypertension	165/115
SC	Hypersomnia	M	52	227	>10	Narcolepsy	150/100
GE	Hypersomnia	M	64	166	>10	Hypothyroid	125/72
RY	Hypersomnia	F	65	228	5	Hypertension/obesity	190/110
HH	Hypersomnia	M	39	175	4	Nasal obstruction	138/98
GL	Hypersomnia	M	33	238	>10	None	142/93
JM	Hypersomnia	M	53	240	4	Hypertension/syncope	135/105
X̄			50.0	217			151/104

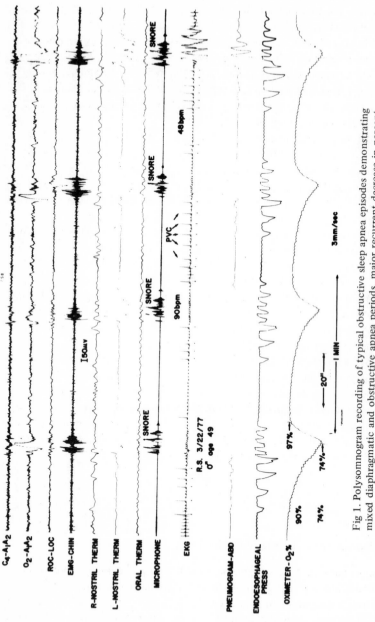

Fig 1. Polysomnogram recording of typical obstructive sleep apnea episodes demonstrating mixed diaphragmatic and obstructive apnea periods, major recurrent decrease in percent oxygen saturation (ear oximetry), associated brady- and tachycardia and multiple premature ventricular contractions.

The following technique was used to obtain an MDVF recording of the upper airway during sleep. The patient was first placed supine on a padded x-ray table with a pillow, and a barium solution was instilled into the nasal passages in order to coat and outline the walls of the nasal, oral, and hypopharyngeal cavities. The room lights were dimmed and several waking baseline video tapes were made during quiet respiration and swallowing. The patient was then allowed to fall asleep in the supine position and a series of video tapes were obtained during several clear episodes of snoring and recurrent obstructive apnea. The patient was then asked to sleep on his side and further video recordings were made. An audio track was recorded simultaneously.

All video tapes were analyzed at full speed, slow motion, and with single stopped frames in both frontal and lateral views. A 14-inch monitor was used. The technique is similar to that described by Sphrintzen et al [11]. The anatomical positions of the lateral pharyngeal walls, soft palate, base of the tongue, and walls of the hypopharynx were identified. The lateral pharyngeal walls were traced on a clear plastic overlay for each of three to five dynamic positional changes during several apneic episodes during sleep. The tracings were then combined to form a composite sequence of changes of the pharyngeal walls (Fig 2).

The technique of fiber-optic examination of the pharynx was as follows. While the patient was awake and lying in bed at night at the usual time of retiring, a Machido fiber-optic endoscope was passed through one side of the nasal cavity to the approximate level of the velum. The tube was held at this position and the patient was then allowed to go to sleep. The fiber-optic image as well as breath sounds were recorded with a Sony color videotape recorder. In some cases a PSG was obtained simultaneously. The fiber-optic scope was repositioned at various levels of the nasopharynx, oropharynx, and hypopharynx. The epiglottis and vocal cords were also observed during sleep in several patients. Patients occasionally complained of mild discomfort during the procedure but because of the hypersomnia usually had little difficulty falling asleep or remaining asleep while the tube was gently repositioned. The fiber-optic recording and examination took approximately two to three hours.

RESULTS

Video Fluoroscopy — Anterior Posterior View

The most important feature observed was the progressive opposition of the right and left lateral pharyngeal walls to each other as the patient was falling asleep during each episode of apnea (Fig 2). The closure first occurred with a constriction in the superior oral pharynx at a point approximately midway between the top of the tongue and the junction between the naso- and oropharynx. This

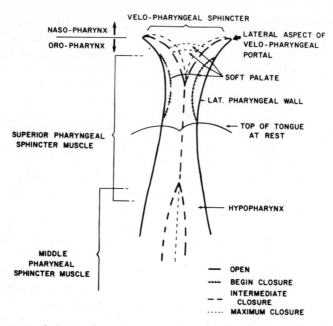

Fig 2. Sequence of closure of oropharynx seen on video fluoroscopy in the anterior-posterior view during an obstructive apnea during sleep. Patient was a 45-year-old male with obstructive sleep apnea documented by polysomnographic recording.

was quickly followed by an intermittent "spasmodic" closure of the lateral pharyngeal walls extending several centimeters above and below the level of the superior surface of the tongue. The timing of this closure was related to inspiratory-expiratory efforts such that closure occurred at the end of expiration just prior to the next subsequent inspiration. At the time of the onset of inspiration, closure was either complete or almost complete. At the beginning of expiration the pharyngeal walls would often partially open, only to close again at the end of expiration and remain closed during the next inspiration. Thus, respiratory diaphragmatic contractions were made during complete or partial closure of the lateral superior pharyngeal walls. A progressive descending wave of closure of the more inferior lateral pharyngeal walls in the hypopharynx was observed to follow the establishment of oropharyngeal obstruction.

Lateral View

The major change seen was a diffuse "darkening" in the region of the super-imposed lateral pharyngeal walls at the time of pharyngeal obstruction. There was no evidence of upward or backward movement of the soft palate. The posterior portion of the base of the tongue did move backward into opposition with the soft palate, but not usually with the posterior pharyngeal wall. In addition, there was an intermittent "down pulling" of the palate, tongue, and pharynx with each strong diaphragmatic inspiratory effort during the interval of superior pharyngeal obstruction.

Fiber-Optic Endoscopic Examination

It was directly observed that the semicircular pharyngeal walls progressively closed in a sphincteric manner during the transition from wakefulness to sleep (Fig 3). The soft palate moved downward and, to a variable extent, posteriorly as well. This active-appearing closure of the velopharyngeal sphincter occurred in a "spasmodic" manner. The timing of the sphincteric closure in relation to the inspiratory-expiratory cycle confirmed the previous fluoroscopic observations. Rapid closure occurred at the transition from expiration to inspiration such that the sphincter was either totally or partially closed at the onset of inspiration and during much of the inspiratory phase. The sphincter often opened partially during expiration only to close again just prior to the next inspiration. However, on many occasions, the sphincter remained totally closed for several inspiratory-expiratory cycles. At the time of a brief arousal and associated with loud snoring and deep breathing, the velopharyngeal sphincter would partially open and rapid vibration of the soft palate could be seen to accompany snoring.

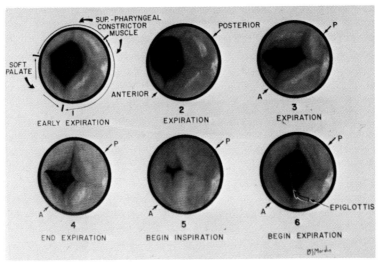

Fig 3. Sequence of closure of velopharyngeal sphincter during an obstructive apnea episode during sleep. View is from above with the fiber-optic positioned at junction of the nasal and oral pharynx. Artist's rendition derived from color videotape.

It was clear that the snoring and snorting noises were due to air moving rapidly through the partially open velopharyngeal sphincter.

Visualization of the epiglottis and vocal cords during the obstructive sleep apneas gave no evidence of obstruction by these structures. The epiglottis did not fully cover the glottis and the vocal cords clearly abducted with each inspiratory effort. These observations plus those on the activity of the pharynx and hypopharynx indicate that the larynx is not the site of upper airway obstruction in the patients with sleep apnea studied by us.

The first report by Kuhlo [9] and recent studies by several Sleep Disorders Centers [1, 12] have demonstrated that establishing a tracheotomy opening during sleep will dramatically and rapidly reverse most of the symptoms of this disorder. At the Sleep-Wake Disorders Unit at Montefiore Hospital, 12 patients have had a therapeutic tracheotomy thus far and we can confirm dramatic improvement. There is a clear and rapid improvement in the hypersomnia and disturbed sleep, a reduction in blood pressure, and a significant decrease in the frequency of sleep-related cardiac arrhythmias. These changes will be reported in subsequent publications from our center.

DISCUSSION

The syndrome of hypersomnia associated with recurrent upper airway obstructive apnea during sleep has been shown to have serious medical and behavioral consequences [1]. Although a wide variety of clinical conditions may be associated with sleep apnea, the patient population outlined in this report forms a fairly distinct and easily diagnosed subgroup. The typical patient is a man between the ages of 40 and 60 years with a long history of loud snoring during sleep who develops progressive daytime sleepiness with increasing frequency of frank and inappropriate sleep episodes. The patient's spouse may describe frequent periods of cessation of airflow during sleep typically followed by loud snoring and snorting sounds. The observations of the dynamic changes in the upper airway made in the present study with video-fluoroscopic and fiberoptic techniques clearly demonstrated that the site of obstruction of breathing is in the oral pharynx. However, it should be emphasized that the velopharyngeal (V-P) sphincter closure is usually associated with a transient cessation of diaphragmatic contraction. This sequence, seen in Figure 1, has been termed "mixed apnea." Our observations indicate that partial or complete closure of the V-P sphincter may occur even if there is a diaphragmatic arrest. Therefore, when diaphragmatic contractions resume the airway is occluded. All of the cases outlined in Table I demonstrated either mixed or obstructive apnea episodes on the polysomnogram. The respiratory cycle sequence of partial to full closure shown in Figures 2 and 3 emphasizes the important participation of the upper

rway musculature in the abnormal respiratory function of this group of
atients. We have directly observed partial closure of the oral pharynx during
spiration and opening during expiration while awake in our patients with the
achido fiber-optic endoscope. Recently Orem et al [13] have described in-
ease in upper airway resistance in normal cats during sleep, although the site(s)
f narrowing was not determined. Sauerland and Harper [14] demonstrated a
ecrease of electromyographic activity of the posterior tongue muscles during
pneic episodes and suggested that this allowed the tongue to fall posteriorly
nd thereby obstruct the airway. While our observations do include a posterior
isplacement of the tongue at the time of the apneic episode, the antero-
osterior (AP) fluoroscopic and fiber-optic visualization demonstrated that the
najor component was the sphincter-like closure of the lateral and posterior
haryngeal walls. Smirne and Comi [15] also reported posterior movement of
1e tongue and soft palate using lateral view cineradiography during obstructive
pnea. However, since AP measurements were not obtained, the important
1teral closure could not be visualized. An early study by Schwartz and Escande
16] on patients diagnosed as having the Pickwickian syndrome demonstrated
losure of the pharyngeal airway during sleep using cineradiographic techniques.
ince the present data indicate that the Pickwickian syndrome patients are ad-
anced cases of the hypersomnia-sleep apnea syndrome, our results conform to
heirs.

Electromyographic recordings of the superior and middle pharyngeal con-
trictor muscles in man and animals during the waking state have shown that, at
est and during quiet breathing, there is no tonic electromyogram (EMG) activity
17, 18]. Basmajian reports that these muscles act in an "all or none" fashion
uring deglutition. However, careful observational and correlative EMG record-
1gs of the pharyngeal muscles during normal waking and sleeping respiration in
nan have not been reported to our knowledge. The mechanism producing the
omplex temporal sequences of velopharyngeal closure, apparently by active
nuscle contraction, as well as cessation of diaphragmatic movements during
leep is unknown. Presumably, complex changes in brain stem neuronal activity
elated to sleep stages are involved. The use of terms such as "peripheral" vs
'central" apnea are misleading since obstructive, diaphragmatic, and mixed
1pneas are therefore all likely to be caused by changes in CNS control of respira-
ory muscles including the diaphragm and pharyngeal muscles. Orem et al have
hown major changes in several pontine and medullary neuronal unit activities in
leep stage and waking states [19]. In addition, sleep apnea has been shown to
1ccur in relation to pathology of the lower brain stem and upper cervical spinal
1ord [20, 21]. Studies in the past have focused primarily on the sleep related
1hanges in the control of diaphragm and intercostal muscles. There are no ex-
1erimental data concerning CNS regional control of upper airway muscles during
espiration in sleep [22].

The incidence of snoring in the general population is high, of course, especially in men [23]. However, the relationship between benign snoring and the malignant snoring found in the hypersomnia-sleep apnea syndrome is unknown. The incidence of the HSA syndrome in the general population is also unknown but, judging from the large number of proven cases seen in our Sleep-Wake Disorders Unit (MHMC), it is probable that the condition is much more common than previously recognized. There are serious medical and psychological consequences of the HSA syndrome including systemic hypertension, cardiac arrhythmias, cor pulmonale, pulmonary hypertension, polycythemia, excessive daytime somnolence, personality changes, and, in some cases, frank myocardial or cerebral infarcts and sudden death in sleep [1]. The important observations by Lugaresi et al on "normal volunteers" with heavy snoring demonstrating a typical obstructive sleep apnea syndrome with hemodynamic abnormalities indicate the potential clinical importance of this "hidden" sleep-related disease [24].

The cause of the severe daytime somnolence found in patients with HSA remains unknown. Two explanations have been suggested. One is that the sleepiness is due to a severe chronic sleep deprivation produced by the major sleep disturbance and disruption occurring night after night by the hundreds of recurring apneas and accompanying arousals. The second is that there is a specific defect in the brain producing both the sleepiness and respiratory abnormalities [1]. We would suggest a third hypothesis, namely that the recurring prolonged and severe hypoxia during the night sleep alters specific brain stem monoamine neuronal regions involved in waking-sleep functions. Studies of brain monoamine synthesis and metabolism during hypoxia have demonstrated a selective sensitivity of catecholamine and serotonin synthesis enzymes [25, 26, 27]. Our observations with ear oximetry indicate that decreases of oxygen saturation down to 70 to 80% are frequent during the obstructive apneic periods. Since it has been shown that decreases of arterial pO_2 to 30 to 50 mm Hg in rats will reduce tryptophan and tyrosine hydroxylation by approximately half in several brain regions [27], it is tempting to speculate that this effect might occur during sleep in patients with obstructive sleep apnea and produce carry-over effects during the next waking day [28]. Some of the major psychological effects of mild to moderate hypoxia are sleepiness, inattention, and memory disturbances, symptoms which are prominant in patients we have seen with HSA syndrome. It is also possible that recurrent hypoxia during sleep could in some way directly alter monoamine-related respiratory and pharyngeal muscle control neurons such that their abnormal temporal functions could lead to increasingly more severe apneic frequency and duration. Evidence that sleep apnea is present with a high frequency in subjects exposed to acute and chronic high altitude environment might support that concept.

The institution of a permanent tracheotomy that is kept open during sleep dramatically reverses most of the symptoms and signs of the HSA syndrome [1,

, 12, 29, 30]. Our own observations on 12 patients successfully treated with tacheotomy at the SWDU at MHMC clearly confirm these reports. The reversal f the hypersomnolence and inattention is certainly the most dramatic change en after surgery and in almost all cases is apparent to the patient and his mily within 48 to 72 hours. Measurement of respiratory function and oxygen turation during sleep with an open tracheotomy demonstrates marked improvement. In addition to the rapid improvement in the daytime hypersomnia nd disturbed sleep, there is usually a reduction in systemic blood pressure and significant decrease in the frequency and severity of the sleep related cardiac rhythmias [29, 31]. It is, therefore, important for all physicians to be aware of is clinical syndrome so that the proper diagnostic and therapeutic recommenations can be made.

EFERENCES

1. Guilleminault C, Tilkian A, Dement WC: The sleep apnea syndromes. Annu Rev Med 27:465–484, 1976.
2. Walsh RE, Michaelson ED, Harkleroad LE, Zighelboim A, Sachner MA: Upper airway obstruction in obese patients with sleep disturbance and somnolence. Ann Intern Med 76:185–192, 1972.
3. Schwartz BA, Escande JP: Respiration hypnique Pickwickienne. In Gastaut H, Lugaresi E, Berti-Ceroni G, Coccagna G (eds): "The Abnormalities of Sleep in Man." Bologna: Gaggi, 1968, pp 209–214.
4. Fruhmann G: Hypersomnia with primary hypoventilation syndrome and following cor pulmonale (Ondine's curse syndrome). Bull Physiopathol Respir 8:1173–1179, 1972.
5. Kravath R, Pollak C, Borowiecki B: Hypoventilation during sleep in children who have lymphoid airway obstruction treated by a nasopharyngeal tube and T and A. Pediatrics 59:865–871, 1977.
6. Levy A, Tabakin B, Hanson J, Narkewicz R: Hypertrophied adenoids causing pulmonary hypertension and severe congestive heart failure. N Engl J Med 277:506–511, 1967.
7. Coccagna G, di Donato G, Verucchi P, Cirignotta F, Montovani M, Lugaresi E: Hypersomnia with periodic apneas in acquired micrognathia. Arch Neurol 33:769, 1976.
8. Weitzman ED, Graziani L: Sleep and the sudden infant death syndrome: A new hypothesis. In Weitzman E (ed): "Advances in Sleep Research," vol 1. New York: Spectrum, 1974, pp 327–344.
9. Kuhlo W, Doll E, Franc M: Exfolgreich behandlung eines Pickwick syndrome durch eine dauertracheal kanule. Dtsch Med Wochenschr 94:1286–1290, 1969.
0. Rechtschaffen A, Kales A: "A Manual of Standardized Terminology, Techniques and Scoring System for Sleep Stages of Human Subjects." Los Angeles: BIS/BRI, UCLA, 1968.
1. Shprintzen RJ, Lencione RM, McCall GN, Skolnick ML: A three dimensional cine fluoroscopic analysis of velopharyngeal closure during speech and non-speech activities in normals. Cleft Palate J 11:412–428, 1974.
2. Lugaresi E, Coccagna G, Mantovani M, Brignani F: Effects of tracheostomy in two cases of hypersomnia with periodic breathing. J Neurol Neurosurg Psychiatry 36:15–26, 1973.

13. Orem J, Netick A, Dement WC: Increased upper airway resistance to breathing during sleep in the cat. Electroencephalogr Clin Neurophysiol 43:14–22, 1977.

14. Sauerland EK, Harper RM: The human tongue during sleep: Electromyographic activity of the genioglossus muscle. Exper Neurol 51:160–170, 1976.

15. Smirne S, Comi G: The obstructive mechanism in Pickwickian syndrome: A serial x-ray study. Sleep Res 4:237, 1975.

16. Schwartz B, Escande J: Etude cinematographique de la respiration hypnique Pickwickienne. Rev Neurol 116:667–678, 1967.

17. Basmajian JV, Dutta CR: EMG of the pharyngeal constrictor and soft palate in rabbits. Anat Rec 139:443–450, 1961.

18. Basmajian JV, Dutta CR: Electromyography of the pharyngeal constrictors and levator Polati in man. Anat Rec 139:561–563, 1961.

19. Orem J, Montplaisir J, Dement WC: Changes in the activity of respiratory neurons during sleep. Brain Res 82:309–315, 1974.

20. Devereux MW, Keane JR, Davis RL: Automatic respiratory failure associated with infarction of the medulla. Arch Neurol 29:46–52, 1973.

21. Krieger AJ, Rosomoff HL: Sleep-induced apnea: Part 1 – A respiratory and autonomic dysfunction syndrome following bilateral percutaneous cervical cordotomy. J Neurosurg 39:168–180, 1974.

22. Garland GM: Pharyngeal respiration. Boston Med Surg J 101:198–199, 1879.

23. Robin IG: Snoring. J Laryngol Otol 62:540–543, 1948.

24. Lugaresi E, Coccagna G, Farneti P, Mantovani M, Cirignotta F: Snoring. Electroencephalogr Clin Neurophysiol 39:59–64, 1975.

25. Davis JN: Adaptation of brain monoamine synthesis to hypoxia in the rat. J Appl Physiol 39:215–220, 1975.

26. Davis JN: Studies of brain monoamine synthesis and metabolism during hypoxia. In Whisnant JP, Sondale BA (eds): "Proceedings of the Ninth Princeton Conference on Cerebral Vascular Disease." New York: Stratton, 1975, pp 301–306.

27. Davis JN, Carlson A: The effect of hypoxia on monoamine synthesis, levels and metabolism in rat brain. J Neurochem 21:783–790, 1973.

28. Semerano A, Bevilacqua M, Battistin L: Blood gas analysis and polygraphic observations in the Pickwickian syndrome. Bull Physiopathol Respir 8:1193–1201, 1972.

29. Tilkian A, Guilleminault C, Schroeder J, Lehrman K, Simmons FB, Dement WC: Sleep-induced apnea syndrome: Reversal of serious arrhythmias after tracheostomy. Circulation 52:II, 131, 1975.

30. Coccagna G, Mantovani M, Brignami F, Parchi C, Lugaresi E: Tracheostomy in hypersomnia with periodic breathing. Bull Physiopathol Respir 8:1217–1227, 1972.

31. Burack B, Pollak C, Borowiecki B, Weitzman E: The hypersomnia-skeep apnea syndrome (HSA): A reversible major cardiovascular hazard. Abstract presented at American Heart Association, November-December, 1977.

DISCUSSION

Dr Severinghaus expressed appreciation for Dr Weitzman's videotape fiberoptic presentation and commented that, although it appeared that the airway was closing and acting like a sphincter, we have no physiologic evidence as yet

lat there is active muscle contraction. He felt subjectively, watching the pictures, that he was not looking at the prime site of the obstruction. For example,
though a closing was seen, at times it remained partially open. He remarked on
he picture of a bubble forming several times during the closing, but it would not
break. He suggested that the pressure difference between the inside and the outside, ie, a negative pressure inside, gives the same visual image as if there were
muscle constriction.

Dr Weitzman explained that the respiration-velopharyngeal closure was paradoxical. The airway often opens during expiration and then immediately closes
during inspiration, this closure appearing to be an active sphincter action by the
superior pharyngeal sphincter muscle. If this inspiratory closure was due to negative pressure, then the site of obstruction must be higher in the airway. There is
no evidence that there is a higher site of obstruction. Although the concept of
the tongue falling posterior presented by Dr Harper is an attractive one, continuous filming in the lateral projection showed that the tongue does not
actually occlude the airway in most instances.

Dr Hill commented on the normal, waking firing activity observed during
swallowing, an action involving the pharyngeal constrictor muscles. One of the
first muscle groups to fire in the sequence is the genioglossus, followed by
marked constriction and rapid firing discharge in the superior, middle, and
inferior constrictors. If a similar action were occurring in sleep apneic patients,
a tremendous firing activity should be recorded in their pharyngeal constrictors,
and this is not the case. The stylopharyngeal, styloglossal, and stylohyoid
muscles are the muscles implicated in opening the pharyngeal tent and extending
the pharynx during active respiration. Dr Hill reported that EMG studies performed at Stanford indicate that these muscles lose tone at an inappropriate
time, and no vector pulls laterally on the pharynx to open it. He suggested a
deficit in a motor loop and raised the question of how to systematically determine whether a sensory deficit exists and if so, its location.

Dr Severinghaus proposed the adaptation to human study of a study that has
been done in dogs. After tracheostomy, a double lumen device can be inserted
through the tracheostomy, one end of which points upwards and serves to inject
a continuous airstream, the other end is directed downwards and through this
the subject breathes. This permits simultaneous recording of EMG, observation
of respiration, and performance of the usual studies.

Dr Guilleminault observed that patients have no feeling of air hunger during
sleep before tracheostomy. Normally, one is acutely aware of an occlusion of the
pharynx, even during sleep, and constant repositioning of the muscles involved
occurs. Sleep apneic patients, however, tolerate this condition during sleep to an
amazing degree. But following surgery, when the tracheostomy was closed
during the course of the night, patients awoke immediately and were acutely
aware of the feeling of being obstructed. This suggests a worsening process, as if

the central mechanisms were gradually closing down. After tracheostomy, patients appear to have lost their tolerance to asphyxia. Dr Severinghaus questioned the roles of sleep, sleepiness, and sleep deprivation in this last observation. As Dr Dement pointed out previously, sleep deprivation depresses reflexes also, the fact that sleep apneic patients are so deeply sleepy may permit them to tolerate the obstruction. But after tracheostomy, and amelioration of the sleep disorder, this tolerance disappears.

16
Fiber-Optic and EMG Studies in Hypersomnia-Sleep Apnea Syndrome

Michael W Hill, Christian Guilleminault, and F Blair Simmons

Patients with hypersomnia-sleep apnea syndrome (HSA) have been documented to suffer partial and total obstruction of their airway during sleep, resulting in hypoxia and cardiovascular arrhythmias [1]. At Stanford, we have focused our research effort on two questions concering HSA which until this time were unanswered. What is the exact level of the obstruction? Is this an active (hypertonic) or passive (hypotonic) obstruction?

We have employed the techniques of fiber-optic endoscopy and electromyographic recording in order to answer these questions. Fiber-optic studies have revealed that obstructions both partial and total occur in the midpharynx just below the oral pharyngeal inlet. Visually, there is a collapse of the lateral pharyngeal walls and to a lesser extent the posterior pharyngeal wall. This sphincteric invagination of the pharyngeal walls is concomitant with each inspiratory effort. The endolarynx, supraglottic larynx, and nasopharynx are not involved in these obstructions. The base of the tongue did not fall posteriorly to produce an obstruction in any of the cases studied.

The abrupt sphincteric and at times rhythmic contraction of the midpharyngeal walls suggested that the obstruction was an "active" (hypertonic) spasm of the superior and middle constrictors of the pharynx during inspiration. This was contradicted by the electromyographic (EMG) recordings. In fact, a hypotonia and at times atonia was found in pharyngeal adductors and abductors during an inspiratory obstruction.

METHODS

Fiber-optic examination of the pharynx and larynx during sleep has provided some important ideas as to the exact mechanisms responsible for obstruction of

Sleep Apnea Syndromes, pages 249–258

the upper airway in sleep apnea patients. Fiber-optic nasal endoscopy has been performed on 11 sleep apneic patients and three control subjects (all male). After achieving topical anesthesia of the nasal mucosa with 4% cocaine or 2% pentocaine, a Machida fiber-optic endoscope was introduced intranasally into the pharyngeal inlet and securely taped to the nose. The scope was left in place during several hours of nocturnal sleep. Patients were acoustically and visually observed continuously and filmed intermittently during the examination. Simultaneous polygraphic recordings were obtained in all cases.

These recurring obstructions were viewed from the nasopharynx, oral pharyngeal inlet, hypopharynx, and supraglottic larynx by advancing and retracting the endoscope. There were no complications resulting from this procedure.

In order to more accurately identify specific muscles responsible for upper airway obstruction in sleep apnea patients, selective EMG recordings have been obtained from the superior, middle, and inferior constrictors, palatoglossus, palatopharyngeus, cricopharyngeus, stylohyoid, stylopharyngeus, and genioglossus muscles. These muscles were selected because of their anatomical importance in maintaining a patient's oropharynx during the respiratory cycles.

Eleven HSA patients and three normal controls were used in the EMG study. They were all male and ranged from 42 to 54 years in age. Electromyographic recordings during wakefulness and nocturnal sleep were obtained in all cases. Bipolar electrodes were used in these recordings. They were fashioned as has been previously described by other investigators [2].

The recording electrodes were placed intraorally when possible. The area chosen for the recording site was topically anesthetized with 4% xylocaine or 4% cocaine. The electrodes were then placed in position using a 22-gauge spinal needle. A minimum distance of 2 mm was obtained between the muscle ends of the recording electrodes to prevent short circuiting. The free ends of the recording electrodes were then brought out either through the mouth or nose and taped to the skin for later recording. The nasal route was safer in terms of accidental dislodgment by the tongue and seemed to be less annoying to the patients. After intraoral placement, the free ends are retrieved by placing a catheter through the nose and into the oropharynx. After securing the wires to the catheter, its withdrawal brings the wires through the nasopharynx and out the external nares.

Certain muscles cannot be implanted accurately and/or safely either intraorally or percutaneously. These muscles (cricopharyngeus, inferior constrictor, and the inferior edges of the middle constrictor) were implanted under direct vision at the time of tracheostomy. The free ends were brought out through the anterior cervical neck skin several centimeters from the tracheostomy site. In these cases the recordings were obtained 36–72 hours after surgery with the tracheostomy open and closed (reproducing the typical syndrome). Good re-

ordings cannot be obtained the first two postoperative nights due to frequent
uctioning required.

During the recording sessions the polygraphic variables related to monitoring
tates of sleep and wakefulness were exactly the same in all patients. The electro-
ncephalogram was always recorded from the standard (C_3/A_2) or symmetrical
$C_4/A_1)$ placements of the international 10-20 system [3]. The electrooculo-
ram was recorded bipolarly from electrodes at the right and left outer canthi.
'wo closely approximated submental electrodes recorded the digastric (chin)
lectromyogram. Respiration was monitored using thoracic and abdominal
train gauges and buccal and nasal thermistors. The subject was grounded with
n electrode on the earlobe. The polygraphic recordings were obtained during
vakefulness and sleep in all subjects. There were no complications from the
EMG studies.

FINDINGS

Fiber-Optic Studies

Under direct visualization the entire pharynx and larynx were viewed during
both unobstructed and obstructed sleep with interval periods of arousal to wakefulness. During quiet sleep one sees a patent pharynx; on inspiration the vocal
cords abduct widely and on expiration return to an intermediate position as
expected.

Obstructive apnea first appears as an invagination of the lateral pharyngeal
walls. Depending on the severity the collapse may be partial or total. What one
sees correlates precisely with what one hears with respect to the patient's
snoring.

This midpharyngeal obstruction is a "mismatch" with the respiratory cycle.
The abrupt collapse occurs at the onset of inspiration. The pharynx contour may
or may not be restored to normal at the end of the inspiratory cycle.

By advancing the scope to the supraglottic area, the laryngeal inlet is seen to
be patent during an obstructive episode. There is clearly no evidence of a glottic
(laryngeal) obstruction. The palate is not pushed posteriorly during an apneic
episode by the tongue. The posterior tongue was observed and filmed and seems
to have very little involvement in the obstruction. The lateral and posterior
pharyngeal walls collapse just below the oropharyngeal inlet and produce the
obstruction.

Electromyographic Studies

Electromyographic recordings obtained from patients with HSA clearly
demonstrate the obstruction is due to a generalized relaxation of the pharyngeal
musculature.

In our group of normal controls we saw repetitive firing in the adductors (middle and superior constrictors) and abductors (stylopharyngeus) of the pharynx which was synchronous with the respiratory cycle both during sleep and wakefulness (Fig 1). In this case electromyographic recording from the superior and middle constrictors showed a burst of activity in midexpiration which continued through midinspiration. This pattern continued in the same rhythmic fashion whether the subject was asleep or in quiet wakefulness.

The same basic pattern of muscle firing is seen in HSA patients during wakefulness and unobstructed sleep (Fig 2). However, during obstructive apnea this motor activity greatly diminishes or completely ceases (Fig 3). In this case motor activity in the middle constrictor abated just prior to the obstructive episode. It is only very late in the apneic episode that we begin to see the first signs of return firing just prior to the return of inspiration. This same pattern was repeated over and over in the various muscles we recorded.

All 11 HSA patients exhibited a marked decrease in electromyographic activity during an obstructive apnea. None of them exhibited any hyperactivity in any of the muscles we recorded during an obstructive episode. This pharyngeal invagination is clearly a "passive" process. Why is the motor pathway to the pharyngeal adductors and abductors altered during sleep?

DISCUSSION

Our observations and recordings reveal the primary defect in obstructive sleep apnea to involve a complex sensory-motor reflex loop. The pharyngeal abductors (ie, stylopharyngeus, etc) clearly represent the motor component of this loop. During normal respiration, a tonic impulse, which begins at midexpiration and ends at midinspiration, is received by the pharyngeal abductors. In this way, a patent pharyngeal airway is maintained during inspiration, and collapse, induced by the negative intrathoracic inspiratory pressure, is avoided.

Electromyographic recordings from the pharyngeal abductors demonstrate an absence of this tonic impulse during an obstructive apnea. This vital sensory-motor reflex arc breaks down in patients with HSA.

Hypotonia, and at times atonia, of the pharyngeal muscles was demonstrated in all of our patients during obstructive sleep apnea. During wakefulness and unobstructed sleep, the normally present "tonic impulse" was recorded in all cases. What factors cause an interruption of this sensory-motor loop? The answer to this question requires a concise knowledge of pharyngeal function and its CNS regulatory neurons.

The basic function of the pharynx is threefold: positional, respiratory, and feeding. The neuromuscular coordination of these processes is highly specific

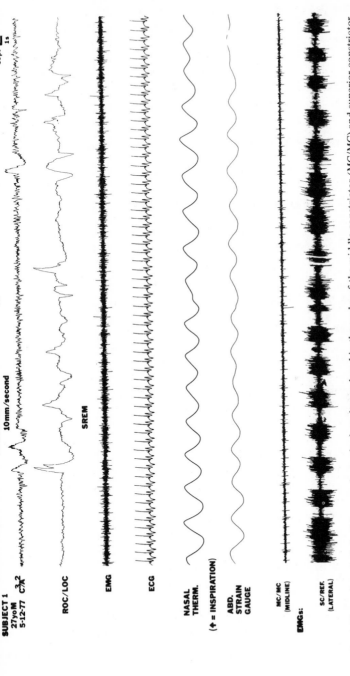

Fig 1. Normal control. In this case, electrodes have been placed in the raphe of the middle constrictor (MC/MC) and superior constrictor (Sc/Ref) muscles. We see repetitive bursts of firing in a cyclic fashion which is synchronous with the respiratory cycle both during sleep and wakefulness. This burst of activity begins in midexpiration and is continued through midinspiration. The basic pattern is the same in both sleep and quiet wakefulness.

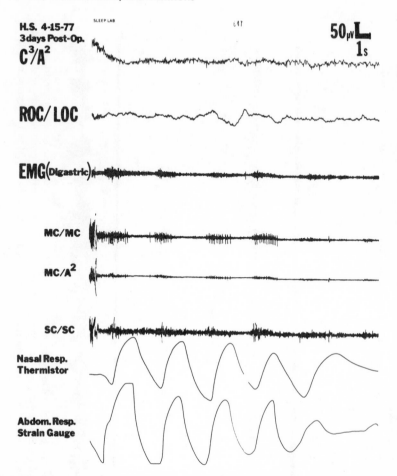

Fig 2. These data were obtained 3 days post-tracheostomy in a patient with HSA. EMG electrodes were placed in the middle constrictor (MC/A^2) close to the midline and laterally (MC/MC). The same cyclic firing, synchronous with the respiratory cycle, is seen during unobstructed sleep.

and necessary for survival. Interestingly, these pharyngeal functions have a common motor effector and separate sensory affectors.

With respect to respiration, the sensory input from the trigeminal, glossopharyngeal, and vagus nerves has been demonstrated to produce profound apnea and even death in animal studies [4–6]. Impulses from sensory afferents (V, IX, X) and changes in pCO$_2$ and pO$_2$ are known to produce alterations in the central regulation of respiration. However, we have observed that the perception

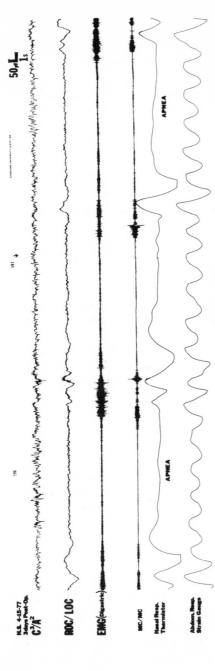

Fig 3. In this case (same patient as in Figure 2) we see the motor activity in MC/MC greatly decreased or completely absent during an obstructive apnea. It is felt, as explained in the text, that this electrode MC/MC is recording the activity of the stylopharyngeus muscle. The motor activity abates just prior to the obstructive episode. It is only very late in the apneic episode that we begin to see the first signs of return firing just prior to the return of inspiration.

of airflow through the pharynx itself plays an important role in maintaining the pharyngeal airway. This is substantiated by soft tissue neck X rays in patients who have undergone permanent tracheostomy. There is a collapse of the pharynx with resultant loss of a pharyngeal air column in these cases.

In addition, we observed an abrupt loss of firing in pharyngeal abductors when the tracheostomy tube was opened. In this case, we were recording medial and lateral portions of the middle constrictor and the medial portion of the superior constrictor. Concomitant with opening the tracheostomy tube, there was a loss of firing in this laterally placed pharyngeal electrode (EMG 1) (Fig 4). However, there was continual firing in the medial one (EMG 2). The lateral electrode was obviously in the stylopharyngeus muscle. This muscle is an abductor of the pharynx. Its origin is the medial aspect of the styloid process, and it passes between the superior and middle constrictors to insert in the lateral pharyngeal wall. Its fibers blend with those of the middle constrictor and some of them lie immediately submucosally in the lateral pharynx. The natural mixing of abductor and adductor fibers in this region requires a second electrode placed more medially for verification of the firing pattern of the adductors. We conclude then that the receptor sites for the perception of airflow must certainly be above the tracheostomy site.

Impulses from upper respiratory sensory afferents interact considerably in the brain stem. Sessle has recently demonstrated a profound suppression of respiratory neurons by upper respiratory tract afferents [7].

The afferent-efferent reflex loop defect in HSA may be complex, involving sensory feedback mechanisms and abnormal inhibition of respiratory neurons in the caudal brain stem. The precise answer must await further research in these areas.

ACKNOWLEDGMENTS

This research was supported by National Institute of Neurological Diseases and Stroke grant NS 10727, Public Health Service Research Grant RR-70 from the General Clinical Research Centers, Division of Research Resources, and by INSERM to Dr Guilleminault.

REFERENCES

1. Guilleminault C, Tilkian A, Dement WC: The sleep apnea syndromes. Annu Rev Med 31: 465–484, 1976.
2. Basmajian JV, Stecko G: A new bipolar electrode for electromyography. J Appl Physiol 17:849, 1962.

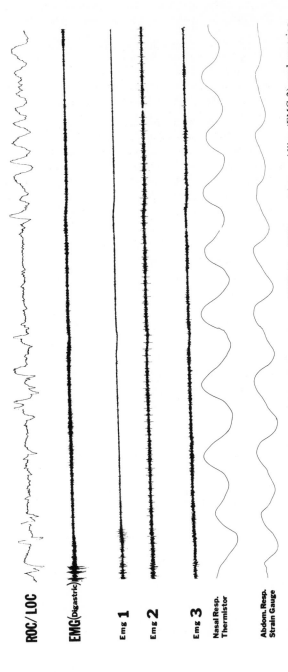

Fig 4. In this case, EMG recordings were obtained from the lateral pharynx (EMG 1), middle constrictor midline (EMG 2), and superior constrictor midline (EMG 3). Upon opening the tracheostomy tube we see an abrupt loss of firing in pharyngeal abductors (EMG 1). Only baseline firing is seen in the middle and superior constrictors. Anatomically and physiologically, this results in a collapse of the pharynx which clinically is what we have observed in these cases. (From top to bottom: EMG 1, channel 4; EMG 2, channel 5; EMG 3, channel 6.)

3. Rechtschaffen A, Kales A: "A Manual of Standardized Terminology, Techniques, and Scoring System for Sleep Stages of Human Subjects." Los Angeles: BIS/BRI, UCLA, 1968.

4. Wealthall SR: Factors resulting in a failure to interrupt apnea. In Bosma JF (ed): "Development of Upper Respiratory Anatomy and Function." Washington, DC: US Government Printing Office, 1975, pp 212–228.

5. Kenny DJ, Holmwood B, Sessle BJ: Regulatory influences on the glossopharyngeal input to the brain stem of cat. J Dent Res 52:100, 1973.

6. Johnson P, Salisbury DM, Storey AT: Apnea induced by stimulation of sensory receptors in the larynx. In Bosma JF (ed): "Development of Upper Respiratory Anatomy and Function." Washington, DC: US Government Printing Office, 1975, pp 160–178.

7. Sessle BJ: Sensory inputs and interactions in single brain stem neurones involved in functional upper and lower respiratory tracts. In Bosma JF (ed): "Development of Upper Respiratory Anatomy and Function." Washington, DC: US Government Printing Office, 1975, pp 131–144.

17
The Bird-Like Face Syndrome (Acquired Micrognathia, Hypersomnia, and Sleep Apnea)

Giorgio Coccagna, Fabio Cirignotta, and Elio Lugaresi

The term "bird-like face syndrome" describes a clinical picture characterized by micrognathia acquired in infancy, hypersomnia, and recurrent apneas during sleep [1]. The syndrome is very rare, but we believe that this rarity is in part due to lack of recognition and the fact that these patients are almost never examined with polygraphic techniques. In fact, in our laboratory in the last ten years we have examined six patients with the syndrome. while only seven other observations were reported in the literature [2–6]. The patients we saw were sent to us because they suffered from hypersomnia and not because of respiratory disturbances during sleep.

CLINICAL PICTURE

Our patients as well as those reported in the literature present a stereotyped clinical picture.

Micrognathia

Micrognathia is the consequence of a pathological process which strikes during infancy, impeding the growth of the mandibular condyles and provoking ankylosis of the temporomandibular joint. The micrognathia gives the patient a typical bird-like profile because of the stunted mental protuberance (Fig 1). In the eight patients for whom the pathology was identified, the mandibular lesion arose between 6 months and 6 years of age. Osteomyelitis was reported in six cases and fracture of the condyles in two cases. Of the 13 patients reported in the literature, nine are males and four are females.

Sleep Apnea Syndromes, pages 259–271

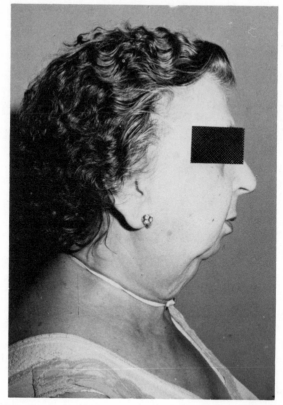

Fig 1. The stunted chin gives the patient a typical bird-like face.

Radiological studies revealed an underdeveloped mandible, often the absence of the condyles which were replaced by fibrous tissue, and complete obliteration of the temporomandibular joint. Aperture of the mouth was extremely limited, varying from 0.5 to 1.5 cm at the level of the anterior dental arch. This created marked difficulty in eating for all patients, and, in the case reported by Hishikawa et al [3], the patient had to have his front teeth extracted to permit food intake.

Respiratory Disturbances

The first respiratory disturbance to appear was invariably heavy snoring. In our patients, who were carefully questioned, snoring appeared at the time micrognathia developed or a few years afterward. The moment when apneas during sleep appeared is more difficult to establish. Usually, the apneas are described, by a spouse or a relative who sleeps near the patient, as respiratory arrests during which the patient seems to be suffocating.

The respiratory arrest is followed by extremely heavy snoring. The patient himself can often establish the period during which apneas became an important syndrome because, from that time on, sleep has been agitated and interrupted by frequent reawakenings provoked by a sensation of suffocation. In our patients, recurrent apneas during sleep appeared at extremely varied intervals after the mandibular lesion — from 3 to 57 years later. Some of our patients breathed noisily even while awake.

One of our patients [1] and the patient reported by Hishikawa et al [3] stopped breathing after administration of preanesthetic medication before surgery to lengthen the mandibular branches. Both patients were tracheotomized and respiration rapidly returned to normal. The tracheal stoma was closed after the emergency had subsided.

Hypersomnia

Hypersomnia may appear at the same time as the apneas, but in four of our patients it developed from 1 to 17 years later. In no case did hypersomnia precede appearance of the apneas. Diurnal hypersomnia is of extremely variable intensity. For many years the episodes of sleep may be brief and occur only in particular situations as after a meal or during monotonous work or intellectual activity. Subsequently, an almost continuous somnolence develops and the patient falls asleep under any circumstances, during conversation and meals and even while standing. In five of our patients hypersomnia and apneas during sleep were suddenly and rapidly aggravated, after years of stability, without apparent reason, except that in one case the change was preceded by a rapid weight gain.

Physical and Laboratory Examinations

Aside from micrognathia, the physical examination of the patients usually did not reveal any other notable peculiarities. None of the patients was obese. In three of our patients the thorax was extremely flattened in an anteroposterior direction and presented a deep transverse depression at the level of insertion of the diaphragm. These same three patients had assumed from infancy a particular positioning of the head which was extended and projected forward. This position, while improving respiration, provoked serious deformation of the cervical spine with inversion of the physiological lordosis and anterior displacement of many vertebral bodies (Fig 2).

Routine laboratory examinations were normal in all patients. Respiratory function tests were either normal [1, 2] or demonstrated slight obstructive or restrictive pulmonary disease [1–3, 5]. Increased inspiratory airway resistance existed in four of our patients and in Valero and Alroy's patient [2].

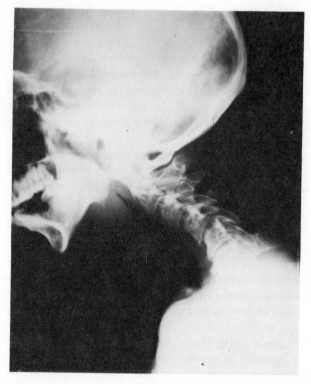

Fig 2. Roentgenogram showing marked mandibular underdevelopment and the absence of the left mandibular ramus which appears to be replaced by fibrous tissue. Serious deformation of the cervical spine is evident.

Alveolar ventilation during wakefulness was normal in some patients [1,3,4], and in others mild alveolar hypoventilation was present [1, 2, 4, 6]. Ventilatory response to hypercapnia was tested in one of our patients by inhalation of a mixture of carbon dioxide in room air. The test demonstrated that the response was diminished overall. In Valero and Alroy's patient results of the rebreathing test also showed that the respiratory center failed to respond to endogenous accumulation of CO_2 [2].

Some patients presented electrocardiographical or radiological signs of right heart overload or hypertrophy or an incomplete bundle branch block [1, 2]. One of our patients had an atrial flutter with unstable block 8/1 to 4/1.

A cineradiographic study during sleep of the oropharynx in two of our patients demonstrated that, during apnea, the oropharyngeal wall collapsed and obstructed the upper airway [1]. Similar studies by Hishikawa et al [3] and by Conway et al [6] showed in their patients the obstruction of the upper airway during apnea was due to a sliding backward of the tongue.

POLYGRAPHIC RECORDINGS

Method

Polygraphic recordings during sleep were carried out for all of our patients and the patients reported by Hishikawa et al, Tammeling et al, Imes et al, and Conway et al [1, 3–6]. In five of our patients the recordings continued without interruption for 24 hours. During diurnal recording the patient was seated in an armchair, and the recording was periodically interrupted to allow the patient to walk around the laboratory.

In addition to the parameters standardly used to identify the stages of sleep [EEG, mylohyoid electromyogram (EMG), horizontal oculogram], we also simultaneously recorded the electrocardiogram, the flow of air through nose and mouth by means of thermistors, and thoracic respiratory activity with an expandable tube placed across the thorax and connected to a piezoelectric transducer. Snoring was recorded by a small microphone placed above the patient and connected to an EEG channel of the polygraph. In some cases an intercostal muscle EMG was also measured by means of superficial electrodes, and in four patients endoesophageal pressure was recorded with a catheter, equipped with a terminal balloon, introduced through a nostril into the lower third of the esophagus.

All of our patients underwent a further polygraphic recording which included simultaneous recording of systemic and pulmonary arterial pressure (two patients), systemic arterial pressure only (three patients), or pulmonary arterial pressure only (one patient). Systemic arterial pressure was recorded directly by percutaneous cannulation of the radial artery with a Teflon needle. The needle was connected to a pressure transducer by Teflon tubing, and a two-way stopcock made it possible to interrupt the recording or the perfusion periodically to take blood samples for immediate gas analysis. In the course of each night an average of 14 arterial blood samples was taken during wakefulness and the various stages of sleep.

Pulmonary arterial pressure was recorded by means of a floating microcatheter introduced into an antecubital vein and pushed into the pulmonary artery. A two-way stopcock was placed between the catheter and the pressure transducer so that the recording could be interrupted periodically and the catheter perfused with heparinized saline solution.

The stages of sleep were identified according to Rechtschaffen and Kales [7], but we preferred to consider the two stages of deep slow wave sleep (stages 3–4) together.

Results

Disturbances of sleep. The presence of marked diurnal hypersomnia was confirmed by the 24-hour polygraphic recordings. In our five patients total sleep time averaged 16 hours. On the average, these patients slept 90% of the recording time at night and 68% of the recording time during the day. Nocturnal sleep was disturbed by frequent reawakenings, some quite protracted. Percentage duration of the individual stages of sleep was quite different during nocturnal sleep and diurnal sleep episodes. During nocturnal sleep, on the average, stages 1–2 represented 70% while stages 3–4 represented 8%. During diurnal sleep, when the patient slept sitting up in an armchair and respiration improved, stages 3–4 reached 17% on the average. Rapid eye movement (REM) sleep stage percentages were almost normal during nocturnal (22%) as well as diurnal sleep (18%). In the patient reported by Hishikawa et al [3] also, sleep was predominantly composed of stages 1 and 2 (66%), while the REM stage represented about 14%.

Respiratory disturbances. Apneas immediately appeared in all patients, as soon as they fell asleep, and continued without interruption for the duration of sleep. The apneas were separated by a few effective respiratory efforts. The respiratory arrests coincided with electroencephalographic signs of falling asleep or deepening of sleep, while resumption of respiration was immediately preceded by signs of electroencephalographic arousal.

Three types of apneas were observed: a) *central* or diaphragmatic, during which there is a simultaneous arrest of airflow through the nose and mouth and an arrest of thoracic movement. These apneas are the least frequent (mean 3%) and the shortest (mean 11 seconds). They occur exclusively during very light sleep and REM sleep; b) *obstructive,* during which thoracic movements persist even when the flow of air through the upper airway ceases. These apneas are the most frequent (mean 86%) and prolonged (mean 28 seconds), and they occur during all stages of sleep; c) *mixed,* during which a central apnea is followed by reappearance of thoracic movements. These apneas represent 11% of the total and occur only during light and REM sleep. Mixed apneas have a mean duration equal to that of obstructive apneas (mean 29 seconds) but individually during REM sleep may be extremely protracted (up to 110 seconds). Our patients spent about 51% of their total sleep time in apnea, but during deep slow wave sleep and REM sleep this figure sometimes rose as high as 77%.

The thoracic movements which characterize obstructive and mixed apneas are the expression of intense respiratory efforts to overcome the upper airway obstruction. They are accompanied by gradual increases in electromyographic activity of the intercostal muscles and in negative endoesophageal pressure, which may exceed 100 cm H_2O during the ineffective inspiratory efforts immediately preceding the resumption of ventilation. Even during the resumption of respiration an incomplete obstruction of the upper airway persists as demonstrated by the persistence of an elevated negative endoesophageal pressure (Fig 3).

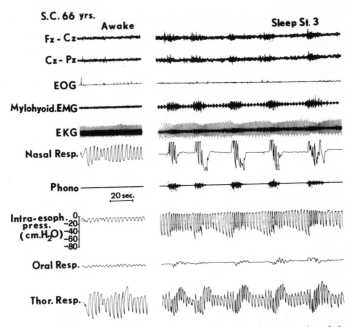

Fig 3. Polygraphic recording including simultaneous recording of nasal, oral, and thoracic respiration and endoesophageal pressure. Left) During quiet wakefulness respiration, negative endoesophageal pressure is slightly higher than normal. Right) During stage 3 of sleep an uninterrupted series of obstructive apneas occurred. Endoesophageal pressure increased progressively during the apneas, reaching a value of 60–70 cm H_2O at the end of the apnea. At the resumption of respiration, partial obstruction of the upper airways persisted, demonstrated by heavy snoring (see phono) and the persistence of an elevated endoesophageal pressure.

During the apneas, especially obstructive or mixed, sinus bradycardia to 22 beats/min appeared; the resumption of respiration was accompanied by tachycardia to 125 beats/min. In one of our patients atrioventricular blocks with periods of asystole up to six seconds appeared frequently. In the patient who had an atrial flutter with incomplete atrioventricular block, the block could reach a ratio of 15/1 during apnea (Fig 4). Disturbances of rhythm and conduction seemed to have a greater relationship to the length of the apnea than to negative endoesophageal pressure values, and they were most marked during REM sleep.

Alveolar ventilation and hemodynamic changes during sleep. These data are summarized for each of our patients in Table I. In all subjects, with the beginning of sleep and the appearance of apneas, a state of alveolar hypoventilation

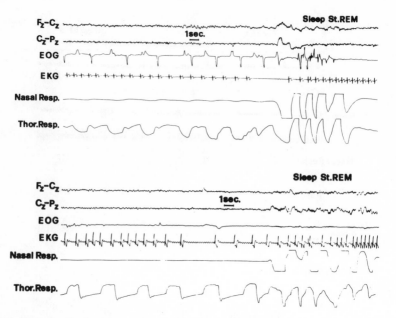

Fig 4. Marked arrhythmia during obstructive apneas in two patients. Above) Complete atrioventricular block with a five-second period of asystole. Below) In the patient with atrial flutter, the conduction ratio increased to 15/1 during apnea.

was established or aggravated, if already present in wakefulness. Alveolar hypoventilation increased progressively during the successive stages of slow wave sleep and reached a maximum during REM sleep.

Alveolar hypoventilation during slow wave sleep was mild or absent in only one patient (DEG) because the obstruction of the upper airway was incomplete and a certain amount of air always passed through the nose or mouth. This patient snored loudly, and the snoring intensified intermittently, coincident with periodic deepening of respiratory efforts. True apneas appeared only during REM sleep, but during this stage, due to technical problems, it was impossible to make any gas analysis determinations.

Pulmonary arterial pressure, which during wakefulness was higher than normal, increased progressively during the successive stages of slow wave sleep and reached highest values during REM sleep. Systemic arterial pressure also increased during slow wave sleep and, except for one case, increased further during REM sleep. Both systemic and pulmonary arterial pressures reached highest values at the end of each apnea (Fig 5).

TABLE I. Systemic and Pulmonary Artery Pressure and Gas Analysis Values During Wakefulness and Sleep (values after tracheostomy are shown in parentheses)

		W	St. 1	St. 2	St. 3–4	St. REM
Obs.1 B.A.	System. Art. Press.	156/90 (130/90)	171/103 (128/91)	193/112 (125/88)	203/111 (124/86)	205/113 (124/86)
	Pulm. Art. Press.	45/23 (33/15)	56/33 (40/20)	68/43 (46/24)	88/57 (48/25)	100/64 (45/24)
	Mean	32 (21)	36 (31)	54 (31)	63 (34)	70 (33)
	$PaCO_2$	52 (30)	–	58.5 (41)	65.6 (45)	66.6 (44)
	PaO_2	74.6 (88)	–	60 (69)	58.6 (80)	53 (80)
	pH	7.36 (7.49)	–	7.34 (7.39)	7.30 (7.35)	7.30 (7.35)
Obs.2 B.G.	System. Art. Press.	125/94 (127/92)	136/99 (120/88)	133/98 (118/85)	133/99 (116/74)	144/102 (120/87)
	Pulm. Art. Press.	46/22 (36/17)	63/30 (36/17)	79/39 (34/15)	84/44 (34/15)	98/58 (35/15)
	Mean	29 (25)	– (25)	– (24)	58 (22)	70 (21)
	$PaCO_2$	59 (38.5)	–	65 (43.3)	68 (41)	70.7 (40.3)
	PaO_2	71 (87.6)	–	58 (79.3)	56 (82)	45 (83.5)
	pH	7.33 (7.40)	–	7.30 (7.36)	7.30 (7.37)	7.27 (7.39)
Obs.3 D.E.G.	System. Art. Press.	226/114	232/118	248/130	258/137	235/127
	$PaCO_2$	40.5	44	44.2	41.6	–
	PaO_2	69.5	58	57	58	–
	pH	7.37	7.33	7.32	7.34	–
Obs.4 T.A.	System. Art. Press.	118/85	134/97	136/101	131/96	154/112
	$PaCO_2$	36.5	–	40	47.4	50.5
	pH	7.38	–	7.33	7.30	7.27
Obs.5 S.G.	System. Art. Press.	167/95 (154/82)	193/107 (148/81)	197/108 (140/74)	192/103 (136/74)	201/109 (147/78)
	$PaCO_2$	51 (40)	53	57.5 (44)	63 (43)	61.3 (41.5)
	PaO_2	73 (87)	70.5	61.2 (80)	60 (82)	48.6 (84)
	pH	7.33 (7.36)	7.32	7.30 (7.36)	7.27 (7.36)	7.28 (7.37)
Obs.6 S.C.	System. Art. Press.	– (142/65)	– (133/60)	– (127/57)	– (119/54)	– (128/55)
	Pulm. Art. Press.	33/17 (26/13)	41/22 (28/13)	54/31 (36/18)	57/33 (36/22)	73/40 (37/19)
	$PaCO_2$	38 (35.5)	–	49 (39.6)	– (41.6)	– (39)
	PaO_2	90 (82.3)	–	56 (79.6)	– (82.3)	– (78)
	pH	7.39 (7.39)	–	7.32 (7.34)	– (7.33)	– (7.36)

TREATMENT

In two of our patients we attempted pharmacological therapy with d-N-methylamphetamine. Initially, there was a reduction of diurnal somnolence, but after a short time the treatment had to be suspended because the patients required too high a dosage level of the drug (60 mg per diem) to maintain modest therapeutic effectiveness. These drugs, however, did not modify the apneas during sleep. Two other patients underwent one or more plastic surgery operations to lengthen the mandibular rami. After surgery, the mouth aperture was larger and eating was easier, but hypersomnia and respiratory disturbances were only slightly modified.

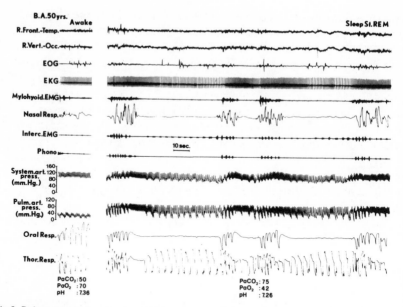

Fig 5. Pulmonary and systemic arterial pressures and gas analysis values during sleep. The gas analysis values were determined immediately after the corresponding fragments of tracings. During wakefulness there was mild alveolar hypoventilation, and pulmonary artery pressure was slightly higher than normal. During REM sleep, an uninterrupted series of mixed and obstructive apneas occurred. Maximum systemic arterial pressure reached 160 mm Hg, and maximum pulmonary artery pressure reached 120 mm Hg. Alveolar hypoventilation worsened markedly. During the obstructive phase of the apneas, marked bradycardia appeared, the EMG activity of the intercostal muscles progressively increased, and oscillations in pulmonary and systemic arterial pressures are observed, synchronous with the ineffective inspiratory movements.

Tracheostomy

Tracheostomy, with insertion of a permanent tracheal cannula, is the only therapeutic measure which permits definitive cure of the syndrome [1, 2, 4–6]. Hypersomnia regresses completely and rapidly in every case, often the same day surgery is performed. Electrocardiographic signs of right heart overload and hypertrophy also regress within a short period of time [1, 2]. In our patient the atrial flutter disappeared the day after the operation [1].

The tracheostomy is well tolerated, and all of our patients (two to eight years after the operation) lead normal lives. The tracheal stoma is kept closed during the day to allow the patient to speak normally, and is opened at night so that the upper airway obstruction can be bypassed.

Four of our tracheostomized patients have undergone repeated nocturnal polygraphic recordings. In all cases, sleep became normal in duration, percentage

f stages, and cyclic organization. Central apneas lasting 6 to 15 seconds per-
sted in two patients during light sleep, but in successive recordings the apneas
radually decreased in number. During polygraphic recordings with the tracheal
toma closed, the obstructive apneas reappeared immediately and progressively
icreased in number during succeeding nights [1]. Nocturnal polygraphic record-
igs in these four tracheostomized patients included simultaneous recording of
ulmonary and systemic arterial pressures and determination of gas analysis
alues. The results are reported in parentheses in Table I. In all patients gas
nalysis values returned to normal during wakefulness and remained normal in
ll stages of sleep. Systemic arterial pressure during wakefulness was markedly
ecreased in patients who were hypertensive before surgery. During sleep, pres-
ure values decreased further, analogous to what occurs in normal subjects [8].
'ulmonary arterial pressure during wakefulness returned to normal or almost
iormal values, but during sleep a degree of hypertension sometimes persisted.

'OMMENT

Acquired micrognathia can be responsible for a clinical picture characterized
y hypersomnia and periodic apneas during sleep identical to what is observed in
ne Pickwickian syndrome [9–11], primary alveolar hypoventilation [11], and
ı patients with an anatomic obstruction of the upper airway due to laryngeal
tenosis [12] or adenoidal or tonsillar hypertrophy [13–15]. In all these syn-
romes, which we have grouped under the heading "hypersomnia with periodic
pnea" (HPA) [16], complete remission is obtained only by elimination of the
iypogenic obstruction of the upper airway (through weight loss, tonsillectomy,
denoidectomy, or tracheostomy).

Micrognathia plays an important role in the development of obstructive
pneas as do other anatomical conditions which provoke an incomplete obstruc-
ion of the upper airway. However, not all individuals who have an anatomic
ibstruction of the upper airway develop HPA. We have, therefore, hypothesized
hat HPA arises when the stenosis of the upper airway is associated with a primi-
ive hypoexcitability of the respiratory center or, more generally, of the reticular
ctivating formation [16]. A hypoexcitability of the respiratory center was
Jocumented in one of our patients and in the patient reported by Valero and
Alroy [2]; both patients experienced a diminished ventilatory response to inha-
ation of CO_2. In addition, small doses of sedative drugs administered as pre-
inesthetic medication provoked complete respiratory arrest in another of our
iatients [1] and in the patient discussed by Hishikawa et al [3].

Obstructive apneas may be caused by marked hypotonia of central origin of
he oropharyngeal muscles which would lead to obstruction of the upper airway
with a valve mechanism due to the collapse of the oropharyngeal walls. This

mechanism has been demonstrated with cineradiography in two of our patients, while in other patients [3, 6], the obstruction seems due to a falling backward of the tongue.

In our patients, as in all cases of HPA regardless of origin, heavy snoring preceded the onset of hypersomnia and periodic apneas by many years. We believe that heavy snoring represents the first step towards development of a true HPA. In fact, certain ventilatory and hemodynamic conditions found in HPA are also found in milder forms in heavy snorers [17]. Heavy snoring may be accompanied by mild hypercapnia which, over the years, may provoke a decrease, or further decrease, in the sensibility of the respiratory center to CO_2, thus favoring the appearance of apneas [1].

REFERENCES

1. Coccagna G, Di Donato G, Verucchi P, Cirignotta F, Mantovani M, Lugaresi E: Hypersomnia with periodic apneas in acquired micrognathia (a bird-like face syndrome). Arch Neurol 33:769–776, 1976.
2. Valero A, Alroy G: Hypoventilation in acquired micrognathia. Arch Intern Med 115: 307–310, 1965.
3. Hishikawa Y, Furuya E, Wakamatsu H: Hypersomnia and periodic respiration. Presentation of two cases and comment on the physiopathogenesis of the Pickwickian syndrome. Folia Psychiatr Neurol Jpn 24:163–173, 1970.
4. Tammeling GJ, Blokzijl EJ, Boonstra S, Sluiter HJ: Micrognathia, hypersomnia and periodic breathing. Bull Physiopathol Respir 8:1229–1238, 1972.
5. Imes NK, Orr WC, Smith RO, Rogers RM: Retrognathia and sleep apnea: A life-threatening condition masquerading as narcolepsy. JAMA 237:1596–1597, 1977.
6. Conway WA, Bower GC, Barnes ME: Hypersomnolence and intermittent upper airway obstruction: Occurrence caused by micrognathia. JAMA 237:2740–2742, 1977.
7. Rechtschaffen A, Kales A: "A Manual of Standardized Terminology, Techniques and Scoring System for Sleep Stages of Human Subjects." Los Angeles: BIS/BRI, UCLA, 1968.
8. Coccagna G, Mantovani M, Brignani F, Manzini A, Lugaresi E: Arterial pressure changes during spontaneous sleep in man. Electroencephalogr Clin Neurophysiol 31: 277–281, 1971.
9. Gastaut H, Tassinari CA, Duron B: Polygraphic study of the episodic diurnal and nocturnal (hypnic and respiratory) manifestations of the Pickwick syndrome. Brain Res 2:167–186, 1966.
10. Kuhlo W: Neurophysiologische und Klinische Untersuchungen beim Pickwick Syndrom. Arch Psychiatr Nervenkr 211:170–192, 1968.
11. Lugaresi E, Coccagna G, Mantovani M, Cirignotta F, Ambrosetto G, Baturic P: Hypersomnia with periodic breathing: periodic apneas and alveolar hypoventilation during sleep. Bull Physiopathol Respir 8:1103–1113, 1972.
12. Coccagna G, Mantovani M, Brignani F, Parchi C, Lugaresi E: Continuous recording of the pulmonary and systemic arterial pressure during sleep in syndromes of hypersomnia with periodic breathing. Bull Physiopathol Respir 8:1217–1227, 1972.
13. Menashe VD, Farrehi C, Miller M: Hypoventilation and cor pulmonale due to chronic upper airway obstruction. J Pediatr 67:198–203, 1965.

4. Luke MJ, Mehrizi A, Folger GM Jr, Rowe RD: Chronic nasopharyngeal obstruction as a cause of cardiomegaly, cor pulmonale and pulmonary edema. Pediatrics 37:762–768, 1968.

5. Ainger LE: Large tonsils and adenoids in small children with cor pulmonale. Br Heart J 30:356–362, 1968.

6. Lugaresi E, Coccagna G, Mantovani M, Cirignotta F: Hypersomnia with periodic apnea. In Guilleminault C, Dement WC, Passouant P: "Narcolepsy." New York: Spectrum, 1976, pp 351–366.

7. Lugaresi E, Coccagna G, Farneti, Mantovani M, Cirignotta F: Snoring. Electroencephalogr Clin Neurophysiol 39:59–64, 1975.

DISCUSSION

Dr Weil asked about the prevalence of the syndrome described by Dr Coccagna, the sex predominance seen, and whether any of these patients were also polycythemic. Dr Coccagna replied that none of the patients were polycythemic and that the sex ratio was five males to one female. No prevalence data are available at this time. One question discussed was whether the anatomic malformation plays the primary role in the appearance of this syndrome. Dr Hill mentioned that otolaryngologists have followed patients with congenital micrognathia, patients with hypolasia of the mandible secondary to radiation therapy for congenital tumors, and patients with macroglossia; heavy snoring and hypersomnia are not seen in these patients. We must assume there are other important factors in addition to the anatomical predisposition. Dr Coccagna agreed that a central factor (central control of muscles or of breathing, for example) may be necessary, and reported two patients who had had reconstruction of the mandible which ameliorated their eating and swallowing difficulties but did not lessen their apneic episodes.

Dr Phillipson commented that patients with bird-like faces develop central as well as obstructive apneas. He mentioned well-described reflexes originating in the pharynx, mediated by the superior laryngeal nerve, which when stimulated produce central (diaphragmatic) apnea and suggested that the sudden closure of the airway, the "sucking in" which occurs, may stimulate these reflexes and result in central apnea.

The genetic factor involved in chemoreceptor response was discussed. A minor mechanical defect may exert greater influence in patients whose other respiratory drives are weakened. It may be instructive to perform ventilatory tests in the family members of these patients.

18
Sleep Apnea Produced by Cervical Cordotomy and Other Neurosurgical Lesions in Man

Abbott J Krieger

Respiratory dysfunction in patients with neurological disease is usually characterized by respiratory muscle weakness and/or irregularity in the respiratory pattern. The syndrome of sleep-induced apnea in association with neurological disease is an uncommon finding but when present is usually associated with significant focal neurological signs. There is no specific treatment for this malady, and if it is not self-limited, the patient usually dies. This clinical syndrome, therefore, is quite different from that which has been described in patients with primary sleep disorders who have no major neurological disease. Like so many other relatively obscure diseases, the syndrome of neurosurgical diseases with sleep-induced apnea has been treated by a relatively few practitioners in the clinical neurosciences because it has rarely been recognized. This report will describe our experiences with this entity as well as related disorders in a descriptive and anecdotal fashion. The clinical disorders to be discussed include sleep-induced apnea after cervical cordotomy and after anterior cervical spine surgery and respiratory insufficiency associated with craniovertebral and hindbrain anomalies. Some experimental observations will also be described.

SLEEP-INDUCED APNEA AFTER CERVICAL CORDOTOMY

Sleep-induced apnea has been observed in 11 patients after bilateral percutaneous cervical cordotomy. A study of the effects of percutaneous cervical cordotomy on respiratory function confirmed previous reports that cordotomy alters respiration, as well as other autonomic functions [1]. Belmusto et al [2] supplied documentation of an intraoperative reduction of tidal volume immediately following section of the ventral quadrant, the majority under general anesthesia. However, two patients operated on under local anesthesia did not

Sleep Apnea Syndromes, pages 273–294

show any respiratory alteration. One of their patients returned two weeks later with cyanosis and a respiratory rate of 2 per minute, precipitated by a single normal dose of a barbiturate. When she recovered from this acute disturbance, her respiratory efforts were ineffective and she required assistance during periods of natural sleep, thus highlighting the problem of sleep-induced apnea. Later in the same year, Nathan [3] made a series of intraoperative bronchospirometric recordings that demonstrated a reduction in tidal volume of the ipsilateral lung, which became profound within two hours after cordotomy. The chest became immobile in the inspiratory position. Movement was restored within a week, but delayed in onset and reduced in range.

The results of our study on percutaneous cordotomy indicate that cervical cordotomy can cause respiratory functional impairment of varying severity depending on the extent of the spinal cord lesions. In the majority of cases there were no symptoms and the condition was clinically occult, the functional impairment being evident only on testing. The dysfunction was greater after a bilateral cordotomy than a unilateral procedure and greater when high levels of analgesia were obtained. It appeared that two distinct but related physiological functions could be affected, namely the respiratory motor function and the control of ventilation. Either or both could be impaired by cordotomy. The respiratory motor function was assessed by the vital capacity, maximum breathing capacity and maximum thoracic pressure. The ventilatory control mechanisms appeared to be affected selectively and independently. There was a reduction of tidal volume on breathing air and CO_2 and an increase in the respiratory rate under these two test conditions. These observations were further amplified in a series reporting the findings in ten patients with sleep-induced apnea [4] as well as another report in which one additional patient was described in greater detail [5].

The characteristic course of this syndrome usually begins with the subjective sensation of asthenia, associated with sighing respirations. At this time objective clinical evidence of functional impairment was not always demonstrable, so the uninitiated might disregard the symptoms by ascribing them to an anxiety reaction. The patient usually went on to hypoventilate and characteristically became apneic when asleep. If the patient was awakened, so called "normal breathing" resumed, but hypoventilation often persisted and the apnea remained a constant danger with the resumption of sleep. If the syndrome was not transient, intubation and control of respiration became necessary. The condition was usually reversible but respiration had to be supported through this period of time. In surviving patients the syndrome lasted from three days to several weeks. All patients complained of vague feelings of lethargy, generalized weakness, and were somewhat confused. Clinically, all these patients experiencing pulmonary dysfunction appeared the same; however, on detailed study of their pulmonary function, two distinct patterns became evident: The first type is manifested by a normal vital capacity and an attenuated CO_2 response; the second type is manifested by a decreased vital capacity and an attenuated CO_2 response.

An example of the first type is a 42-year-old man who had a number of percutaneous cordotomies for intractable back pain. On admission, pulmonary function studies showed a marked reduction in the vital capacity and a normal CO_2 response (Fig 1). The reduced vital capacity probably was related to the presence of pain during the testing procedure. After the cordotomy the pain was relieved, the vital capacity improved. The CO_2 response was unaffected in the immediate postoperative period, but when tested again three months later was found to be somewhat decreased. Pain recurred and a repeat cordotomy was performed with transient relief of his pain. The vital capacity remained unaffected but the CO_2 response decreased further. Another cordotomy six days later was followed by adequate pain relief. This time while on the operating table, he complained of the feeling that he had a heavy weight on his chest. Later that afternoon he was lethargic and confused. That evening, his pain re-

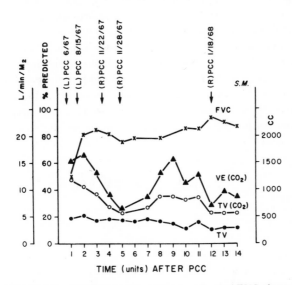

Fig 1. Results of pulmonary function tests showing an unchanged FVC after several cordotomies despite fall of the VE (CO_2). L/min/m$_2$, liters per minute per square meter of body surface area; VE (CO_2), minute ventilation breathing 5% carbon dioxide; FVC, forced vital capacity as a percentage of predicted; TV, tidal volume in ml; TV (CO_2), tidal volume breathing 5% carbon dioxide. Percutaneous cervical cordotomy (PCC) procedures are indicated by arrows. The abscissa is calibrated in arbitrary time units indicating the interval between pulmonary function tests. Reprinted from J Neurosurg 40:168–180, 1974, by permission of the publisher.

turned. On sensory testing, analgesia was spotty and his breathing was less labored. At this time pulmonary function studies showed an unaffected vital capacity and a marked decrease in his ventilatory response to inhaled CO_2. Repeated pulmonary function studies indicated a gradual return of the CO_2 response towards normal with a consistently unaffected vital capacity. Still another cordotomy was performed six weeks later because of recurrence of pain; once again this was effective. Following the procedure he again became lethargic and dyspneic. This continued into the evening, and he was placed in the intensive care unit for closer observation. During the night his breathing was uneven and irregular (Fig 2) and several times he became totally apneic. On each apneic occasion he was awakened and adequate respiration resumed. The next day his original pain recurred; with its return his breathing and state of consciousness improved. Pulmonary function studies performed the afternoon after the cordotomy and preceding the sleep-induced apnea showed another marked decrease in the CO_2 response and a normal vital capacity.

An example of a patient in whom both the vital capacity and CO_2 response diminished after cordotomy is that of a 48-year-old woman with a long standing rheumatoid arthritis with intractable joint pain. Pulmonary function studies prior to cordotomy were essentially normal (Fig 3). With each stage of the bilateral cordotomy she sustained a marked reduction of both vital capacity and CO_2 response. Following the second cordotomy she had a transient period of hypotension and that night she was found to be apneic while asleep. After a short period of assisted ventilation she recovered. No further episodes of respiratory arrest occurred. Follow-up pulmonary function studies during the next nine months revealed a gradual recovery of the vital capacity to near precordotomy levels with persistently impaired CO_2 response; however, during the recovery phase starting with test 3 a dissociation between the vital capacity and the

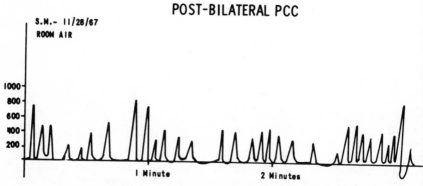

POST-BILATERAL PCC

S.M.- 11/28/67
ROOM AIR

Fig 2. Postcordotomy respiration pattern showing irregularity in rate and depth of breathing. Reprinted from J Neurosurg 40:168–180, 1974, by permission of the publishers.

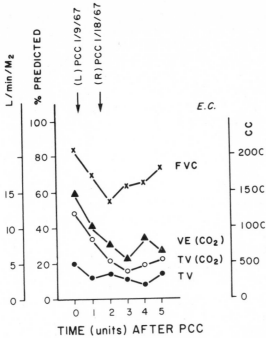

Fig 3. Pulmonary function studies showing a parallel fall in FVC and VE (CO_2) after each cordotomy. However, during the recovery starting with test 3, dissociation between these two functions becomes apparent. Abbreviations as in Figure 1. Reprinted from J Neurosurg 40:168–180, 1974, by permission of the publishers.

ventilatory response to CO_2 is apparent, indicating these mechanisms are carried in different pathways.

Another example of this syndrome is that of a 44-year-old woman who had a bilateral cervical cordotomy for intractable hip pain after complications of surgery for osteoarthritis. This patient had 23 episodes of respiratory arrest during a four-month period until her death. The length between these respiratory arrests varied from 1 to 5 days; the longest interim was 17 days. At the beginning of a typical cycle, the patient was mentally and physically alert with vital signs within normal limits. She gradually became listless, confused, and hostile. She slept poorly during the night and had short sleep periods during the day. Her cardiac pattern alternated between tachycardia (140–160) and bradycardia (60–80); blood pressure varied widely (60–200 systolic); respiration became increasingly irregular in rate and depth. She then began to fall asleep for 10- to 30-second periods, during which she assumed an increasingly blank expression with her mouth falling open and her eyes closed; her hands, forearm, and legs would twitch slightly and then her musculature relaxed visibly. At the end of such a sleep interval, she would jerk herself awake and become alert for a moment or two, but soon lapsed back into an unconscious state. As these episodes became more frequent, her mental status deteriorated and she began to hallucinate about her husband coming to the hospital room and demanding that she come home with him. Usually quite soon after the husband hallucinations began, her blood pressure fell to hypotensive levels (90–100 systolic) and she became increasingly difficult to arouse even with painful stimuli. Then her breathing would stop initially with her chest in an inspiratory position. This apneustic state lasted for about one to two minutes before she could be placed on a Byrd respirator (which was then the common type of assisted ventilatory machine used) because her intrapulmonary pressure was so high that no air could be exchanged. During the initial episodes of respiratory arrest, her tracheostomy tube was changed several times because of the difficulty in initiating supportive ventilation — which was attributed erroneously to a blocked tube On a number of occasions she had a cardiac arrest coincident with the respiratory arrest. They were all very brief and required short periods of external cardiac massage. During the time she was unconscious she could be aroused for short periods of time after which she lapsed back into an unconscious state. She remained this way for as long as 12 hours, and upon awakening was at the beginning of the cycle again. She could not be resuscitated from the last episode and died. Her respiratory pattern most of the time was a cluster-type breathing at rest which was worsened with the inhalation of 100% O_2 (Fig 4).

One last observation in this interesting syndrome is that the patients themselves know intuitively when they can be extubated and function normally again. This woman was intubated 14 days when she wrote this note: "I'm really fine. Much better. Why why don't they take it all out. I bet I'll do fine." And she did (Fig 5).

SLEEP-INDUCED APNEA AFTER ANTERIOR CERVICAL SPINE SURGERY [6]

Four patients who developed respiratory failure after anterior spine surgery had many similarities in their clinical course. Three had surgery at the C3-4 interspace and the fourth had surgery at the C4-5 interspace. All had high sensory levels of analgesia postoperatively. Two had distal upper limb weakness. All had periods of confusion postoperatively. All had overt respiratory dysfunction at night. The two patients in whom this condition was unrecognized died. Death occurred in one patient during sleep, and in the other death occurred during tracheostomy. Both surviving patients had impaired respiratory function immediately after surgery. Both patients became apneic during sleep and both required assisted ventilation at night for several days.

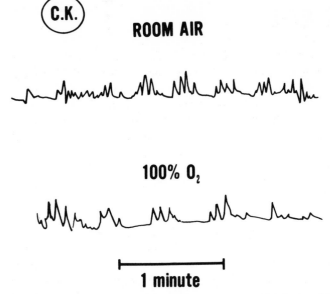

ROOM AIR

100% O$_2$

1 minute

ig 4. Note cluster-type breathing pattern in upper trace. During 100% O$_2$ breathing respira-
ory rate decreased with increased irregularity. Reprinted from Crit Care Med 2:91–95,
974, by permission of The Williams & Wilkins Co, Baltimore, copyrighters.

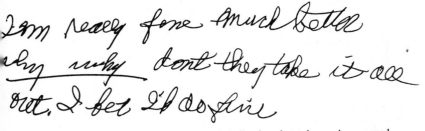

Fig 5. Intubated sleep-induced apneic patient's indication that tube can be removed.

In one patient, DH, the tidal volume in the recovery room postoperatively
varied between 100 and 150 ml and he, therefore, was maintained on a ventila-
or for several hours at which time his tidal volume was 500 ml with a respira-
ory rate of 20 breaths per minute resulting in a minute ventilation of 10 liters
per minute. Pulmonary function studies were performed daily. The studies performed included his ventilatory response to 5% CO$_2$ and vital capacity. The improvement in his vital capacity and minute ventilation breathing CO$_2$ are shown
in Figure 6. On the sixth postoperative day his minute ventilation breathing

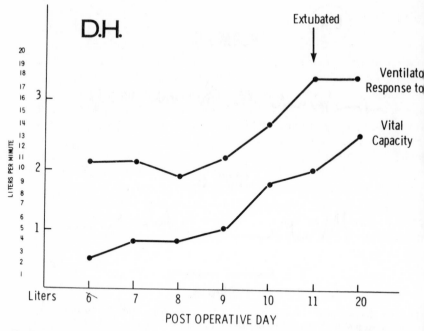

Fig 6. Pulmonary function was measured daily from the 6th to the 11th postoperative day. On the ordinate the small-number scale refers to minute ventilation breathing CO_2 and the large numbers refer to vital capacity. Breathing was normal by the 20th postoperative day. Reprinted from J Surg Res 14:512–517, 1973, by permission of the publishers.

room air was 10.6 liters, which was not changed by 5% CO_2 inhalation. His pCO_2 went from 46 torr breathing room air to 55 torr breathing 5% CO_2. His vital capacity was 800 ml. By the 11th postoperative day his ventilation breathing 5% CO_2 increased to 18 liters per minute and his pCO_2 went from 39 to 42 torr and his vital capacity was 1,800 ml. He was extubated and did quite well. On the 20th postoperative day, his respiratory rate was 16, tidal volume 560 ml, minute ventilation 8.9 liters per minute, pH 7.45, pCO_2 44, and pO_2 79.

RESPIRATORY ABNORMALITIES IN PATIENTS WITH CRANIOVERTEBRA AND HINDBRAIN ANOMALIES

Respiration in patients with the Arnold-Chiari malformation [7], the Dandy-Walker syndrome [8], and Reye syndrome [9] illustrate aspects of respiratory abnormalities that may be relevant to the syndrome under discussion. Respiration was measured in 15 patients with myelomeningocele and hydrocephalus in which shunts were performed for the control of hydrocephalus. This study was

dertaken because a small percentage of infants with the Arnold-Chiari mal-
rmation developed respiratory dysfunction which is most dramatically accom-
nied by laryngeal stridor. The stridor often appears precipitously and is
sely correlated with increased intracranial pressure. In most cases the stridor
relieved by shunt revision since this reduces the increased intracranial pressure.
espiration was measured in one patient who developed laryngeal stridor asso-
ated with this syndrome. This occurred at the age of 2 months at which time
tracheostomy was performed. At the age 4–5 months breathing was tested and
corded every day for three weeks. The respiratory pattern was characterized
irregularity of tidal volume and rate with interspersed short periods of apnea
ig 7). The ventilatory response to CO_2 remained normal. During this period of
servation the ventriculoperitoneal shunt became obstructed. At the time of
e surgical revision the ventricular pressure was elevated to 300 mm of water.
espite shunt revision with relief of increased pressure no change in breathing
ttern occurred. Other patients tested have had a decreased ventilatory response
CO$_2$ with regular respiratory patterns.

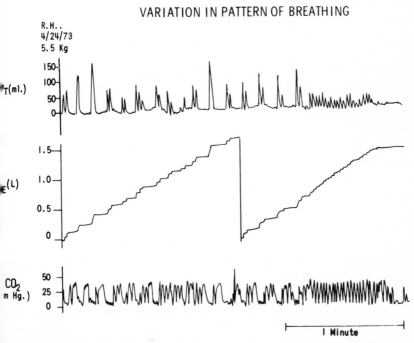

VARIATION IN PATTERN OF BREATHING

ig 7. Note irregular breathing pattern on the top line. The second trace is that of minute
entilation. The bottom trace is end tidal CO_2. Reprinted from Laryngoscope 86:718–
23, 1976, by permission of the publishers.

Respiration was measured in one patient with a Dandy-Walker syndrome. Th[Dandy-Walker syndrome is characterized by hydrocephalus associated with a cystic fourth ventricle and hypoplasia and agenesis of the cerebellar vermis. Th[patient's respiration was examined 12 times between age 8 hours and 26 days. The pattern of respiration was normal when the infant was breathing 100% O_2 before a shunting operation was performed (Fig 8). One day following surgery, there was prolonged inspiratory spasms (apneustic-like breathing) when 100% O_2 was inspired. This pattern of respiration continued for three days when the pattern changed to a cluster type breathing with recurring apneic periods of variable duration. By the 24th postoperative day breathing had become and remained normal.

The respiratory function of a 6½ year-old child with Reye syndrome was studied. The clinical course of this patient's illness was a complicated one. Importantly, for purposes of the present presentation, there were abnormal physical features signifying involvement of the medulla oblongata: loss of function

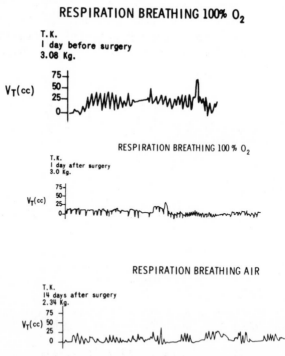

Fig 8. Patterns of respiration one day prior to surgery (top trace), apneustic breathing one day after surgery, cluster breathing 14 days after surgery. Reprinted from Neurology 24: 1064–1067, 1974, by permission of The New York Times Media Company, Inc, copyrighters.

f the seventh through the twelfth cranial nerves bilaterally, tetraparesis, recur-
ng convulsive disorders, and prolonged periods of apnea necessitating mechani-
al ventilatory support. Artificial ventilation was necessary for approximately
ix weeks. For an additional three weeks, there was decreased ventilatory
esponse to CO_2 inhalation and irregularly recurring periods of sleep-induced
pnea. The use of a rocker bed decreased the frequency of these spells; however,
hallow respirations during sleep persisted for ten weeks before relatively normal
espiration was established. Of particular interest is the demonstration of the
oluntary and automatic patterns of respiration as the comparison of her spon-
aneous breathing pattern to the breathing patterns with maternal coaching
lustrates (Fig 9).

None of the various respiratory abnormalities encountered was specific for a
articular type of pathophysiological process that results in alteration in breath-
ng. In the instance of hydrocephalus with associated Arnold-Chiari syndrome, it
ppeared that laryngeal stridor may be precipitated by increased intracranial
ressure, since it is often favorably influenced by reducing the pressure with a
urgical shunt. This implies partial physiological interruption of vagal function.
A similar mechanism might explain the changing respiratory pattern in the
atient with the Dandy-Walker syndrome, influenced in part by movement of
he brain stem resulting from the decreased ventricular size produced by the
hunting procedure.

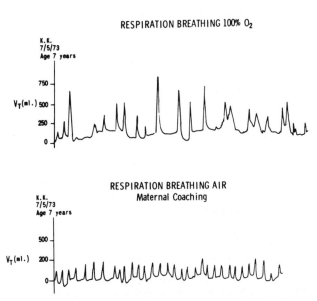

Fig 9. Top trace) spontaneous respirations; bottom trace) respiration with maternal coaching. Note voluntary mechanism of driving respiration to a relatively normal pattern.

A 45-year-old man was admitted for treatment of syringomyelia [10]. The patient underwent a posterior fossa exploration. At surgery the spinal cord was widened, the cerebellar tonsils were located beneath the arch of the first cervical vertebra indicative of an Arnold-Chiari malformation, as well as syringomyelia. The central canal was packed with muscle and a Silastic tube was placed in the fourth ventricle and brought down to the cervical subarachnoid space to promote drainage from the ventricular system. This resulted in the spontaneous emptying of the central canal with a narrowing of the cervical spinal cord. Several hours postoperatively, he was noted to have decreased minute ventilation, and reintubation and ventilation was assisted for the first postoperative night. During the ensuing week it was noted that although his blood gases returned to normal his ventilation decreased at night requiring assisted ventilation until the fifth postoperative day when he was extubated; however, on the seventh postoperative day the patient became psychotic, manifested by hallucinations and delusions. Because of this continued sleep-induced apnea a tracheostomy was performed and his ventilation was assisted at night for approximately three weeks. The patient was then started on an active program of rehabilitation and was discharged from the hospital.

REGULATION OF RESPIRATION

A brief discussion of mechanisms responsible for regulation of respiration may be helpful in understanding the respiratory derangements observed clinically. As early as 1923, Lumsden [11] showed that serial transections of the brain stem do not produce marked changes in respiration as long as transections are rostral to the level of pons. Later, Pitts et al [12] reported that the portion of CNS caudal to inferior colliculi is of paramount importance for the regulation of respiration. Within the pons and medulla, three centers have been defined as primary sites of respiratory control. These three centers are the pontile pneumotaxic and apneustic centers and the medullary respiratory centers. The apneustic center drives the medullary inspiratory center and eupenic respiration results by intermittent inhibition of the apneustic center by the vagi and the pneumotaxic center [13]. Transection at the midpontine level [14] or discrete bilateral destruction of the pontile pneumotaxic centers [15] produces a diminution of respiratory rate and concomitant increase in tidal volume. If the vagi are cut bilaterally in either of these acute preparations, a respiratory pattern characterized by prolonged inspiratory phases is produced. This pattern of respiration is termed apneusis.

Another afferent feedback mechanism was suggested by Krieger et al [16] on the basis of their experiments on cats. A variety of slow respiratory patterns were observed in cats with ventrolateral cervical cord lesions when an additional idpontine transection or a bilateral vagotomy was performed. In many cases, pattern of breathing was produced that was similar to apneusis (Fig 10).

The integrated phrenic nerve activity was compared after ablation of the arious feedback mechanisms. The normal envelope of the phrenic discharge as altered by each ablation procedure as shown in Figure 11. After vagotomy aere was a slight increase in slope of the rising phase, while after midpontine ansection in ventrolateral cervical cord lesions there was a decrease. The disharge tended to plateau in all of them at an approximately steady level until returned to the baseline. The shape of the phrenic discharge after these selective ablations showed an inspiratory shift of phase of respiration. This finding as expected since apneusis, the most marked inspiratory shift, results from the ombination of any two of these ablations. These observations indicated that an nportant afferent pathway is present in the ventrolateral cervical cord which eriodically inhibits the apneustic center and affects the inspiratory neuronal nd phrenic discharge.

Although the brain stem centers caudal to the level of the inferior colliculi re vital for the maintenance of a normal pattern of respiration, there are other reas of brain which participate in regulation of respiration. Portions of cerebral ortex, the basal ganglia, the limbic system including hypothalamus, and the erebellum are known to influence respiration. Suprapontine structures may ontain important compensating mechanisms for some deficits in the pontobul-

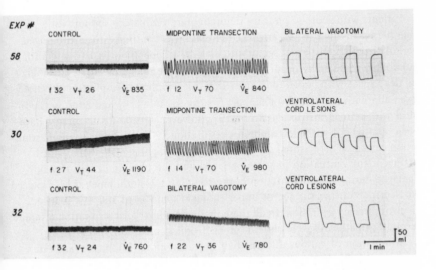

Fig 10. Apneustic breathing produced by various combinations of ventrolateral cord lesions and either midpontine transection or bilateral vagotomy. Reprinted from J Appl Physiol 33:431–435, 1972, by permission of the publishers.

PHRENIC NERVE ACTIVITY AFTER SELECTIVE LESIONS

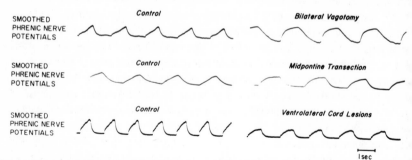

Fig 11. Integrated phrenic activity after selective ablation of feedback mechanisms. Note the changes in slope of the rising phase after each selective ablation and the increased duration of the plateau which indicates lengthened inspiratory phase.

bar respiratory mechanisms. Indeed, St. John et al [17] have shown that unanesthetized cats with chronic pneumotaxic center lesions can maintain a normal pattern of respiration. Under anesthesia, bilateral vagotomy produced apneusis in these animals.

Use of Stimulators for Ventilation

Patients with acute respiratory failure require ventilatory support for a variable period of time. When artificial ventilation is continued for a prolonged period of time retention of secretions, atelectasis, pneumonitis, and interstitial pulmonary edema may occur. These changes result in an increase in physiological dead space with impaired oxygenation. Electrophrenic respiration was used as an alternative to respirator support first by Sarnoff [18] and later by Glenn et al with refined instrumentation [19]; however, several disadvantages have been pointed out with electrophrenic respiration [20]. Unilateral phrenic stimulation can cause mediastinal shift, movement of diaphragm alone may not be sufficient for ventilation in some patients, and the phrenic nerves may be damaged during the implantation of the stimulator. Osterholm et al [21] placed an electrode on the surface of upper thoracic spinal cord and this induced electrothoracic respiration. In all these methods of artificial respiration efferent respiratory pathways were chosen for electronic stimulation.

Stimulation of various afferent pathways can either inhibit or facilitate respiration [22]. For example, stimulation of midthoracic intercostal nerves can inhibit respiration [23]. The afferent pathway in the ventrolateral spinal cord demonstrated by Krieger et al [16] may arise from the upper thoracic wall. It is an intriguing question as to whether stimulation of selected afferent pathways in correct or ameliorate some respiratory derangements observed clinically. For example, in some patients an apneustic pattern of breathing has been observed 5, 8]. As pointed out earlier apneusis is characterized by prolonged inspirations. Since the presence of an inhibitory pathway has been demonstrated in the entrolateral cervical spinal cord [16], which arises from the upper thoracic wall [23], it is logical to expect that stimulation of upper intercostal nerves would interrupt the prolonged inspiration during apneusis. On the basis of this assumption, we carried out the following experiments. Cats of either sex, weighing 3—4 g, were decerebrated at midcollicular level. The cats were immobilized with flaxedil and artificially ventilated. Phrenic nerve activity was recorded before and after production of apneusis (Fig 12). The latter was induced by ablation of pneumotaxic center and vagi bilaterally. The external intercostal nerves at T5 and T6 were exposed and stimulated (5 V, 50 Hz); this stimulation interrupted the prolonged inspiration (Fig 12). Similar observations have been made by Remmers [24]. In another series of experiments, the sciatic nerve was stimulated (5—6 V, 50 Hz) in order to interrupt the apneusis (Fig 12).

Obstructive upper airway apnea has been observed in some patients during sleep [25, 26]. In this disorder, persistent diaphragmatic movement fails to achieve ventilation because of a functional obstruction in the upper airway. It is well known that the activity in the recurrent laryngeal nerve either opens or

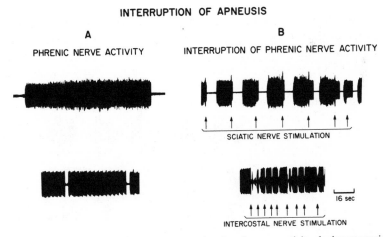

INTERRUPTION OF APNEUSIS

A
PHRENIC NERVE ACTIVITY

B
INTERRUPTION OF PHRENIC NERVE ACTIVITY

SCIATIC NERVE STIMULATION

16 sec

INTERCOSTAL NERVE STIMULATION

Fig 12. Effect of afferent nerve stimulation on the phrenic nerve activity during apneusis. Top trace: A) Prolonged burst of phrenic nerve activity during apneusis; B) The apneustic burst was interrupted by stimulation of afferent fibers in the sciatic nerve (5 V, 50 Hz). Bottom trace: A) Phrenic nerve activity during apneusis in another cat; B) Interruption of the phrenic nerve activity was produced by stimulation of afferent fibers in the fifth external intercostal nerve (5 V, 50 Hz).

closes the larynx through contraction of corresponding musculature. The role of recurrent laryngeal nerve in the respiratory mechanisms has not been investigated as extensively as other components of respiratory regulatory mechanisms. That intrinsic laryngeal muscles play a role in respiration is widely accepted but there is disagreement concerning mechanisms which regulate the flow of air through the larynx. It has been consistently reported that the abductor muscle, posterior cricoarytenoid, exhibits bursts of activity in phase with eupenic inspiration [27]; however, the role of adductors, thyroarytenoid, and lateral cricoarytenoid muscles, remains controversial [28]. Reports of an absence or paucity of cyclic respiratory activity of laryngeal adductors in eupnea may be in part due to use of barbiturate anesthetics [29]. In our preliminary experiments, we recorded activity from the recurrent laryngeal nerves in decerebrate cats. The latter were immobilized with Flaxedil and artificially ventilated. Activity of the recurrent laryngeal nerve was correlated with the phrenic nerve activity. This model has the following advantages: 1) Use of anesthetics is eliminated, 2) the afferent activity which may be present in recurrent laryngeal nerve [28] can be distinguished from the efferent inspiratory activity which is expected to be in phase with phrenic nerve firing, and 3) activity in phase with the expiratory center, if present, can be observed between phrenic nerve bursts. Figure 13 shows a typical recording from a whole recurrent laryngeal nerve. There is a burst of activity in phase with phrenic nerve firing which has been shown to be associated with abduction of posterior cricoarytenoid muscle. A burst of activity which appears as a mirror image of phrenic nerve burst appears as soon as phrenic nerve stops firing. This recording suggests adduction of laryngeal muscles is not a passive motion but is actively regulated by expiratory centers in the medulla. A similar suggestion has been made by Kurozumi [30].

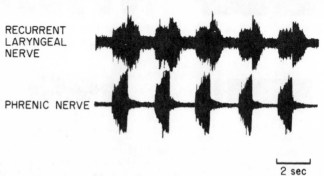

RECURRENT
LARYNGEAL
NERVE

PHRENIC NERVE

2 sec

Fig 13. Correlation of recurrent laryngeal and phrenic nerve activity. Top trace: recurrent laryngeal nerve activity; bottom trace) phrenic nerve activity. Initially both nerves fire simultaneously; however, there is a burst of activity in the recurrent laryngeal nerve during the expiratory phase when the phrenic nerve is silent.

roper functioning of the intrinsic laryngeal muscles, especially the timing of
their abduction and adduction in relation to phrenic nerve activity, may be of
importance in preventing an upper airway obstruction. The changes in the
activity of laryngeal nerve and the muscles it innervates under various conditions
of respiratory disorders need further investigation.

Clinical Pulmonary Function Testing

In some systemic conditions there is a poor correlation between the degree of
mechanical defects in respiration and the levels of dyspnea, hypercapnia, and
hypoxia. Defects in the central respiratory control mechanism may predispose
some patients to respiratory dysfunction during stressful situations. This can be
clearly seen in two clinical manifestations of emphysema, ie, the "pink puffer"
and the "blue bloater" [31], as well as between obese subjects who have normal
blood gases and breathing pattern and those who display signs of dyspnea,
hypercapnea, hypoxia, and an irregular breathing pattern [32–34].

The "blue bloater" is a patient with relatively minor obstruction to ventilation who is cyanotic and is liable to worsen with infection. The "pink puffer,"
on the other hand, despite a great deal of disease manages to maintain ventilation near normal levels. The obesity hypoventilation syndrome is likewise
blurred, as the majority of obese people have no respiratory problems although
pulmonary functions may show substantial restriction, obstruction, and perfusion abnormalities, while other patients with similar clinical presentations
show alveolar hypoventilation and irregular breathing patterns which are accentuated during sleep. It remains to be clarified whether these contrasting clinical
pictures are due to abnormalities in the central respiratory control mechanism,
altered central chemosensitivity, or mechanical changes which distort the
afferent-efferent information affecting the central respiratory control mechanism. The following procedures have been used to assess alterations in chemosensitivity and mechanics of respiration in these patients. Upper airway obstruction in obese patients was simulated by the use of threshold loads during wakefulness. We chose threshold loads because we felt that upper airway obstruction
was best modeled by a fixed inspiratory pressure or opening pressure. This
method of altering the work of breathing may be an important challenge to the
respiratory center perhaps on both the afferent and efferent level. The characteristics of this load are illustrated in Figure 14. As can be seen airflow is
absent until the threshold pressure is exceeded at which point tidal exchange
proceeds. Threshold pressure was produced by counterweighting a 120-liter
tissot spirometer with 10, 20, and 30 pounds. This produced threshold loads
of -3.5, -7.0, and -10.0 cm H_2O (Fig 15). Inspiring a liter of gas from the
drum required raising a weight of known amount; thus a fixed amount of additional work is imposed on the subject per liter of gas independent of frequency

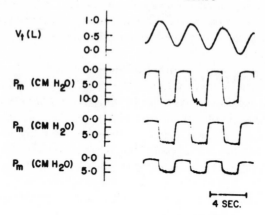

CHARACTERISTICS OF THRESHOLD

LOADS

14

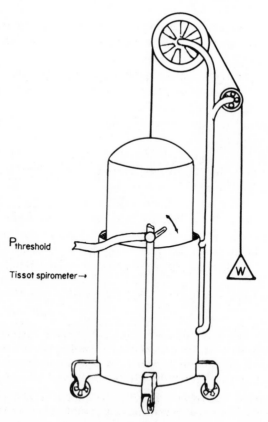

15

Respiratory Load

r tidal volume (Fig 16). When this loading technique was imposed on the
espiration of an obese somnolent patient during wakefulness the breathing pat-
ern became more irregular than it was in the control period. This observation
vas closely correlated with the degree of loading. Normals tested with this load
nd even greater loads show no irregularities in breathing, although the fre-
uency of respiration decreased.

Threshold-loaded CO_2 responses were performed in patients with and without brain stem pathology in order to determine if a correlation exists between
espiratory function and the aforementioned neurological impairment. Responses
neasured consisted of unloaded responses and responses with three graded
hreshold loads during CO_2 rebreathing. In normals, loaded ventilatory responses
o CO_2 were found to be incrementally reduced. In patients with brain stem
pathology further reduction in the loaded CO_2 response was noted.

CONCLUSION

From the foregoing discussion, it is evident that the mechanisms of respira-
ory derangements observed clinically are far from clear. In this paper a variety

EFFECT OF THRESHOLD LOADS

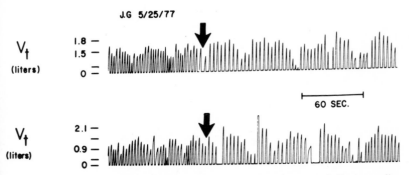

Fig 16. Note increased irregularity with increased threshold loads. Arrow indicates application of load; top trace: −7 cm water; bottom trace: −10 cm of water.

Fig 14. Tidal volume V_t and mouth pressure P_m with the application of three inspiratory
threshold loads are known. Inspiration is in a downward direction. Mouth pressures of −10
cm H_2O, −7 cm H_2O, and −3.5 cm H_2O are illustrated. Note that the onset of inspiration
occurs when the preset threshold pressure is obtained.

Fig 15. A tissot spirometer counterweighted with a weight (W) produces a fixed pressure
threshold load. The threshold pressure is proportional to the weight (W). Inspiring a liter of
gas from the drum raises the weight a known distance resulting in a fixed quantum of work.

of respiratory disorders and possible mechanisms involved in the genesis and/or exacerbation of some of these malfunctions has been described. In addition to the known feedback mechanisms that influence respiration, namely the pneumo taxic center and the vagi, a third afferent pathway in the ventrolateral cervical spinal cord may play an important role in the regulation of respiration. Damage to this pathway may be partially responsible for respiratory distress observed in some patients, particularly after cordotomy. A deficit in one or more components of the respiratory regulatory mechanisms may be compensated for by suprapontine structures of the central nervous system. Indeed, St. John et al [17] have shown that cats with pneumotaxic center lesions can maintain a normal pattern of respiration. In these animals apneusis developed only under anesthesia and bilateral vagotomy.

At the present time, positive pressure ventilation remains the safe and effective means in the management of patients with respiratory disorders. Electrophrenic and electrothoracic respiration has also been attempted. In these studies stimulation of efferent pathways has been used to ventilate patients. The present paper discusses the possibility of stimulating some afferent pathways to revert some abnormal patterns of respiration to a normal breathing pattern. Preliminary experiments in our laboratories have shown that apneustic pattern of breathing in cats can be interrupted by stimulation of upper external intercostal nerves. Detailed investigations in this direction may offer a novel approach for ameliorating at least some respiratory disorders.

ACKNOWLEDGMENTS

This research was supported by the General Medical Research Service of the Veterans Administration.

REFERENCES

1. Rosomoff HL, Krieger AJ, Kuperman AS: Effects of percutaneous cervical cordotomy on pulmonary function. J Neurosurg 31:620–627, 1969.
2. Belmusto L, Woldring S, Owens G: Localization and patterns of potentials of the respiratory pathway in the cervical spinal cord in the dog. J Neurosurg 22:277–283, 1965.
3. Nathan PW: The descending respiratory pathway in man. J Neurol Neurosurg Psychiatry 26:487–499, 1963.
4. Krieger AJ, Rosomoff HL: Sleep-induced apnea, part 1: A respiratory and autonomic dysfunction syndrome following bilateral percutaneous cervical cordotomy. J Neurosurg 40:168–180, 1974.
5. Krieger AJ, Standish MS, Rosomoff HL: Respiratory and autonomic dysfunction following percutaneous cervical cordotomy. Crit Care Med 2:91–95, 1974.

6. Krieger AJ, Rosomoff HL: Sleep-induced apnea, part 2: Respiratory failure after anterior spinal surgery. J Neurosurg 40:181–185, 1974.
7. Krieger AJ, Detwiler JS, Trooskin SZ: Respiratory function in infants with Arnold-Chiari malformation. Laryngoscope 86:718–723, 1976.
8. Krieger AJ, Detwiler JS, Trooskin SZ: Respiration in an infant with the Dandy-Walker syndrome. Neurology 24:1064–1067, 1974.
9. Krieger AJ, Trooskin SZ, Detwiler JS: Reye's syndrome with respiratory failure. Postgrad Med 59:239–243, 1976.
10. Krieger AJ: Respiratory failure as a surgical risk in patients with hindbrain anomalies. Heart Lung 2:546–551, 1973.
11. Lumsden T: Observations on the respiratory centers in cats. J Physiol 57:153–160, 1923.
12. Pitts RF, Majoun HW, Ranson SW: The origin of respiratory rhythmicity. Am J Physiol 127:654–670, 1939.
13. Wang SC, Ngai SH: General organization of central respiratory mechanisms. In "Handbook of Physiology." Washington, DC: American Physiology Society, 1965, pp 487–505.
14. Ngai SH, Wang SC: Organization of central respiratory mechanisms in the brain stem of the cat: Localization by stimulation and destruction. Am J Physiol 190:343–349, 1957.
15. Glasser RL: Vagal inhibition of cardiovascular activity in the decerebrate cat. Am J Physiol 203:449–452, 1962.
16. Krieger AJ, Christensen HD, Sapru HN, Wang SC: Changes in ventilatory patterns after ablation of various feedback mechanisms. J Appl Physiol 33:431–435, 1972.
17. St. John WM, Glasser RL, King RA: Rhythmic respiration in awake vagotomized cats with chronic pneumotaxic area lesions. Respir Physiol 15:233–244, 1972.
18. Sarnoff SJ, Hardenbergh E, Whittenberger JL: Electrophrenic respiration. Am J Physiol 155:1–9, 1948.
19. Glenn WWL, Hageman JH, Mauro A, Eisenberg L, Flanigan S, Harvard M: Electrical stimulation of excitable tissue by radiofrequency transmission. Ann Surg 160:338–350, 1964.
20. Bergofsky EH: Mechanism for respiratory insufficiency after cervical cord injury. Ann Intern Med 61:435–447, 1964.
21. Osterholm JL, Lemmon WM, Hooker TB, Pyneson J: Electrorespiration by stimulation of thoracic spinal cord. Surg Forum 17:421–423, 1966.
22. Kao FF: An experimental study of the pathways involved in exercise hyperpnoea employing cross-circulation techniques. In Cunningham DJC, Lloyd BB (eds): "The Regulation of Human Respiration." Oxford: Blackwell, 1963, pp 461–502.
23. Remmers JE: Inhibition of inspiratory activity by intercostal muscle afferents. Respir Physiol 10:358–383, 1970.
24. Remmers JE, Marttila I: Action of intercostal muscle afferents on the respiratory rhythm of anesthetized cats. Respir Physiol 24:31–41, 1975.
25. Gastaut H, Tassinari C, Duron B: Etude polygraphique des manifestations episodiques (hypniques et respiratoires) diurnes et nocturnes du syndrome de Pickwick. Rev Neurol 112:573–579, 1965.
26. Guilleminault C, Tilkian A, Dement WC: The sleep apnea syndromes. Annu Rev Med 27:465–484, 1976.
27. Sherrey JH, Megirian D: Spontaneous and reflexly evoked laryngeal abductor and adductor muscle activity of cat. Exp Neurol 43:487–498, 1974.
28. Murakami Y, Kirchner JA: Respiratory movements of the vocal cords. An electromyographic study in the cat. Laryngoscope 82:454–467, 1972.

29. Sherrey JH, Megirian D: Analysis of the respiratory role of intrinsic laryngeal motoneurons of cat. Exp Neurol 49:456–465, 1975.

30. Kurozumi S, Tashiro T, Harada Y: Laryngeal responses to electrical stimulation of the medullary respiratory centers in the dog. Laryngoscope 81:1960–1967, 1971.

31. Howell JBL: Effects and associations of disturbed airways resistance and ventilatory control. In Pengelly LD, Rebuck AS, Campbell EJM (eds): "Loaded Breathing." Edinburgh: Churchill Livingstone, 1974, pp 3–9.

32. Cullen JH, Formel PF: Respiratory defects in extreme obesity. Am J Med 32:525–531, 1962.

33. Bedell GN, Wilson WR, Seebohm PM: Pulmonary functions in obese persons. J Clin Invest 39:1049–1060, 1958.

34. Zwillich CW, Sutton FD, Pierson DJ, Creagh EM, Weil JV: Decreased ventilatory drive in the obesity-hypoventilation syndrome. Am J Med 59:343–348, 1975.

19
Sleep Study and Respiratory Function in Myotonic Dystrophy

Joseph Cummiskey, Patricia Lynne-Davies, and Christian Guilleminault

Myotonic dystrophy is a genetic disorder supposedly inherited as an auto-somal dominant trait. It has been known to be associated with endocrine dys-function, skeletal abnormalities, cardiac abnormalities, polar cataracts, frontal baldness, and testicular atrophy. Coccagna et al [1] reported a patient with myotonic dystrophy who had hypersomnia and alveolar hypoventilation. Benaim and Worster-Drought [2], Bashour et al [3], Gillam et al [4], and Kohn et al [5] have already described alveolar hypoventilation in patients with myo-tonic dystrophy.

We review six patients with myotonic dystrophy who were studied during sleep for evidence of sleep apnea. Respiratory function was studied during the day. Abnormalities of central control of respiration were looked for by means of hypoxic and hypercarbic studies.

PATIENT POPULATION AND COMPLAINTS

The patients were six young adult men, with a mean age of 25.5 years (range 17 to 34) who had given informed consent to participate in the study. Their mean weight was 61.3 kg (range 50.2 to 68.2 kg), and mean height was 173 cm (range 168 to 188 cm).

The severity of the muscular disease has been classified into four grades [4]: grade I, disease mild; grade II, disease moderately severe but patient still able to do a light job; grade III, patient severely incapacitated; grade IV, patient bed-ridden. All patients presented grade I myotonic dystrophy syndrome and had noted symptoms for a mean of 12 years (range 6 to 18 years). They had been followed at Stanford University Hospital for a mean of 3.6 years (range 1 to 5) (Table I).

Sleep Apnea Syndromes, pages 295–308
© 1978 Alan R. Liss, Inc., 150 Fifth Avenue, New York, NY 10011

TABLE I. Clinical Features of Patients With Myotonic Dystrophy (MD)

Patient	A	B	C	D	E	F
Sex	M	M	M	M	M	M
Age (years)	28	26	28	17	20	34
Weight (kg)	68.2	59.1	65.9	65.9	50.2	58.5
Height (cm)	170	168	170	188	171	172
Age onset (years)	14	13	15	11	11	16
Functional grade	I	I	I	I	I	I
Daytime somnolence	Yes	Yes	Yes	Yes	Yes	Yes
Smoking history	No	No	No	No	No	Moderate
Chest X ray	Normal	Normal	Normal	Normal	Normal	Normal
12-Lead ECG during wakefulness	Normal	Normal	Normal	Normal	Normal	Normal
Family history of MD	Mother; 2 half-brothers; 4 uncles (maternal)	Brother; father	Brother; father	Half-brother; mother; 4 uncles (maternal)	Half-brother; mother; 4 uncles (maternal)	Aunt, 2 cousins
Endocrine dysfunction	No	No	No	No	No	No
Skeletal abnormalities	No	No	No	No	No	No
Eye examination	Normal	Normal	Normal	Normal	Normal	Normal
Frontal baldness	No	Yes	No	No	No	No
Testicular atrophy	No	No	Yes	No	No	No

Sleep Complaint

Four of the six patients had been seen and followed at the Sleep Disorders Clinic for a complaint of daytime somnolence. The two remaining patients also reported daytime somnolence, but this was not the cause of the referral and was not of major concern to them since they lived on a farm and could sleep during the daytime as needed. Sleepiness was subjectively a major problem for patients A, E, and F and impaired their social and professional lives. It had led to the discovery of myotonia dystrophica in patients A and F.

EXPERIMENTAL PROTOCOL

Patients were required to keep track of their sleep schedules before coming to the Medical Center and to obtain a normal amount of sleep for the week prior to the experimental protocol. On the morning of day 1, they were asked to come to the Clinical Research Center where a neurological evaluation and standard blood and urine tests were performed. A respiratory study (see below) followed. An intraarterial oxygen electrode (International Biophysics Corporation Model #625-001, Irvine, California) which continuously records arterial pO_2 was placed through the femoral artery into the lower part of the aorta. The pO_2 electrode recorded values were regularly verified by direct blood gases measurement obtained through the femoral catheter.

Overnight sleep monitoring included Holter electrocardiogram (ECG) recording, and a separate ECG (lead II) continuously recorded on paper simultaneously with recordings of electroencephalogram ($C_3/A_2 - C_4/A_1$ from the international 10-20 system), electrooculogram, digastric electromyogram, and thoracic and abdominal movements. Oral and nasal thermistors monitored air movement, and the intraarterial electrode continuously monitored arterial pO_2. Lights-out time was 2230 hours (10:30 PM), the patients' normal bedtime. The nocturnal recording lasted for nine hours, and patients were awakened at 0730 hours, also in accord with their usual daytime routine. In fact, four of the six patients acknowledged getting up earlier, usually having only eight hours of dark time; nine hours was the longest acknowledged dark time given by one patient. After awakening, the arterial pO_2 electrode was disconnected and the patient had breakfast.

Patients were continuously monitored polygraphically during day 2 and night 2 and through the beginning of day 3, until 1030 hours. Dark time for night 2 was similar to that of night 1. Patients were free to move about within the limits of a large room and could watch television or read except for specific testing periods. Several dynamometric studies were performed from 1000 to 1100 hours. At 1100, 1400, 1600, and 1900 hours patients were asked to stop all activities, close the window drapes, turn off television or radio, lie down on their beds, close their eyes, and try to sleep for a 15-minute period. State of alertness and type of sleep were polygraphically monitored. If they did not fall asleep, patients could resume activity after this 15-minute trial until the next scheduled tentative nap.

Respiratory Study During the Daytime

The following lung functions were measured in these six patients.

1. Spirometry was performed, using a bell spirometer. From the tracing, values were obtained for the forced vital capacity (FVC), forced expiratory volumes at one and three seconds (FEV$_1$ and FEV$_3$), maximum expiratory flow rate (MEFR), and maximum midexpiratory flow rate (MMRF). Maximum voluntary ventilation (MVV) was measured by asking the patient to breathe as rapidly and deeply as possible for 15 seconds.

2. Total lung capacity and its subdivisions were measured by helium dilution and from the spirometer measurements.

3. Diffusion was measured by the single-breath carbon monoxide method.

4. Arterial blood gases were measured from an arterial line in the radial artery.

5. The ventilatory response to hypoxia was measured by the steady-state method [6].

6. The ventilatory response to carbon dioxide was measured by a steady-state method [7]. Inspiratory CO_2 concentrations of 2, 4, 6, and 8% were breathed for ten minutes. An F_1O_2 of 21% was present with the remainder made up with nitrogen. The expiratory volume was measured for five minutes, and arterial gases and pH were measured during this collection.

RESULTS

Evaluation of Sleep and Sleepiness

Mean nocturnal total sleep time was 412 minutes (range 326 to 477). All patients presented some stages 3–4 non-rapid eye movement (NREM) sleep; however, patients A and F, who had the smallest amount, presented 1 and 6%, respectively, of stages 3–4 NREM sleep. This is a reduced amount for their ages and a reduced amount compared to the rest of the group which had a mean of 21.5% stages 3–4 (range 18.5–23.8%).

During the scheduled daytime naps, patient F presented one sleep onset rapid eye movement (REM) period (defined by the appearance of REM sleep within 15 minutes after sleep onset); none was recorded in any other patient. All patients fell asleep during the daytime naps and slept from five minutes (patient

B) to 100 minutes (patient F). Patients B, C, and D fell asleep during only one of the four daily scheduled naps in contrast to patients A, E, and F. The shortest sleep latencies were six and seven minutes seen in patients E and F respectively.

In summary, patients with the greatest complaint of sleepiness had, objectively, the largest amount of daytime sleep. Patients F, A, and E (rank-ordered by decreasing objective findings) apparently had a more severe problem than the others.

Sleep Apnea and Arterial Oxygen Measurements During Sleep (Table II)

Patients A, F, and C had more than five sleep apneic episodes per sleep-hour (for Apnea Index, see Chapter 1). Patient C was borderline, but patients A and F were definitely pathological. Apneas were predominantly mixed and obstructive in these three cases. Patient E had an Apnea Index of 4 and predominantly central apnea (Fig 1). Patient D's Apnea Index was 0; however, his arterial pO_2 progressively dropped during sleep. From an awake value of 93 mm Hg just before sleep onset, the reading progressively dropped to 60 mm Hg during the first five hours of sleep with a mean drop of 5 mm Hg per hour, and then stabilized at 60 mm Hg until morning awakening. As seen in Table II, all patients had some lowering of arterial pO_2 during sleep compared to values recorded just before sleep onset. The lowest recorded arterial pO_2 values during sleep were seen in patients A and F (40 mm Hg in both) during REM sleep.

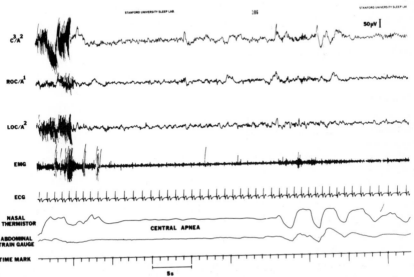

Fig 1. Example of a central apnea in patient E. This apnea follows a short movement and can be considered a posthyperventilation type of apnea with decrease in $PaCO_2$.

TABLE II. Analysis of Apnea

Patient	Degree of somnolence	Apnea index (apnea/sleep-hour)	Arterial PaO$_2$ (mm Hg)		
			Awake supine	Asleep	Lowest value recor
A	Severe	36	89	40	REM sleep
B	Moderate	0.8	91	75	REM sleep
C	Moderate	6.4	87	65	REM sleep
D	Mild	0	93	60	End of night
E	Moderate	4	86	55	REM sleep
F	Severe	16	85	40	REM sleep

Respiratory Function Tests (Tables III–VII)

Total lung capacity (TLC) was reduced in all subjects, averaging $81.2 \pm 8.7\%$ of the value predicted on the basis of the individual's age and height. While only patient E had an obvious restrictive defect, this trend towards small lung volumes was statistically highly significant ($P < 0.005$ by two-tailed t test). The major reason for the reduction in TLC was the consistently compromised inspiratory capacity ($P < 0.001$). Vital capacity was also lower than normal ($P < 0.002$), but the impact of the reduced values for inspiratory capacity was minimized somewhat by a concomitant reduction in residual volume ($P < 0.02$). Functional residual capacity was similarly low in absolute terms ($P < 0.05$), with the result that the only lung volume that showed no significant change from predicted values was expiratory reserve volume. When functional residual capacity was expressed as a percentage of the measured total lung capacity, it was within normal limits for the subject's age group in five individuals ($48.4 \pm 3.4\%$ TLC) but was abnormally low, at 35%, in Patient E. Since functional residual capacity represents the resting volume of the respiratory system between breaths, when the elastic recoil of lungs and chest wall are balanced, this observation suggests that five of the six subjects had relatively normal elastic properties.

Similarly, airway dynamics appeared normal, as evidenced by normal values for the forced expiratory volume in one second, expressed as a percentage of vital capacity (mean $85.3 \pm 5.8\%$). Flow rates were significantly lower than predicted, but this reflects the reduction in vital capacity, since normal flow rates are predicted on normal volumes. More interestingly, the MEFR, which represents the voluntary part of the expiratory flow, was decreased by an average of 20% in five of the patients (excluding patient D), while the involuntary MMFR was increased (mean 70%) in six of the six patients. This finding, with the decreased MVV (mean $72 \pm 17\%$ of predicted) in the six patients, is strongly suggestive of alveolar hypoventilation secondary to their muscular disease.

The marginally reduced PaO$_2$ of five of the five patients is significant ($P < 0.01$). The PaCO$_2$, although low, is not significantly reduced.

TABLE III. Lung Volumes (liters) in Patients With Myotonic Dystrophy (predicted values in parentheses)*

Patient	TLC	RV	FRC	VC	IC	ERV
A	4.91	0.61	2.40	4.30	2.51	1.79
	(5.96)	(1.31)	(2.86)	(4.62)	(3.10)	(1.53)
B	4.82	1.13	2.24	3.69	2.58	1.11
	(5.80)	(1.25)	(2.75)	(4.56)	(3.06)	(1.51)
C	5.09	1.07	2.38	4.02	2.71	1.31
	(5.96)	(1.31)	(2.86)	(4.62)	(3.10)	(1.53)
D	6.26	1.02	2.85	5.24	3.41	1.84
	(7.36)	(1.53)	(3.48)	(5.80)	(3.89)	(1.91)
E	3.86	0.82	1.35	3.03	2.51	0.52
	(6.05)	(1.24)	(2.79)	(4.85)	(3.25)	(1.60)
F	5.57	1.33	3.01	4.25	2.57	1.68
	(6.19)	(1.42)	(3.05)	(4.69)	(3.14)	(1.55)

*Abbreviations: TLC, total lung capacity; RV, residual volume; FRC, functional residual capacity; VC, vital capacity; IC, inspiratory capacity; ERV, expiratory reserve volume.

TABLE IV. Airflows in Patients With Myotonic Dystropy (predicted values in parentheses)*

Patient	FVC (L)	FEV_1[a]	FEV_3[a]	MEFR[b]	MMFR[b]	MIFR[b]	MVV[b]
A	4.30	77	95	317	252	230	105
	(4.62)	(> 72)	(> 95)	(402)	(192)		(169)
B	3.69	94	100	271	239	258	111
	(4.56)	(> 72)	(> 95)	(327)	(114)		(169)
C	4.02	84	100	297	205	236	150
	(4.62)	(> 72)	(> 95)	(366)	(156)		(169)
D	5.20	85	100	629	272	512	179
	(5.80)	(> 72)	(> 95)	(432)	(192)		(207)
E	3.03	89	100	329	201	198	84
	(4.85)	(> 72)	(> 95)	(246)	(260)		(131)
F	4.25	83	100	427	224	294	142
	(4.69)	(> 72)	(> 95)	(396)	(180)		(173)

*Abbreviations: FVC, forced vital capacity; FEV, forced expiratory volume (one and three seconds); MEFR, maximum expiratory flow rate (corrected for volume); MMRF, maximum midflow rate (corrected for volume); MIFR, maximum inspiratory flow rate; MVV, maximum voluntary ventilation.
[a]In percent of FVC.
[b]In liters per minute.

All four patients tested responded to the hypoxic stimulus by increasing their respiratory rate. Two patients also increased their minute ventilation. The failure of two patients to increase their minute ventilation was due to a decrease in tidal volume.

TABLE V. Respiratory Function in Patients With Myotonic Dystrophy (predicted values in parentheses)

| Patient | Age (years) | Arterial blood gases on room air | | | | | Diffusion D_{LCO} (ml/min/mm Hg) | Helium mixing time (min) |
		pH	pO_2 (torr)	pCO_2 (torr)	HCO_3^- (mEq/L)	A-a Difference (torr)		
A	28	–	–	–	–	–	29 (31)	3
B	26	7.40	87 (93)	43	27	10	29 (31)	2
C	28	7.43	85 (92)	37	24	20	33 (31)	4
D	17	7.42	95 (96)	37	23.8	10	54 (43)	2
E	20	7.43	87 (95)	36	24.1	19	33 (34)	2
F	34	7.37	84 (89)	40	22	17	46 (30)	4
Predicted		(7.38–7.42)		(38–42)	(23–25)	(<15)		(<5)

TABLE VI. Ventilatory Studies in the Resting Supine Position on Room Air and With Hypoxia

Patient	F_1O_2	F_1CO_2	pH	pO_2 (torr)	pCO_2 (torr)	HCO_3^- (mEq/L)	f (per min)	V_T (L)	$\dot{V}_E$ (L/min)
A	0.210	0.00	7.41	101	36	23.0	12	0.48	5.75
	0.124	0.00	7.41	44	37	23.7	19	0.39	7.42
B	0.210	0.00	7.40	79	40	25.4	10	0.74	7.40
	0.124	0.00	7.40	41	40	24.3	19	0.31	5.90
C	0.210	0.00	7.43	85	37	24.0	9	0.74	6.68
	0.124	0.00	7.61	64	25	24.6	16	0.68	10.92
E	0.210	0.00	7.43	87	36	24.1	13	0.51	6.95
	0.124	0.00	7.43	41	40	26.3	22	0.28	6.16

TABLE VII. Ventilatory Response to Hypercarbia
in the Resting Supine Position

Patient	Ventilatory response to 1 torr increase in $PaCO_2$ (L/min)
A	1.10
B	0.77
C	0.70
D	1.35
E	1.35
F	4.80

DISCUSSION

During the past few years, the relationship between mytonic dystrophy, the origin of hypersomnia observed in some of these patients, and disorders of breathing during wakefulness and sleep has been questioned. Leygonie-Goldenberg et al [8] have found after monitoring the nocturnal sleep of 15 myotonic dystrophic patients that one-third of them had polygraphic abnormalities during sleep, particularly a REM onset sleep period. These authors raised the question of the relationship between the complaint of sleepiness and a central nervous system defect similar to that involved in narcolepsy. Kilburn et al [9], after studying nine patients with myotonic dystrophy, suggested that a combination of weakness of the chest bellows, the increased effort of breathing due to myotonia, and possibly a central neurogenic alteration, resulted in the alveolar hypoventilation syndrome and the secondary development of daytime somnolence. Coccagna et al [1], who studied one patient with the combination of myotonic dystrophy, alveolar hypoventilation, hypersomnia, and sleep onset REM periods, also supported the hypothesis of a primary central disturbance to explain the hypersomnia and some anomalies of sleep structure such as the abundance and precocity of REM sleep.

The frequent occurrence of ventilatory insufficiency in progressive muscular dystrophy is well known. However, the complaint of excessive daytime sleepiness (EDS) is far less prominent than in mytonic dystrophy. During the past 28 months in our clinic, we have seen ten patients with myotonic dystrophy (nine of the ten of grade I type) and a complaint of EDS. In comparison, we have seen one very impaired muscular dystrophy patient with a similar type of complaint. Despite the possibility of recruitment bias, this finding may suggest that excessive daytime sleepiness is not necessarily solely related to ventilatory insufficiency secondary to muscular wasting.

Leygonie-Goldenberg [8] found that myotonic dystrophy patients may present excessive daytime somnolence with or without polygraphic documentation o

REM onset sleep periods. In our own patient group, one patient presented only one REM onset sleep period during a daytime nap. Considering these data, the question arises whether REM onset sleep periods may simply be indices of sleep deprivation secondary to the respiratory disturbance [10]. Favoring such an hypothesis, we must stress that sleep onset REM periods are frequently recorded in sleep apneic patients but are no longer seen after tracheostomy although a marked REM rebound phenomenon is observed in children [11] as well as in adults.

Our patients not only presented sleep apnea, but two of the five (patients A and F) had a predominance of mixed and obstructive apneas during sleep. Their arterial pO_2 swings at the end of each apneic episode were similar to those seen in obstructive sleep apneic patients (Fig 2). In these two cases, the most severe desaturation was seen during REM sleep. This is in contrast to findings noted in patient D who had no apnea, developed a slight decrease in PaO_2 during sleep —

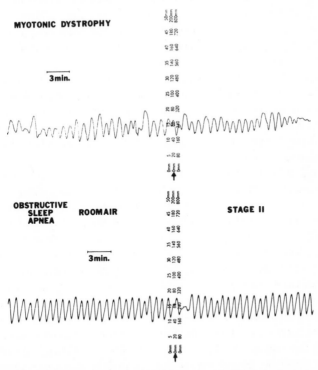

Fig 2. Continuous oxygen tracing obtained with intraarterial IBC electrode during stage 2 NREM sleep. Top tracing was obtained in patient F, bottom tracing from a classical obstructive sleep apnea patient. The duration of each apneic episode can be easily evaluated by measuring the intrapeak distance. Oxygen drops with each apnea and return to higher values with resumption of breathing. Arrow indicates the PaO_2 scale.

from the beginning to the end of the night (decreasing from 90 to 60 mm Hg at the end of nocturnal sleep), and has minimal sleepiness and normal ventilatory measurements.

Can we explain the daytime sleepiness of myotonic patients by the combination of disrupted nocturnal sleep and alveolar hypoventilation as proposed by Semerano et al [12] and by our group [13] in obstructive sleep apneic patients as an hypoxic action on the brain neurotransmitters involved in sleep and wakefulness? This seems logical, but one wonders why obstruction during sleep is associated with a greater complaint of sleepiness than in central apnea or alveolar hypoventilation secondary to muscle weakness of the chest bellows.

Another question is the relationship between the daytime pulmonary test abnormalities and the positive polygraphic finding of sleep apnea. These myotonic dystrophy patients had pulmonary function tests suggestive of mild alveolar hypoventilation. Their response to a hypoxic stimulus was an increase in frequency suggesting that the afferent side of the response is intact. The efferent side is abnormal. This was manifested by a failure of the patients to increase their minute volume due to a decrease in tidal volume. Patient D had no evidence of sleep apnea. He was also the only one with a normal maximum expiratory flow rate, and a normal PaO_2. His ventilatory responses to hypoxia and hypercarbia were normal.

The five other patients are divided into mild, moderate, and severe sleep apnea. Mild sleep apnea was less than one apneic episode per sleep-hour and a PaO_2 greater than 70 torr; moderate sleep apnea was between three and ten sleep apneic episodes per sleep-hour with the lowest PaO_2 between 65 and 55; severe sleep apnea was greater than 15 apneic periods per sleep-hour and a PaO_2 less than 55 torr.

Patients B and E have an Apnea Index compatible with that of normal controls (see Chapter 1). However, patient B had carbon dioxide retention ($PaCO_2$ — 43) despite his decreased PaO_2 of 5 torr below predicted; this patient was one of the two with the most blunted hypoxic and hypercarbic responses during wakefulness. Patient E had the most severe restrictive lung disease of the entire group; his Apnea Index, however, was within the normal range (borderline high). Patients E and C had an elevated alveolar-arterial oxygen difference but had Apnea Indices of 4 and 6, respectively. Again, these two patients could scarcely be considered to have a pathological sleep apnea syndrome.

Only two patients (F and A) presented a sleep apnea syndrome. Their Apnea Indices were between 15 and 40 (moderate sleep apnea syndrome; see Table I, Chapter 11 for comparison), and their apneas were predominantly obstructive and mixed. These two patients had nothing on their tests of lung volumes or mechanics to differentiate them from patients B, C, and E. F was one of the patients noted to have a $PaCO_2$ at the upper limit of normal, relative to the low PaO_2. This suggests alveolar hypoventilation. Both the hypoxic and the hyperarbic studies were blunted in patient A, but the latter study was above the normal mean in patient F. The only major difference during sleep in these two patients was the low arterial pO_2 which can be interpreted as the result of recurrent sleep apnea.

Although some abnormalities were noted during ventilatory daytime testing, some of them related to muscle impairment, these do not explain the nocturnal findings. Different mechanisms may be involved in respiratory dysfunctions during sleep. Ventilatory abnormalities may lead to the disclosure of the sleep apnea syndrome or worsen it, but it is our feeling that a direct central nervous system dysfunction is responsible for the sleep apnea syndrome in myotonic dystrophy, and that daytime sleepiness is greatly exacerbated by the sleep apnea syndrome.

ACKNOWLEDGMENTS

This research was supported by National Institute of Neurological Diseases and Stroke grant NS 10727, Public Health Service Research Grant RR-70 from the General Clinical Research Centers, Division of Research Resources, and by INSERM to Dr Guilleminault.

REFERENCES

1. Coccagna G, Mantovani M, Parchi C, Mironi F, Lugaresi E: Alveolar hypoventilation and hypersomnia in myotonic dystrophy. J Neurol Neurosurg Psychiatry 38:977–984, 1975.
2. Benaim S, Worster-Drought C: Dystrophia myotonica (with myotonia of the diaphragm causing pulmonary hypoventilation with anoxaemia and secondary polycythaemia). Med Illustr 8:221–226, 1954.
3. Bashour F, Winchell P, Reddington J: Myotonia atrophica and cyanosis. N Engl J Med 252:768–770, 1955.
4. Gillam PMS, Heaf PJD, Kaufman L, Lucas BGB: Respiration in dystrophia myotonica. Thorax 19:112–120, 1964.
5. Kohn NN, Faires JS, Rodman T: Unusual manifestations due to involvement of involuntary muscle in dystrophia myotonica. N Engl J Med 271:1179–1183, 1964.
6. Dripps R, Comroe J Jr: The effect of the inhalation of high and low oxygen concentrations on respiration, pulse rate, balistocardiogram, and arterial oxygen saturation (oximeter of normal individuals). Am J Physiol 149:277–291, 1947.
7. Lambertsen CJ: Carbon dioxide and respiration in acid-base homeostasis. Anesthesiology 21:642–651. 1960.
8. Leygonie-Goldenberg F, Perrier M, Duizabo P, Bouchareine A, Harp A, Barbizet J, Degos JD: Troubles de la vigilance et de la fonction respiratoir dans la maladie de Steinert. In "Proceedings of the Third European Congress on Sleep." Basel: Karger, in press.

9. Kilburn KH, Eagan JT, Sieker HO, Keyman A: Cardiopulmonary insufficiency in myotonic and progressive muscular dystrophy. N Engl J Med 261:1088–1096, 1959.

10. Carskadon MA: The role of sleep-onset REM periods in narcolepsy. In Guilleminault C, Dement WC, Passouant P (eds): "Narcolepsy." New York: Spectrum, 1976, pp 491–519.

11. Guilleminault C, Tilkian AG, Dement WC: Sommeil et respiration dans le syndrome "apnée au cours du sommeil" chez l'enfant. Electroencephalogr Clin Neurophysiol 41:367–378, 1976.

12. Semerano A, Bevilacqua M, Battistin L: Blood gas analysis and polygraphic observations in the Pickwickian syndrome. Bull Physiopathol Respir 8:1193–1201, 1972.

13. Guilleminault C, Eldridge FL, Simmons FB, Dement WC: Sleep apnea syndrome: Can it induce hemodynamic changes? West J Med 123:7–16, 1975.

14. Phillipson EA: Regulation of breathing during sleep. Am Rev Respir Dis 115(Suppl): 217–224, 1977.

20

Sleep Apnea Syndrome as a Long-Term Sequela of Poliomyelitis

Christian Guilleminault and Jorge Motta

Abnormalities in the central regulation of respiration in acute and convalescent poliomyelitis were adeptly described as early as 1958 by Plum and Swanson [1]. In this pioneer report the role of sleep in the appearance or exacerbation of respiratory distress was emphasized. One group of reported patients presented "apneic events" (4 to 12 seconds in duration) only during sleep.

Since the advent of systematic immunization, poliomyelitis occurs relatively infrequently in North America and Western Europe. However, we have had the opportunity to study five patients (in Paris and at Stanford University) between 1970 and 1976 who were referred for a complaint of inappropriate and excessive daytime sleepiness (EDS). All of them had experienced an attack of poliomyelitis between 1948 and 1954, a minimum of 16 years before consultation.

PATIENTS

All patients were male; their mean age was 39.2 years (range 34–48 years). Most of them had had poliomyelitis during their late teens or early twenties. All had some involvement of bulbar musculature at the time of the attack. Two of the five were kept under a ventilator for four and seven months, respectively, at the time of the acute phase. All patients had undergone rehabilitation, and four of the five were able to walk — two with the help of crutches and braces on one leg; one used a wheel chair. All of them were socially active and employed in professions ranging from physician, accountant, to business representative; four of the five were married and had children.

Sleep Apnea Syndromes, pages 309–315

These patients had been followed for some years after rehabilitation (mean number of follow-up years after acute attack, five years), and all of them had been considered stabilized for many years, without neurological abnormalities except for the atrophy of limb muscles and the absence of deep tendon reflexes. None of them had marked kyphoscoliosis, severe chest malformation, or apparent loss of chest or abdominal muscle strength when seen during wakefulness All of them were able to chew, swallow, and breathe adequately on command. Excessive daytime somnolence had appeared insidiously a mean of two years before referral (range one to three years). Irresistible urges to sleep occurred primarily when patients were inactive — sitting quietly, reading, or driving.

Interviews with the families eliminated histories of continuous heavy snoring or abnormal movements during sleep. However, observation of stop-breathing episodes during sleep in recent years was noted by the spouses of two patients.

PROCEDURES

All patients underwent nocturnal standard polygraphic monitoring which included the use of strain gauges and thermistors to assess respiration. Pulmonary function was assessed during wakefulness; spirometry and arterial blood gases were measured in all cases. Hypercarbic response was measured by the steady-state method. An F_1CO_2 of 0.03, 0.05, and 0.07 was breathed for ten minutes; F_1O_2 of 0.21, with the remainder made up of nitrogen, was used. In patients 4 and 5, brachial arterial gases and pH were also measured during the test. During sleep, patients 1–4 were monitored with an ear oximeter (Waters Instrument Co). Patient 5 underwent a more intensive investigation which included hemodynamic study during sleep and wakefulness (see Chapter 11 for description of technique), continuous arterial pO_2 recording, and 24-hour Holter monitoring (see Chapter 12). In two cases (patients 4 and 5), polygraphic monitoring was repeated with the patient under currass.

RESULTS

Pulmonary Function Tests

Total lung capacities and vital capacities in all patients were less than predicted. Three patients (1, 3, and 5) were at the lower limit of normal and had a significant restrictive effect. The maximum voluntary ventilation (MVV) and maximum expiratory flow rate (MEFR) were reduced in all patients. The partial pressure of arterial oxygen (PaO_2) was also reduced in all patients (range 74–83 torr); the partial pressure of arterial carbon dioxide ($PaCO_2$) was at the

per limit of normal relative to PaO_2 in three of the five patients and was ele-
ted in two cases (see Table I). Ventilatory responses in patients 4 and 5 were
ater than 2.3 liters/min to 1 torr elevation in $PaCO_2$.

eep

The mean nocturnal sleep time in all five patients was 482 minutes (range
5–522). All patients had short nocturnal sleep latencies (mean, 3 minutes 37
conds). All patients had very disturbed sleep, similar to that observed in
tients with other types of the sleep apnea syndrome. Sleep was continuously
terrupted by short bursts of alpha waves at the end of each apneic episode.
ese bursts were seen in both rapid eye movement (REM) and non-rapid eye
ovement (NREM) sleep, resulting in extremely low sleep efficiency. No stages
-4 NREM sleep were recorded in any of the five patients. Two patients had a
EM period at onset of nocturnal sleep.

All patients were monitored during an afternoon nap the following day (mean
p duration, 42 minutes; range 25–71 minutes); again, short sleep latencies
ere seen (mean, 4 minutes 10 seconds).

espiration During Sleep

All patients had multiple apneic episodes during sleep; their mean Apnea
dex (number of apneas per sleep-hour) was 96 (range 80–104). A predomi-
nce of central apnea (mean 52%) was monitored, but mixed (mean 32%) and
re obstructive (mean 16%) apneic episodes were also recorded. All patients
perienced their longest apneic episodes during REM sleep concomitant with
rsts of rapid eye movements. Oxygen desaturation occurred during sleep in
sociation with repetitive apneas, and the lowest desaturations were observed
so during REM sleep, at the end of long apneas — particularly those of mixed
pe. As this parameter was assessed with an ear oximeter during sleep in
atients 1–4, only relative oximetric values could be obtained. More accurate
easurements were taken in patient 5 with an indwelling arterial pO_2 electrode
BC). Patient 5 desaturated to 30–22 torr during REM sleep compared to a

TABLE I. Blood Gases in the Supine Position During Wakefulness

Patient	pO_2 (torr)	pCO_2 (torr)
1	78	42
2	81	40
3	76	45
4	83	41
5	74	51

mean of 45 torr during NREM sleep (sample blood gases during NREM sleep: pO_2, 48 torr, pCO_2, 73 torr, pH, 7.30). Large swings of SaO_2, related to apnea and postapneic hyperventilation, were recorded during sleep in patients 1 to 4. The lowest mean oxygen saturation during REM sleep was 72% (±5% for instrument error).

Pressure Measurements in Patient 5

Cyclical systemic and pulmonary hypertension during sleep in patient 5 was similar to that seen in other sleep apnea patients (see Chapter 11). Systemic pressure showed a gradual rise during hypoxemia and a further brief rise at onset of respiration; mean pulmonary arterial pressure (PAP) rose with the development of hypoxemia. A cyclic pattern of marked sinus arrhythmia appeared with repetitive apnea (see Chapter 12). Rapid eye movement sleep had a dramatic impact on this patient, producing further worsening of hypoxemia, hypercapnia and acidosis, with concomitant increases in pulmonary and systemic pressure. Table II presents measurements obtained in patient 5.

THERAPEUTIC TRIALS AND FOLLOW-UP MONITORING

Medroxyprogesterone (20 mg daily for six weeks) in patient 5 led to no symptomatic improvement.

All patients received mechanical respiratory assistance, hooking themselves to a currass at night, just before sleep onset. This therapy brought symptomatic improvement, ie, decrease in daytime somnolence, to all patients. Satisfactory use of the currass requires that the patient obtain a perfectly fitted, custom-made apparatus. We also learned that an appropriate respiratory rate setting for each patient was vital. All our patients required a low frequency setting point (8 to 10 cycles/minute); a higher frequency setting (12 to 14 cycles/minute) resulted in complaints of marked discomfort and multiple arousals. Follow-up recording under currass in patients 4 and 5 after nightly respirator use for 12 and 6 weeks, respectively, demonstrated an increased number of obstructive apneas during sleep under the higher frequency, and a worsening of sleep disruption

TABLE II. Measurements Obtained During Sleep and Wakefulness in Patient 5

Apnea index	FAP (mm Hg)		PAP (mm Hg)		PaO_2 (mm Hg)	
	Awake supine	Asleep	Awake	Asleep	Awake	Asleep
104	150/90	160/100	20/10	53/37	74	30

sulting in complete awakening secondary to obstructive apnea, confirming the objective complaint. Follow-up recordings of patients 4 and 5 included monitoring of oxygen saturation (Waters Instrument Co ear oximeter in patient 4 and C intraarterial oxygen electrode in patient 5). During the course of the recording of patient 5, while he slept, the currass was disconnected, and a dramatic op in arterial oxygen pressure was observed. Comparison of these recorded lues with baseline values obtained during sleep six weeks earlier (before treatment) showed a much more pronounced oxygen drop at the time of the second cording. This decrease was significant during NREM sleep and became alarming ring REM sleep when PaO_2 of 22 torr and $PaCO_2$ of 79 torr were recorded d did not lead to the patient's awakening.

ISCUSSION

All of our patients were referred for excessive daytime sleepiness and all prented documented sleep disturbances similar to those observed in typical sleep neic patients with no apparent neurological lesion. These poliomyelitis tients, interestingly enough, presented not only central apnea — the predominant type — but also mixed and obstructive components, indicating an upper rway involvement also in these centrally lesioned patients. Rapid eye movement sleep led to lengthening of apnea and a secondary increase in oxygen desturation similar to that observed in a large and well-defined group of sleep neic patients free from neurological symptoms. Cardiovascular impact, similar that previously described in predominantly central sleep apnea patients (see apter 11) also was monitored in one of these patients who underwent a comete nocturnal hemodynamic study.

The similarities between these patients with neurological sequelae and the eep apneic patient population previously described raise the question of a relaonship: Is there a similar defect in both instances? Also, why is there such a ng silent phase between the acute disease and the onset of EDS?

The effect of central nervous system disease on respiration has been extenvely studied. In 1963, Plum and Brown [2] reported a series of patients with rain insult and abnormal control of breathing. Little attention has been given, owever, to the role of sleep state on the control of breathing in neurological atients and even less to the long-term — ie, several years — in patients with ntral nervous system lesions, and to the possibility of progressive deteriora on of their control of breathing, particularly during sleep. It is possible that me centrally lesioned patients may have initially, or may retain after the acute nd convalescent phases of their disease, abnormal control of breathing only uring REM sleep, during which state chemical stimuli seem to lose most of their rive (see Chapters 4 and 8). If hypoxemia is marked at the end of REM sleep periods, disturbances may gradually appear during NREM sleep also and then lengthen with time.

The long silent phase should be carefully evaluated, and neurologists should be cautioned about the possibility of the central nervous system lesion acutely disrupting control of breathing after long periods of time. Extended follow-up including continuous all-night polygraphic monitoring is performed only except tionally on this type of patient. Nonetheless, some of these patients may be at risk for progressive deterioration, ie, gradual development of vascular impairment and/or arrhythmias secondary to hypoxia, during sleep.

Neurological literature contains reports supporting this possibility. In 1957, Efron and Kent [3] reported the case history of a patient who had encephalitis in 1917 at age 17 and, with the exception of abnormal response to general anesthesia noted in 1938, had no clinical symptoms until 1940. She deteriorate thereafter, developing excessive daytime somnolence, cyanosis, ankle edema, a right heart failure. In this case, 20 years elapsed between the original brain insu and the appearance of secondary symptoms. This patient's abnormal response t anesthesia could have raised questions as early as 1938 about the integrity of th central control of breathing. The reported clinical symptomatology raises the question of whether this patient was a sleep apnea case.

A final comment on our studies concerns the use of the respirator. The currass is infrequently used now, and diaphragmatic pacing (see Chapter 23) may be a more satisfactory mode of treatment for these patients in the future. Howeve physicians and patients using the respirator should be cautioned about potentia dangers should power failure or mechanical failure occur during sleep. Six week after the beginning of nocturnal mechanical ventilation, patient 5 had apparent lost the capability to respond to levels of hypoxia and hypercapnia lower than those observed during baseline monitoring. This lack of response was particular striking during REM sleep. Was this lack of response due to an increased central nervous system defect developing in less than two months or to a change in some defense mechanism during sleep after the short use of the currass? Or did we "surprise" the already lesioned respiratory control system by abrupt change in some "set point" when mechanical assistance was suddenly interrupted in a sleepy patient? These questions remain unanswered. In this one particular patient, however, polygraphic recording demonstrated a greater lack of response during REM sleep — greater than we anticipated — than we had ever previously recorded.

ACKNOWLEDGEMENTS

This research was supported by National Institute of Neurological Diseases and Stroke grant NS 10727, Public Health Service Research grant RR-70 from he General Clinical Research Centers, Division of Research Resources, and by NSERM to Dr Guilleminault.

REFERENCES

. Plum F, Swanson AG: Abnormalities in central regulation of respiration in acute and convalescent poliomyelitis. Arch Neurol Psychiatry 80:267–285, 1958.

2. Plum F, Brown HW: The effect on respiration of central nervous system disease. Ann NY Acad Sci 109:915–931, 1963.

3. Efron R, Kent CD: Chronic respiratory acidosis due to brain disease. Arch Neurol Psychiatry 77:575–587, 1957.

21
Shy-Drager Syndrome and Sleep Apnea

Jonathan G Briskin, Kenneth L Lehrman, and Christian Guilleminault

Shy-Drager syndrome is a rare combination of a Parkinsonian motor disorder and autonomic insufficiency associated with degenerative changes of the extrapyramidal and autonomic nervous system [1]. Afflicted patients present with disturbances of all autonomic functions progressing toward autonomic arreflexia.

A patient with Shy-Drager syndrome has been reported [2] who manifested an ataxic respiratory pattern while awake and asleep — and who ultimately died of respiratory arrest. Recently, we have polygraphically monitored three patients with Shy-Drager syndrome presenting with upper airway sleep apnea. Two also underwent overnight hemodynamic monitoring.

CASE REPORTS

Patient 1 [3] was a 59-year-old white male with a five-year progressive history of urinary incontinence, incomplete emptying of the bladder, impotence, and perianal numbness. He had noted increasing light-headedness on standing or exercise and two episodes of orthostatic syncope had occurred. During the two years prior to consultation, the patient frequently fell asleep during the day; reports of disturbed nocturnal sleep with loud snoring were obtained from the spouse. During the daytime, hoarseness and slurring of speech were noted. The combination of increasing orthostatic symptoms and daytime hypersomnolence had severely limited his ability to work.

Patient 2 was a 61-year-old white male with a seven-year history of orthostatic hypotension and progressive worsening of extrapyramidal symptoms. Beginning three years prior to referral to the Sleep Clinic, severe daytime somnolence had progressively appeared. Nocturnal sleep had been observed to be disturbed for the prior five years and was characterized by abnormal respiration during sleep associated with snorting and loud snoring.

Sleep Apnea Syndromes, pages 317—322

Patient 3 was a 59-year-old locomotive engineer who began to experience daytime somnolence approximately five years prior to consultation. During the following four years he had gradually become impotent and had developed urinary and fecal incontinence and severe postural hypotension. His wife reported a long history of heavy snoring "like the honking of a flock of geese." During sleep he had been observed to stop breathing briefly and had required resuscitation twice (in 1975 and 1977). During the six months before referral, the patient had appeared not only somnolent but also confused and disoriented, and his family believed his mental capability was impaired.

In all cases, some neurological findings were noted during initial evaluation. These were slight in patient 1 (mild intention tremor), more marked in patient 2, who presented pyramidal and extrapyramidal symptoms, and in patient 3 pyramidal symptoms were associated with cerebellum involvement resulting in upper and lower level hypermetria and dysmetria.

Pulmonary function tests in all three cases were consistent with mild distal obstruction and air trapping. Patients 1 and 2 had normal responses to hypoxemia and hypercarbia while awake. Patient 3 had normal response to hypercarbia but severely blunted response to hypoxia.

Polygraphic Monitoring

As all patients were clinically suspected of sleep apnea syndrome, polygraphic monitoring and cardiovascular studies during sleep and wakefulness were scheduled. Patient 2 died abruptly during sleep before undergoing the protocol. Patients 1 and 3 underwent all night polygraphic monitorings which included the following variables: electroencephalogram (EEG) $(C_3/A_2 - C_4/A_1$, from the international 10-20 system), electrooculogram (EOG), digastric electromyogram (EMG), and electrocardiogram (ECG). Thoracic and abdominal movements and oral nasal thermistors were used to gauge movement of air. During one 24-hour period the study also included Holter (ambulatory) ECG.

Hemodynamic Study

After several nocturnal monitorings, patients 1 and 3 also underwent hemodynamic monitoring studies. The right heart catheterizations were performed by the Seldinger technique using a #7.0 F Swan-Ganz thermodilution catheter and a PE 160 femoral arterial catheter. Pulmonary and arterial pressures, cardiac output, respiration, and arterial oxygen levels were recorded continuously during wakefulness and sleep and were measured by analysis of EEG, EOG, and chin EMG. Arterial blood gases were obtained periodically during wakefulness and sleep; this allowed recalibration of the PaO_2 intraarterial electrode (IBC). An endoesophageal pressure transducer was also continuously monitored to better identify the type of apnea.

To evaluate autonomic reflexes, interventions tested baroreceptors and afferent nerves (tilt table, Valsalva maneuver, amyl nitrite, and carotid sinus massage), central integrative centers (Valsalva maneuver and mental arithmetic), sympathetic outflow (Valsalva maneuver, cold pressor test), organ responsiveness (norepinephrine and angiotensin infusion), and presence of functioning nerve endings (metaraminol). Between interventions, control measurements were repeated to confirm return to baseline values.

RESULTS

During wakefulness, both patients demonstrated essentially normal hemodynamics. The heart rate responded minimally to all intervention except atropine infusion, which caused a subnormal heart rate increase (64 to 69 and 66 to 70 beats/min, in patients 1 and 3, respectively). Reflex tachycardia did not occur during orthostatic hypotension or amyl nitrite inhalation. With Valsalva maneuver, the decreased venous return caused hypotension without the expected reflex tachycardia or the postrelease hypertension in patient 1, and led to a very mild heart rate increase (from 63 to 71 beats/min), with a further slight rise (to 75) upon release in patient 3. Finally, both patients had an exaggerated hypertensive response to levarteranol and metaraminol (see Table I).

Sleep Data From Overnight Recording

While sleeping, both patients developed upper airway obstruction resulting in increased respiratory effort and progressive increase in endoesophageal pressure. Sleep data obtained prior to the hemodynamic studies showed markedly decreased stages 3 and 4 NREM sleep in both patients (see Table II). Rapid eye movement sleep was even more severely impaired, representing 0.8% total sleep time in patient 1 and 4.6% in patient 3 (normal, 20%). Both patients averaged over 430 apneic episodes per night, and their mean Apnea Indices (see Chapter 1 for definition) were 75 and 79, respectively. Over 70% of the total number of apneic episodes were obstructive.

Hemodynamic Monitoring During Sleep

Resting pulmonary and femoral arterial pressures were normal during wakefulness. While sleeping, both patients developed obstruction with increased respiratory effort and wide swings in pulmonary arterial pressure. Systemic arterial pressure elevations were, however, severely blunted (Fig 1). The PaO_2 pressures dropped to 36 and 38 mm Hg, respectively, and oscillated between 40 and 60 mm Hg during the course of sleep. Heart rates cycled only slightly

TABLE I. Hemodynamics in Shy-Drager Syndrome and Sleep Apnea

Intervention	Patient	Heart rate (beats/min)	Femoral artery (S/D/M, mm Hg)	Pulmonary artery (S/D/M, mm Hg)	Cardiac index (liters/min/m^2)
Control	1	64	155/80/100	20/16/20	2.7
	3	63	152/76/84	40/14/19	–
Carotid sinus	1	62	130/75/100	32/20/25	–
massage	3	63	154/76/–	40/14/–	–
Valsalva	1	72	90/65	–	1.0
	3	70	90/64	48/38	–
Cold pressor	1	64	150/75/100	30/20/23	2.4
test	3	73	134/72/94	35/13/19	–
Amyl nitrate	1	65	85/40/60	25/15/18	1.9
	3	79	60/32/–	30/19/–	–
Norepinephrine	1	62	190/90/120	38/22/28	2.2
	3	61	182/106/126	62/20/25	–
Metaraminol	1	62	240/105/140	52/26/32	2.2
	3	70	220/100/142	64/23/–	–
Atropine	1	78	200/100/135	–	2.9
	3	76	150/76/82	42/12/18	–

TABLE II. Sleep Data*

	NREM sleep			REM sleep
	Stage 1	Stage 2	Stages 3–4	
Patient 1	26	71	2	0.8
Patient 3	0.1	95.3	0	4.6
After tracheostomy				
Patient 3	0.1	97.8	0	2.2

*Given in percentage of total sleep time.

during obstructive sleep apnea in both cases (60 to 90 beats/min with apneic episodes).

Follow-Up Course

Both patients were placed under medications including 9-α-fluorohydrocorti-sone, L-dopa, and cyproheptadine daily. Despite medical treatment, two weeks after investigation patient 1 suffered a respiratory arrest while sleeping and expired before arriving at the hospital.

In view of the two previous cases, a tracheostomy was scheduled and performed on patient 3. Twenty-four hours after surgery, confusion and disorientation had completely disappeared. Daytime somnolence decreased and the patient was soon able to handle his personal business. A follow-up monitoring performed two weeks after surgery demonstrated considerable improvement of oxygen saturation during sleep but persistence of some central apneic episodes. No change in total REM time was noted, confirming that the abnormal REM sleep decrease was unrelated to the obstructive sleep apnea syndrome. The patient had a fairly normal life at home, despite his neurological symptoms, during the first three months after surgery. Central apneic episodes during sleep progressively increased thereafter, and he expired four and a half months after surgery, suffering a respiratory arrest during sleep.

COMMENTS

Three patients with Shy-Drager syndrome, two of whom were extensively investigated, presented with severe obstructive sleep apnea. These two patients both demonstrated marked blunting of the normally expected reflex tachycardia in response to hypotension and minimal response to atropine. Despite absence of peripheral pressure changes during sleep apneic episodes with PaO_2 as low as 38 mm Hg, there were marked rises in pulmonary arterial pressure, suggesting the important role of local hypoxemia and acidosis in causing cyclic pulmonary hypertension.

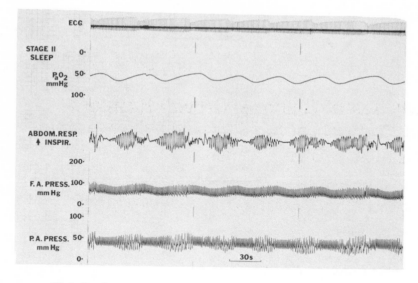

Fig 1. Simultaneous recordings in patient 3 during obstructive sleep apnea.

Sleep apnea syndrome, a complication ordinarily unsuspected in patients with Shy-Drager syndrome, may be responsible for some of the daytime symptoms such as confusion, disorientation, decreased intellectual performance, and day-time somnolence; it may reduce the life expectancy of these patients. A combination of tracheostomy and a diaphragmatic pacemaker may be suggested in these cases.

ACKNOWLEDGMENTS

This research was supported by National Institute of Neurological Diseases and Stroke grant NS 10727, Public Health Service Research grant RR-70 from the General Clinical Research Centers, Division of Research Resources, and by INSERM to Dr Guilleminault.

REFERENCES

1. Shy GM, Drager GA: A neurologic syndrome associated with orthostatic hypotension. Arch Neurol 2:511, 1960.
2. Lockwood AH: Shy-Drager syndrome with abnormal respirations and antidiuretic hormone release. Arch Neurol 33:292, 1976.
3. Lehrman KL, Guilleminault C, Schroeder JS, Tilkian A, Forno LS: Sleep apnea in a patient with Shy-Drager syndrome. Arch Intern Med 138:206–209, 1978.

Secretion of Glucose, Growth Hormone, and Cortisol During Sleep in Patients With Obstructive Sleep Apnea

Laughton E Miles, Suzanne Austin, and Christian Guilleminault

PATIENTS AND METHODS

Eight male patients diagnosed with predominantly obstructive sleep apnea syndrome gave informed consent to undergo continuous blood withdrawal during wakefulness and sleep for determination of possible abnormal levels of hormonal secretion during sleep and/or circadian rhythm disturbances of the secretory pattern related to their sleep apnea syndrome.

All patients had complete physical examinations, detailed neurologic and otolaryngologic examinations, routine chemistries and hematologic studies, pulmonary function studies, chest X rays, and resting electrocardiograms. Their mean age was 55 years (range 34–62), and their mean weight was 106 kg (range 75–163). Two subjects had mild, maturity-onset diabetes. All had been previously monitored during nocturnal sleep and their mean Apnea Index (see Chapter 1 for definition) was 85 (range 62–140). A mean of 91% of their apneic episodes were obstructive, and they spent a mean of 59% of total sleep time without air exchange.

Polygraphic monitoring included simultaneous recording of electroencephalogram ($C_3/A_2 - C_4/A_1$ from the international 10-20 system), electrooculogram, digastric electromyogram, electrocardiogram (lead II), oral and nasal thermistors, and thoracic and abdominal movements. Gas-sterilized polyethylene tubing (PE-50) (Clay-Adams Inc, Parsippany, New Jersey) was inserted intravenously in the right or left forearm through a 16-gauge Abbocath-T intravenous Teflon catheter (Abbot Laboratories, North Chicago, Illinois). Blood was withdrawn continuously, using a Minipuls II pump (Gilson Medical Electronics Inc, Middleton, Wisconsin), at the rate of 15 ml/hr, and collected in six-minute aliquots. The blood withdrawal system had previously been treated with heparin and

© 1978 Alan R. Liss, Inc., 150 Fifth Avenue, New York, NY 10011

tridodecylmethylammonium chloride (TDMAC) (Polysciences Inc, Warrington, Pennsylvania) to enable the blood to be withdrawn without the use of soluble anticoagulants, but each aliquot of blood was mixed with EDTA. Blood plasma was stored frozen for subsequent assay for glucose (Beckmann Glucose Analyzer, Beckmann Instruments Inc, Palo Alto, California), cortisol (radioimmunoassay) (Micromedic Diagnostics Inc, Horsham, Pennsylvania), and growth hormone (HGH) (two-site immunoradiometric assay) [1].

The blood withdrawals were carried out for varying durations and with variable start times, because the patients were admitted primarily for other diagnostic or therapeutic procedures. Nevertheless, the blood withdrawals always included the early portion of nocturnal sleep when obstructive apnea was severe. On one occasion (patient PT), severe venous spasm resulted in the blood withdrawal being prematurely terminated after four hours. One patient (FL) was simultaneously receiving intermittent boluses of intravenous heparin because of preexisting recurrent thrombophlebitis.

RESULTS

Results of all eight patients are shown in Figures 1 through 8. The HGH and cortisol patterns consist of an unusually large number of experimental determinations plotted on a relatively extended time axis. These factors allow assay variance and minor fluctuations in plasma concentrations to become especially evident.

The overall results can be summarized as follows. Growth hormone secretion was minimal and, when present, was usually associated with stress. Five secretory episodes occurred at catheter insertion and two at catheter removal. Three secretory episodes were temporally related to the occurrence of chest pain or difficulty with the blood withdrawal during the night. Six episodes appeared to be associated with REM sleep and, in three subjects, minor episodes occurred less than one hour after final wake. Only three subjects (FL, PT, MC) had brief episodes of stage 3 slow wave sleep. In two of these subjects (PT and MC), the slow wave sleep had a temporal relationship with very minor episodes of HGH secretion; in both subjects HGH secretion elsewhere during the night was of greater magnitude. Overall, only three episodes of HGH secretion were greater than 1.5 ng/ml, and none was over 4 ng/ml. In normal adult males HGH usually rises to greater than 10 ng/ml during nocturnal sleep.

The plasma cortisol patterns generally appeared to be within normal limits. In some subjects, the morning cortisol values were unusually low, and there was

ome indication of a phase shift in the circadian acrophase or nadir. This pos-
ibility could not be confirmed without obtaining frequent samples over a more
xtended period. On at least seven occasions, plasma cortisol secretion was
pparently associated with mild stress of either catheter insertion or manipula-
ion, or chest pain; there appeared to be a tendency for cortisol to show fluctua-
ions which were reciprocal to the changes occurring in plasma growth hormone.

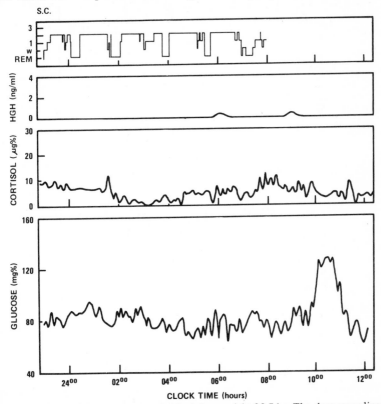

Fig 1. Patient SC: male, age 52 years, height 1.8 m, weight 90.7 kg. The sleep recording
showed findings typical of severe obstructive sleep apnea, including absence of slow wave
sleep. HGH secretion was minimal (less than 50 pg/ml) throughout the night except for
two very small secretory episodes at 0600 (immediately following an REM period) and 0900
during wakefulness. The plasma cortisol nadir was at about 0300 and the probable circadian
acrophase at about 0800 (wake onset). Other secretion might have been associated with
catheter insertion (2300) and disrupted sleep before an REM period (0130). Plasma glucose
fluctuated from 65 to 90 mg% except for a rise following breakfast. There was some tendency for the glucose to fall throughout the night, but there was no evidence of hypoglycemia.

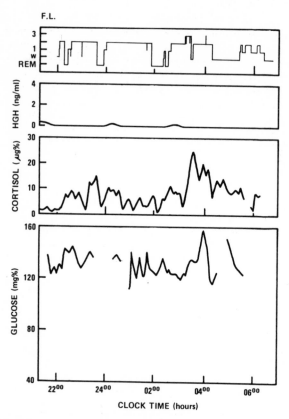

Fig 2. Patient FL: diabetic male, age 54 years, height 1.7 m, weight 115.8 kg. The diabetes was treated by diet alone. This was an abnormal study owing to the necessity for hourly administration of intravenous heparin. Sleep recording showed only two brief periods of slow wave (stage 3) sleep at about 0330 and findings were typical of severe obstructive sleep apnea. HGH secretion was minimal (less than 50 pg/ml) throughout the night except for two very small episodes at 2400 and 0230, each of which followed an episode of REM sleep. There was also a very small rise of HGH at the time of catheter insertion. Plasma cortisol was lowest at 2200 and highest at 0400 with a secondary peak at 2330. Plasma glucose was chronically elevated and fluctuated from 110 to 160 mg%.

Plasma glucose tended to fluctuate throughout sleep with the values varying about 20%. Consistent rises occurred following meals, and there were no episodes of hypoglycemia. Two subjects with maturity onset diabetes showed generally elevated plasma glucose levels.

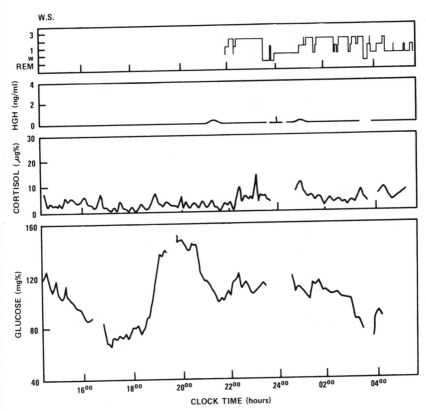

Fig 3. Patient WS: male, age 34 years, height 1.9 m, weight 163.3 kg. Sleep recording showed no slow wave sleep, long periods of wakefulness, and findings typical of severe obstructive sleep apnea. HGH secretion was minimal (less than 50 pg/ml) throughout the night except for two very small episodes at 2130 and 0100 which both occurred during wakefulness. The second episode may also have been associated with stress during temporary difficulty with the blood withdrawal. Plasma cortisol showed a possible phase-lead shift of the circadian nadir (1800) and acrophase (2300-0100), but the clock time of usual acrophase (0800) was not seen. There was significant secretion of cortisol associated with sleep onset (2200) and possible stress (0100). Plasma glucose fell to normal levels with fasting (1700 and 0400) and was elevated for several hours after meals (2000). WS is known to be an untreated mild maturity-onset diabetic.

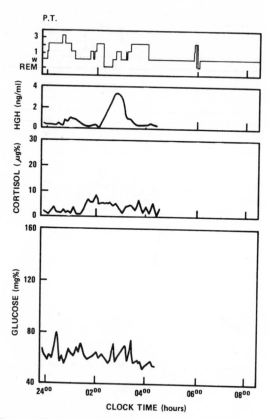

Fig 4. Patient PT: male, age 57 years, height 1.7 m, 137.2 kg. Study terminated prematurely owing to difficulty with blood withdrawal. Sleep recording showed one brief episode of slow wave sleep at 0030, long periods of wakefulness, and findings typical of severe obstructive sleep apnea. HGH showed a small rise (0.9 ng/ml) which may relate to the episode of slow wave sleep. There was a later rise to 3.3 ng/ml without a conclusive association. Cortisol was lowest at 0100 and maximal at 0200 after long wake and possible stress; the plasma glucose remained within normal limits at 55 to 75 mg%.

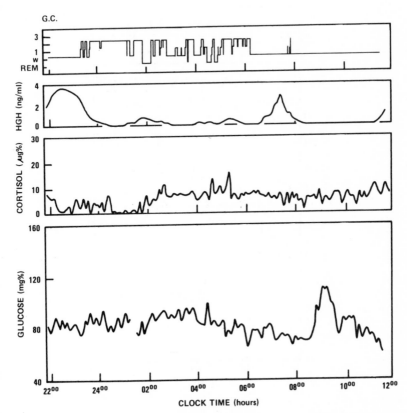

Fig 5. Patient GC: male, age 57 years, height 1.7 m, 74.8 kg. Sleep recordings showed no slow wave sleep, many brief awakenings, and findings typical of severe obstructive sleep apnea. HGH showed a stress rise at catheter insertion and removal. There were several very minor secretory episodes throughout the night without conclusive associations, and an unexplained rise at about 0700 after final awakening. Plasma cortisol showed a nadir at about 0100, a probable circadian acrophase at about 0500, and a possible stress rise at the time of catheter removal. Plasma glucose appeared normal with a gradual fall (80–95 to 70–75 mg%) throughout the night, followed by a normal rise after breakfast.

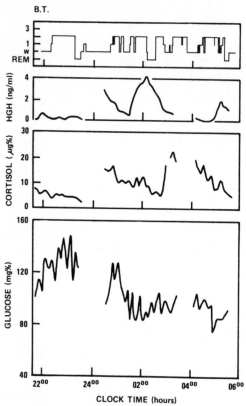

Fig 6. Patient BT: male, age 62 years, height 1.85 m, weight 108.9 kg. Difficulties with blood withdrawal at midnight and about 0330 due to venous spasm. The sleep recordings showed no slow wave sleep, many long awakenings, and findings typical of severe obstructive sleep apnea. HGH showed a probable stress rise to 3 ng/ml due to catheter manipulations about midnight. There was also a rise to 4 ng/ml at 0200, just before the second REM period, not obviously associated with any particular sleep stage. There was also a small HGH peak just before the final REM period and near the time of final wake. Plasma cortisol showed a nadir at about 2330, a probable stress rise at 0030, and major secretory activity at 0300-0500. This might indicate a minor phase shift in the circadian acrophase. Plasma glucose showed a rise following the evening meal to 145 mg% and values which fluctuated from 80 to 100 mg% during the night.

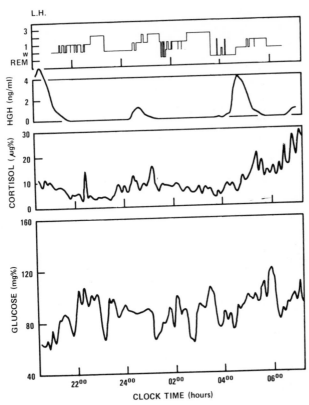

Fig 7. Patient LH: male, age 62 years, height 1.7 m, weight 78.7 kg. Sleep recordings showed no slow wave sleep, multiple brief awakenings, and one long awakening associated with anginal chest pain which was terminated by sublingual nitroglycerine. There were also findings typical of severe obstructive sleep apnea. HGH showed stress rises on intravenous catheter insertion and removal, and a small rise to 1.2 ng/ml associated with either stress or the nitroglycerine. There was also a rise to 4 ng/ml at 0500 which coincides with sleep stage REM. Plasma cortisol showed a nadir at about 2330 and was still rising towards an acrophase at 0700, with a secondary peak at about 0100 and 0530. Plasma glucose varied fairly widely from 70 to 115 mg% with no obvious associations.

ACKNOWLEDGMENTS

This research was supported by National Institute of Mental Health grant MH 29861; National Institute of Neurological Diseases and Stroke grant NS 10727; Public Health Service Research grant RR-70 from the General Clinical Research Centers, Division of Research Resources; and by the Institute for Medical Research of Santa Clara County, California.

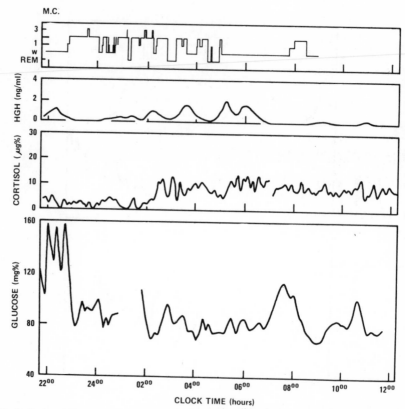

Fig 8. Patient MC: male, age 58 years, height 1.8 m, weight 83.0 kg. Sleep recordings showed only transitory episodes of slow wave (stage 3) sleep at about 2330, 0115, and 0200; multiple brief awakenings, one long wake between 0500 and 0740, and findings typical of severe obstructive sleep apnea. HGH showed small secretory peaks associated with catheter insertion and final awakening. In addition, there were four small peaks of progressively increasing amplitude during sleep. At no time did the amplitude exceed 2 ng/ml, and there was no obvious relationship to any sleep stage. Plasma cortisol showed minimal values between 2300 and 0130 and an apparent circadian acrophase at about 0600. Plasma glucose showed rises following the evening meal and breakfast, and fluctuated from 70 to 90 mg% during sleep.

REFERENCES

1. Miles LEM: Immunoradiometric (IRMA) and 2-site IRMA assay systems. In Abraham GE (ed): "Handbook of Radioimmunoassay." New York: Macmillan, 1977, pp 131–177.

23
Diaphragm Pacing in the Management of Central Alveolar Hypoventilation

William WL Glenn, Mildred Phelps, and Larry M Gersten

BACKGROUND

Electrical stimulation of the phrenic nerves as a method of artificial respiration began about 200 years ago in the second half of the 18th century. Static electrical machines were used as the source of electricity for therapeutics in the mid 18th century followed early in the 19th by electrical discharges from the voltaic battery. After the discovery of inductive electricity by Faraday in 1834 stimulation of excitable tissue by this technique became popular. Around the middle of the 19th century artificial respiration by electrical stimulation of the phrenic nerve was an accepted method in at least some French hospitals for the treatment of respiratory arrest. By 1875 the location of the phrenic nerve in the neck was well-known and its stimulation transcutaneously was a standard practice among electrotherapeutists [1]. As a method of artificial ventilation this was a temporary expedient at best, and when more efficient means of artificial ventilation using negative pressure body chambers and endotracheal positive pressure breathing devices were developed early in the 20th century, phrenic nerve stimulation was set aside.

Artificial respiration by phrenic nerve stimulation was briefly revived by Sarnoff in 1948 for the treatment of patients with bulbar poliomyelitis [2]. In his patients Sarnoff stimulated the nerve in the neck either through a wire passed percutaneously around the nerve or transcutaneously through skin electrodes placed over the nerve. He gave the technique the name of electrophrenic respiration or EPR. As with the earlier use of phrenic nerve stimulation by these techniques, artificial respiration could be sustained for hours or, at most, a few days. With the isolation of the poliomyelitis virus and development of an effective vaccine in the early 1950s, interest in phrenic nerve stimulation for artificial respiration again waned.

Sleep Apnea Syndromes, pages 333–345

Our interest in artificial respiration by phrenic nerve stimulation evolved from our work in 1958 with Mauro [3] on the development of an implantable electrical cardiac pacemaker employing radiofrequency (RF) induction. Neural tissue was stimulated through RF induction by Lafferty and Farrell [4] in animal experiments using splanchnic nerve stimulation. We adapted the RF technique to the phrenic nerves in our laboratories in 1962. As the end organ was the diaphragm, we deemed it appropriate to speak of electrical pacing of the diaphragm. The technique was first applied to a patient with acute ventilatory insufficiency in 1964 [5] and to a patient with the chronic form in 1966 [6]. Since that time a diaphragm pacemaker has been implanted in 153 patients in this country and abroad, 48 of whom were operated upon at Yale-New Haven Medical Center.

THE DIAPHRAGM PACEMAKER

The diaphragm pacemaker consists of four parts: a radiofrequency generator and transmitter, an external coil or antenna, a radiofrequency receiver, and neural electrodes. The programmed RF pulse is transmitted via the antenna through the intact skin to the RF receiver in the subcutaneous tissue where it is converted to electrical pulses delivered via wire electrodes to the phrenic nerve. The details of the electronic apparatus and the method of its application have been described elsewhere [6, 7].

Technique of Implantation of Receiver-Electrode Assembly

The radio receiver and neural electrode are implanted subcutaneously under local anesthesia. The phrenic nerve is identified in the neck as its passes over the anterior scalene muscle. Only minimal dissection is undertaken for placement of the neural electrode to avoid injury to the nerve. The electrode can be either monopolar (cathode) or bipolar, though we prefer the monopolar, entailing less dissection of the nerve. An indifferent (anode) electrode is implanted subcutaneously, usually through the same incision on the anterior chest wall as that made for inserting the radio receiver.

The system is activated when the externally located antenna attached to the transmitter is placed on the skin overlying the receiver.

CLINICAL APPLICATION

Indications

Diaphragm pacing is indicated in chronic ventilatory insufficiency without significant impairment of phrenic nerves, lungs, or diaphragm. Pacing is contrandicated if insufficiency is due to a lesion of the lower motor neurons of the phrenic nerve, to a muscular dystrophy affecting the diaphragm, or to extensive parenchymal lung disease. Also, acute ventilatory insufficiency such as follows acute poisonings, surgical operations, or other conditions that give rise to short-term hypoventilation are better treated by conventional methods, ie, endotracheal intubation and positive pressure respiration.

Clinical Material

Specifically, four categories of patients have been successfully treated by diaphragm pacing (Table I).

The first category consists of patients with quadriplegia secondary to a lesion of the cervical cord above the level of the phrenic nerve cell bodies (C3-5). Such patients are totally paralyzed from the neck down but have viable lower motor neurons below the site of cord transection [7].

We have placed pacemakers in 12 patients in this category. In nine instances quadriplegia resulted from traumatic injury to the cord, in seven above C-3 and in two between C-3 and C-5. In three cases quadriplegia developed as a complication of meningitis.

TABLE I. Diaphragm Pacing in the Management of Chronic Hypoventilation*

	Respiratory center involvement		Parenchymal lung disease		Incomplete cervical cord lesion		Complete cervical cord lesion (quadriplegia)	
Etiology	Encephalitis	7	COPD	1	Poliomyelitis	2	Trauma	9
	CVA	5			Atlanto-occipital deformity	2	Meningitis	3
	Unknown	5			Bilateral cervical			
	Trauma	4			cordotomy	1		
	Leigh disease	4			Syringomyelia	1		
	Brain stem cyst or tumor	3						
	Shock therapy	1						
Total cases		29		1		6		12
Duration of pacing (mean, months) through June 30, 1977		36		35		29		32
Range (months)		1–99		35		7–47		4–79

*Yale series, 48 cases (as of June 30, 1977).

The second category comprises patients with hypoventilation secondary to organic lesions of the spinal cord or brain stem that interrupts afferent or efferent neurons to the respiratory center or involves the respiratory center directly. There is commonly other manifestation of neurologic disease, such as partial paralysis of skeletal muscle groups.

Six of our patients were in this category. In two, an incomplete cord lesion was caused by poliomyelitis. Two had an atlanto-occipital deformity, one a bilateral cervical cordotomy, and one a syringomyelia.

A third category contains those patients with chronic obstructive lung disease who are oxygen sensitive and in whom the function of the lungs and diaphragm can be improved by diaphragm pacing. Thus far we have paced only one patient in this category [8].

The fourth, and thus far the largest, category is that of patients with central alveolar hypoventilation (Ondine's curse). Characteristically these patients exhibit CO_2 retention and hypoxemia, most markedly during sleep, cor pulmonale with right heart failure, near normal ventilatory capacity (Fig 1), and diminished or absent ventilatory control responses to induced hypoxemia and hypercapnia.

Twenty-nine patients in our series fall into this category. The etiology of their hypoventilation was usually not definite at the time of initial referral for treatment. In our series of 29 there was a history at least suggestive of encephalitis in seven patients. In five, a cerebrovascular accident (CVA) was documented involving the brain stem. Four patients gave a history of trauma to the brain and in four others a presumptive diagnosis of Leigh's disease was made. In three patients a tumor or cyst involving the medulla was diagnosed, and in one patient loss of ventilatory control followed shock therapy. No etiology was apparent in five patients.

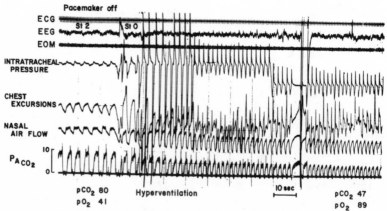

Fig 1. Central alveolar hypoventilation. This patient developed marked hypoventilation during sleep but was able to return his arterial blood gases to near normal through hyperventilation.

ESULTS

Quadriplegia. Eleven of the 12 patients in this category underwent bilateral acemaker implantation; the 12th, who had a C-4 transection of the cord and as left with minimal viability of his phrenic nerves, had a pacemaker implanted n only one side. Eight have achieved full-time ventilatory support for 1 to 74 nonths, an average of 29 months. Two patients achieved part-time support for nore than 50% of the time. The two other patients whose spinal cords were raumatized in the region of the phrenic nerve outflow (C3-5) could only be aced on one side and were supported by pacing for only a few hours each day.)ne of these latter two died of respiratory insufficiency, and another patient vho was fully supported by pacing died because of meningitis.

Incomplete spinal cord injury. Four of the six patients in this category re- eived unilateral pacemakers for nocturnal support of ventilation. Two have equired bilateral pacing, one with syringomyelia, another with an atlanto- ccipital deformity. The group has been paced for 7 to 47 months, an average f 29 months. One patient, in whom ventilatory insufficiency was secondary to ilateral cervical cordotomy, died of metastatic sarcoma 20 months after pacing egan.

Chronic obstructive lung disease. The one patient has been paced unilaterally luring sleep. Pacing-protected oxygenation has been possible for 35 months.

Central alveolar hypoventilation. Nocturnal pacing has been carried out in 29 atients for 8 to 12 hours daily for two weeks to 99 months, an average of 36 nonths. There have been seven deaths, five due to the underlying disease, one o pacemaker failure, and one to sedation.

In summary, 48 patients with chronic ventilatory insufficiency have been reated in our institution by diaphragm pacing (Table I). There were 29 with he diagnosis of central alveolar hypoventilation, 12 with quadriplegia, six with ncomplete cord lesions, and one with chronic obstructive pulmonary disease nd oxygen sensitivity. Their ages ranged from 2 to 71 years, and the mean age vas 42.75 years. Successful pacing of one hemidiaphragm for nocturnal support f ventilation has been carried out for more than eight years and of both hemi- liaphragms for total ventilatory support for more than six years.

COMMENT

In the process of caring for these individuals a number of problems have arisen and some new information has been acquired. The problems can be divided into those related to: first, the electronic apparatus, second, the direct effect of long-term electrical stimulation on neural and muscular tissue, specifi- cally the phrenic nerve and diaphragm; and third, the alteration of the normal respiratory cycle by the electrical pacing of the diaphragm.

Beyond a brief mention, the first two problems do not concern us here. The electronic apparatus has on the whole performed with a minimum of difficulty except for the RF receiver. Due to the ingress of body fluid, failure of the internal components of the receiver was a frequent complication early in our experience. Now, using an integrated circuit that can be sealed hermetically, receiver failure is uncommon.

As regards damage to the phrenic nerve tissue by electrical stimulation, we believe that none results from the minimal current required in diaphragm pacing. The cumulative charge to the phrenic nerve in 24 hours at 15 respirations/min with 35 electrical impulses/respiration is 0.567 coul, well below that shown to be safe for the brain in short-term experiments [9]. Histopathologic studies of human phrenic nerves which were stimulated two to four years support the belief that any phrenic nerve injury must be due to surgical trauma rather than to the electrical stimulus and thus is probably preventable [10]. Our information on the effects of pacing on the diaphragm muscle is incomplete. One might expect maximal contraction over a long period to cause muscular hypertrophy, and we have seen this, but further investigation is necessary.

Of particular interest in the investigation of patients prone to sleep apnea is the effect of pacing on respiratory function. We have recently reported our early experience with pacing as it relates to sleep apnea [11], and the present account is an extension of that work.

Effect of Pacing on Respiratory Function

Bilateral phrenic stimulation is more physiologic than unilateral as adequate ventilation is possible with submaximal contraction of both hemidiaphragms, but such stimulation places both phrenic nerves at risk of injury and is not justified for part-time pacing at the present time.

The electrical impulses that stimulate the phrenic nerve can be programmed to mimic the patient's normal flow vs volume curve, but attaining an adequate minute ventilation while stimulating only one phrenic nerve requires maximum contraction of the hemidiaphragm. Fatigue of the diaphragm under these circumstances occurs quickly unless the ratio of the duration of inspiration to expiration is maintained at about 1:2. If inspiration is prolonged, fatigue results and, if it is shortened, inspiration is abrupt and tidal volume decreases. At a respiratory rate of 15/min each cycle lasts four seconds and inspiration is about 1.3 seconds in duration. The effect of maximal contraction of the hemidiaphragm occurring over such a short period is to create a sudden increase in negative intrapleural and intrathoracic pressure (Fig 2). If the patient is sleeping at the time, and, particularly if he is prone to upper airway obstruction, the effect of the increase in negative pressure on flaccid pharyngeal muscles is to cause them to collapse, producing obstruction to air flow. In the presence of partial or complete upper airway obstruction this effect of pacing would be markedly accen-

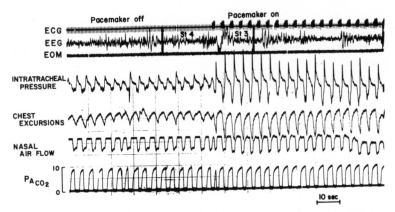

Fig 2. The effect of maximal contraction of the hemidiaphragm during pacing. Note increase in chest excursions and in positive and negative intratracheal pressures. In other studies using an intraesophageal balloon an increase was shown in intrathoracic negative pressures during diaphragm pacing.

tuated, resulting in an increase in the frequency and duration of obstruction (Fig 3). Pacing-induced obstruction may also be related to an interruption of the normal reflex that controls patency of the upper airway during normal respiration.

Sleep Apneas

Sleep studies were carried out in all of the patients with central alveolar hypoventilation (CAH) who required pacing except two small children. Early in our experience only an arterial blood gas study was made. The methodology of these sleep studies has been described in detail elsewhere [11].

Some patients with CAH, in contrast to individuals with normal sensitivity to hypoxia and hypercapnia, may not vigorously resist apnea of central origin or that due to obstruction. In several patients, an upper airway obstruction (UAO) was not suspected until a sleep study was carried out with the pacemaker operating. The ventilatory responses to hypoxia or inhaled CO_2 in all of the patients we studied were without exception subnormal or absent [12]. The usual patterns of sleep apneas were identified: central, obstruction, a combination of these and, in addition, several patterns of pacer-induced apneas.

In the course of our studies on 29 patients with CAH who required pacing of one hemidiaphragm, we have detected upper airway obstruction in 15, about one-half the total group. The incidence is probably higher as all of these patients were not specifically studied for UAO. Thirteen of the 15 patients with UAO have required a tracheostomy. Eleven of these patients have had a repeat overnight study. In three patients the repeat study showed only moderate hypoventilation during spontaneous respiration after tracheostomy. In two of them the

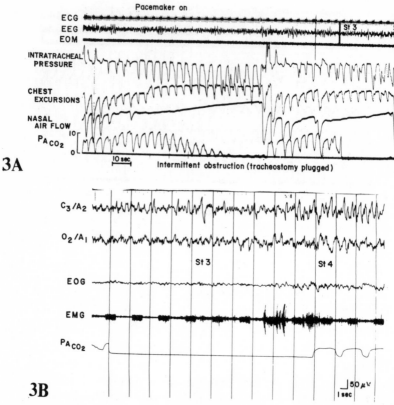

3A

3B

Fig 3. A) An increase in the duration and frequency of upper airway obstruction was demonstrated in patients who had evidence of obstruction before pacing was instituted. Note the prolonged period of obstruction (about 80 seconds) during pacing. The intratracheal pressure becomes increasingly negative as the obstruction persists. The pacemaker artifact is superimposed on the ECG recording. B) This recording represents the time between the two vertical lines in A. The patient was in stage 3 and 4 sleep. (from Glenn WWL, PACE, 1978, with permission).

ventilatory control studies are still abnormal and pacing is being continued. In the other eight, although there was some improvement in ventilation following tracheostomy with the patient breathing spontaneously, there is still significant hypoventilation as evidenced from the grossly abnormal arterial blood gases, indicating the persistence of CAH and the need for ventilatory support by diaphragm pacing (Table II). In four of these patients ventilatory responses to hypoxia and CO_2 inhalation continue to be suboptimal or absent following tracheostomy. The remaining four have not been restudied [11].

Of particular interest was the effect of diaphragm pacing on apnea of central origin or apnea due to obstruction. Usually pacing prevented central apnea but

TABLE II. Arterial Blood Gas Study in Patients With CAH and UAO Before and After Tracheostomy

Patient number	Condition	Pretracheostomy				Posttracheostomy			
		pH	pCO_2	pO_2	(sat %)	pH	pCO_2	pO_2	(sat %)
2	Awake	7.52	36	74	95	7.36	50	71	92
	Asleep	7.38	62	33	61	7.35	52	43	76
3	Awake	7.35	66	30	57	7.34	58	40	72
	Asleep	7.35	70	26	46	7.33	60	42	74
5	Awake	7.32	89	64	88	7.49	52	73	95
	Asleep	7.25	100	60	85	7.37	72	52	85
6	Awake	7.42	60	38	74	7.39	50	60	89
	Asleep	7.40	63	36	68	7.24	74	40	67
9	Awake	7.37	48	62	90	7.33	54	40	83
	Asleep	7.33	53	37	70	7.31	57	45	79
11	Awake	7.42	38	59	89	7.53	28	96	97
	Asleep	7.31	55	31	60	7.36	42	36	71
14	Awake	7.46	33	70	94	7.39	42	62	91
	Asleep	7.32	59	43	75	7.35	51	46	80
16	Awake	7.34	55	54	86	7.41	36	66	92
	Asleep	7.26	76	45	80	7.30	55	56	85

in three patients with prolonged and frequent episodes of central apnea and who had shown no evidence of UAO, pacing caused obstruction. In one patient the development of obstruction when paced during episodes of central apnea appeared to be related to the stage of sleep. In stage 4, pacing caused obstruction, while in stage 1 pacing relieved central apnea without causing obstruction (Fig 4).

Postpacing apnea has been a constant finding in patients with CAH (Fig 5). Usually the apneic periods are of short duration, 10–20 seconds, but in some patients apnea was prolonged when pacing was discontinued, lasting for a minute or more. On the basis of available data we suspect that the arterial carbon dioxide level at the time of pacing is discontinued, correlated with the patient's ventilatory response to inhaled CO_2, and is the determining factor in the duration of postpacing apnea. The stage of sleep may also be a factor.

CONCLUSIONS

1. Electrical pacing of the diaphragm by modern techniques is a safe and effective method for prolonged artificial respiration.

2. Many patients with sleep apnea or hypoventilation of central origin also have at least the potential for UAO.

3. Effective treatment of individuals with both CAH and UAO is tracheostomy and diaphragm pacing.

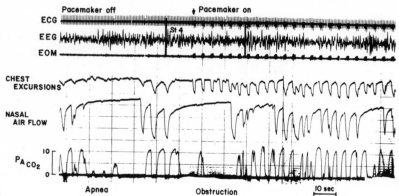

ECG · EEG · EOM · CHEST EXCURSIONS · NASAL AIR FLOW · $P_{A_{CO_2}}$

Pacemaker off · Pacemaker on · St 4 · Apnea · Obstruction · 10 sec

4A

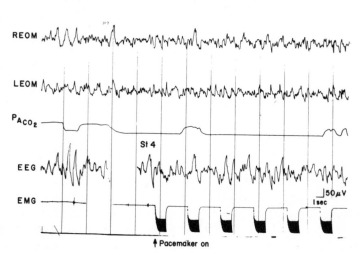

REOM · LEOM · $P_{A_{CO_2}}$ · EEG · EMG

St 4 · 50 μV · 1 sec · Pacemaker on

4B

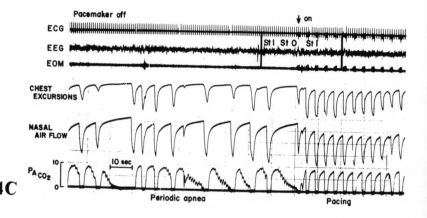

ECG · EEG · EOM · CHEST EXCURSIONS · NASAL AIR FLOW · $P_{A_{CO_2}}$

Pacemaker off · on · St I St O St I · 10 sec · Periodic apnea · Pacing

4C

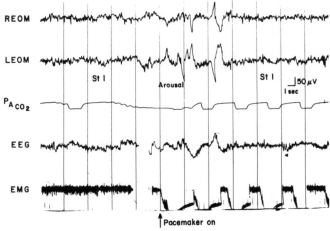

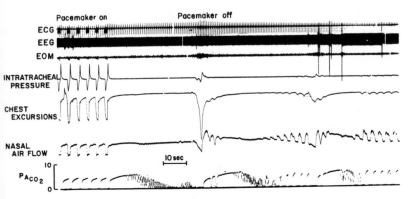

Fig 4. A) This patient with central alveolar hypoventilation developed repeated episodes of prolonged apnea. When the diaphragm pacemaker was activated episodes of upper airway obstruction replaced central apnea. B) Note that he was in stage 3 to 4 sleep during this period. C) Later in the night the above study was repeated. This time the patient was in a lighter stage of sleep (stage 1) and when the pacemaker was turned on the pattern of periodic central apnea was broken. Upper airway obstruction did not develop. D) Sleep stage 1.

Fig 5. Postpacing apnea in a patient with central alveolar hypoventilation and upper airway obstruction. The tracheal stoma was open; the patient was breathing room air. The arterial blood gases just prior to turning off the pacemaker were $PaCO_2$ 29, PaO_2 67, pH 7.47. Earlier in the evening with the patient breathing spontaneously and the tracheostomy stoma plugged the arterial blood gases with $PaCO_2$ 60, PaO_2 50, pH 7.26. Upper airway obstruction was not evident at this time.

ACKNOWLEDGMENTS

I gratefully acknowledge the assistance of Mr James Hogan, and Mr Jack Gorfien. I am also appreciative of the assistance of Mrs L Jacobs in the preparation of this manuscript .

This study was supported by grants HL-04651 from the National Heart and Lung Institute and RR-00125 of the National Institutes of Health and by the Culpeper Foundation.

REFERENCES

1. Beard GM, Rockwell AD: "A Practical Treatise on the Medical and Surgical Use of Electricity." New York: William Wood & Co, 1878, Chap 35.
2. Sarnoff SJ, Hardenbergh E, Whittenberger JL: Electrophrenic respiration. Science 108: 482, 1948.
3. Glenn WWL, Mauro A, Longo E, Lavietes DH, Mackay FJ: Remote stimulation of the heart by radiofrequency transmission. N Engl J Med 261:948–952, 1959.
4. Lafferty JM, Farrell JJ: A new technique for chronic remote stimulation. Science 110 140–141, 1949.
5. Glenn WWL, Hageman JH, Mauro A, Eisenberg L, Flanigan S, Harvard M: Electrical stimulation of excitable tissue by radiofrequency transmission. Ann Surg 160:338– 350, 1964.
6. Glenn WWL, Holcomb WG, Hogan J, Matano I, Gee JBL, Motoyama EK, Kim CS, Poirier CS, Forbes G: Diaphragm pacing by radiofrequency transmission in the treatment of chronic ventilatory insufficiency. J Thorac Cardiovasc Surg 66:505–520, 1973.
7. Glenn WWL, Holcomb WG, Shaw RK, Hogan J, Holschoh K: Long-term ventilatory support by diaphragm pacing in quadriplegia. Ann Surg 183:566–577, 1976.
8. Glenn WWL, Gee JBL, Schachter EN: Diaphragm pacing: Application to a patient with chronic obstructive lung disease. J Thorac Cardiovasc Surg 75:273–281, 1978.
9. Rowland V, MacIntyre WJ, Bidder TG: The production of brain lesions with electric currents. II. Bidirectional currents. J Neurosurg 17:55–69, 1960.
10. Kim JH, Manuelidis EE, Glenn WWL, Kaneyuki T: Diaphragm pacing: Histopathological changes in the phrenic nerve following long-term electrical stimulation. J Thorac Cardiovasc Surg 72:602–608, 1976.
11. Glenn WWL, Gee JBL, Cole DR et al: Combined central and obstruction alveolar hypoventilation: Treatment by tracheostomy and diaphragm pacing. Am J Med 64:39–49, 1978.
12. Farmer WC, Glenn WWL, Gee JBL: Alveolar hypoventilation syndrome: Studies of ventilatory control in patients selected for diaphragm pacing. Am J Med 64:50–60, 1978.

DISCUSSION

Dr Severinghaus inquired whether transected patients ever retained a central respiratory rhythm differing from the pacer-induced rhythm or if, as soon as pacing began, the central rhythm disappeared. Dr Glenn responded that quadplegics with complete transection, although they have normal respiratory centers, become very anxious when they are not paced and not getting enough oxygen, but there is no peripheral evidence (flaring of the nostrils, etc) of central rhythm. A very cooperative patient breathed enough CO_2 to reach a very high level, and he described a tremendous desire to breathe but there was no visible evidence of it. This is in contrast to the classical experiment by Campbell who curarized himself and, although his pCO_2 rose to approximately 70 mg, he reported absolutely no desire to breathe. Dr Phillipson recalled a reported case of a Toronto woman with a C2-C3 transection. Despite the fact that great care was taken so that there would be no change in blood gases, minute volume, or tidal volume, when the pacing was switched from the right to left side the patient complained of "shortness of breath" lasting for 30 seconds to one minute. In this case the only connection between trunk and brain was the vagus nerves. Dr Glenn noted that he had seen similar cases.

The participants expressed the need to test chemoreceptor sensitivity during sleep in both central and obstructive sleep apneic patients. Dr Weil recalled the standard "Kinney technique," wherein a large box encloses the patient's head and, with a reasonable seal around the neck, a stream of air is pushed continuously into the box. Using newer technology it is possible not only to measure ventilation noninvasively, but also to measure oxygen consumption and CO_2 production.

Dr Dement noted the need to consider both the risk of pace maker implantation in a patient with intermittent periods of central sleep apnea and the long-term potential risks of the disorder itself. Dr Glenn felt that technically it is possible to obtain good results in patients with central sleep apnea although the indications for surgery in these patients are not as well defined as they are for patients with classical Ondine's curse.

24
Tracheostomy and Sleep Apnea

Michael W Hill, F Blair Simmons, and Christian Guilleminault

OTOLARYNGOLOGICAL EVALUATION

Over 150 patients (adults and children) have been seen at the Sleep Disorders Clinic for a sleep apnea syndrome. Eighty-five of them presented respiratory obstruction during sleep. All patients in whom continuous polygraphic recordings during sleep revealed a predominantly upper airway apnea syndrome are given complete otorhinolaryngological examinations. The majority of these patients have no obvious anatomical cause for their sleep pathology. Laryngoscopy has been normal in all cases, except in one child an anterior laryngeal web was found. The common denominator in this group is a short, thick neck with normoglossia, and an occasional relative macroglossia secondary to a mild mandibular hypoplasia [1].

If an obvious airway obstruction is discovered, ie, enlarged tonsils, hypertrophied adenoids, markedly deviated nasal septum, laryngeal web, etc, it is surgically corrected and the patient is then restudied with an all-night polygraphic recording. These were the findings in 25 cases: enlarged tonsils and hypertrophied adenoids in 16 children and four adults, markedly deviated septum in five adults. In those cases where minor surgery was unsuccessful (two children and six adults, including the five patients whose deviated septums were repaired) or no anatomical obstruction was found, the patient became a candidate for permanent tracheostomy.

SURGICAL MANAGEMENT OF AIRWAY OBSTRUCTION DURING SLEEP

Tracheostomy is performed only as a last resort where cardiovascular parameters and social factors dictate [2]. Upper airway apnea patients present some challenging medical, surgical, and social problems with respect to tracheostomy.

Sleep Apnea Syndromes, pages 347–352

Preoperatively, there are two issues which the surgical-anesthetic team must discuss. In our experience, the use of barbiturates or other sedative preoperatively is extremely dangerous. It has been documented that these patients are much more susceptible to the respiratory depression associated with these medications. A fatal apneic episode might well be precipitated [3]. With proper counseling a relaxed and sleepy patient will arrive in the operating room.

The second issue is that there is no such entity as a "routine tracheostomy" in a sleep apnea patient. An anesthesiologist without previous experience with hypersomnia-sleep apnea (HSA) patients must sometimes be convinced of this. We are prepared to treat each of these as if an emergency tracheostomy might be necessary. These short-, thick-necked individuals represent a difficult intubation. Emergency airway obstructions have been precipitated in two patients by competent anesthesiologists early in our study who were simply unable to intubate them. In both instances, emergency local tracheostomies had to be performed. In these cases, the anesthesiologist was unable to intubate the patient, after induction in one case and supraglottic edema and bleeding resulting from intubation trauma in the other.

Most intubations are under general anesthesia. The tracheostomy is then performed in an orderly fashion. A general anesthetic is preferred in these usually thick-necked individuals.

Utilizing a generous transverse cervical incision, a standard tracheostomy is performed with the following modification: A permanent tracheal fenestration is created. This has been done satisfactorily by utilizing tracheal and cervical flaps. Creation of two horizontal, laterally based cervical flaps and an H incision in the anterior tracheal wall results in a permanent but easily reversible tracheal stoma [4]. Some defating may be necessary prior to flap advancement. Closure of skin to tracheal mucosa enhances healing and reduces granulations. An antibiotic ointment is placed on the closure line until complete healing has taken place. Sutures are removed in 10–14 days.

We have observed that some of these obstructive apnea patients have small tracheas with respect to other individuals of comparable size. Selection of an appropriate tracheostomy tube with respect to size and curve is critical to avoid the long-term sequelae of indwelling tracheostomy tubes. Our choice in most cases is a #6 Moore Silastic tracheostomy tube. This tube is soft and flexible and adapts nicely to the neck-tracheal contours encountered in sleep apnea patients. The tube may or may not be fenestrated prior to initial placement (Fig 1). Without this fenestration, some of the patients are unable to ventilate comfortably with the tracheostomy tube plugged during waking hours. Routinely, we fenestrate the tracheostomy tube three to four days after surgery. The Moore tracheostomy tubes should be completely replaced every four months. They undergo a change in their chemical properties with time, becoming brittle, and then may fragment and become lodged in the tracheobronchial tree. By replacing them at the proper interval, this problem can be easily prevented. A protocol

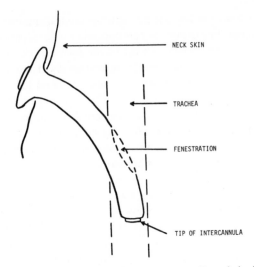

Fig 1. Fenestration of a tracheostomy tube (lateral view).

or postoperative management of the tracheostomy tube with respect to suction and mist is included at the end of this chapter.

Since June 6, 1973, 30 tracheostomies for upper airway sleep apnea syndrome have been performed, 28 in adults and two in children. Twenty-seven of these patients presented upper airway sleep apnea, two adult patients had a combination of upper airway sleep apnea and narcolepsy, and one adult patient had a combination of Shy-Drager syndrome and sleep apnea (see Chapter 21). The decision to perform tracheostomies in these cases was made only after multiple investigations which included not only cardiovascular and pulmonary evaluations during wakefulness and sleep, but also placement of a short pharyngeal airway tube which did not relieve the sleep related disorder, and intubation of patients followed by complete reevaluation during sleep. Surgical indications in the special cases are difficult. The narcoleptic sleep disorder and concomitant cataplexy are, of course, not relieved by this procedure. However, there was a decrease in daytime somnolence in our two patients with sleep apnea associated with narcolepsy, as well as in the sleep-apnea-related symptoms — particularly nocturnal asystole and daytime hypertension in one case. In all cases, tracheostomy has been successful in relieving the symptoms of upper airway obstructive apnea. These patients have, more importantly, benefited from a significant improvement in their cardiovascular parameters as documented by postoperative polygraphic recordings (see Chapters 11 and 12).

Our standard long-term follow-up, including nocturnal polygraphic monitoring in all cases with one every six to nine months for our first ten tracheostomized patients (the two children are included in this group), has been essentially free of serious complications. Immediate postoperative complications have been limited to atelectasis (in one patient) and pneumonia (two patients) in our series. Coughing is present in all patients to some degree postoperatively; however, severe paroxysmal coughing signals an improperly fitting tracheostomy tube. In these cases, immediate replacement with an appropriate substitute is of paramount importance.

Depression is the most common delayed complication, and as previously mentioned, preoperative counseling is of utmost importance. The patient and spouse are forewarned that this is normal and may last several months. This has not been a chronic problem in any of our patients, and most adjust in a much shorter time. In addition, detailed explanations of the surgical procedure; demonstration of the tracheostomy tube and its care with respect to mist and suction; and presentation of photographs of masked, tracheostomized patients for understanding of the cosmetic effect of the surgery are all important details which facilitate rapid adjustment. We have found that direct contact between volunteer patients who had had a tracheostomy for sleep apnea and the patient scheduled for surgery has given the best results. Children have even more difficulties in adjusting to this surgery, and interaction between the parents, the medical team — which may include a child psychiatrist if warranted — and teachers is of great importance. Unfortunately, we did not involve the school teachers in our first child case, and the child's normal social reintegration was considerably delayed.

Careful evaluation, sufficient therapeutic indication, preoperative psychological counseling, and in-hospital, postoperative patient training for tracheostomy care allow the patient and physician to deal with any long-term problems much more effectively. However, some caution is necessary to temper our optimism as our longest follow-up is only five years.

ACKNOWLEDGMENTS

This research was supported by National Institute of Neurological Diseases and Stroke grant NS 10727, Public Health Service Research Grant RR-70 from the General Clinical Research Centers, Division of Research Resources, and by INSERM to Dr Guilleminault.

REFERENCES

1. Simmons FB, Guilleminault C, Dement WC, Tilkian AG, Hill M: Surgical management of airway obstructions during sleep. Laryngoscope 87:326–338, 1977.
2. Guilleminault C, Eldridge FL, Simmons FB, Dement WC: Sleep apnea syndrome: Can it induce hemodynamic changes? West J Med 123:7–16, 1975.

Simmons FB, Hill MW: Hypersomnia caused by upper airway obstructions: A new syndrome in otolaryngology. Ann Otol Rhinol Laryngol 83:670–673, 1974.
Fee WE Jr, Ward PH: Permanent tracheostomy: A new surgical technique. Presentation at the Meeting of the American Broncho-Esophagological Association, Boston, Massachusetts, May 9–10, 1977 (in press).

PROTOCOL

Postoperative Care of the Sleep Apnea Patient After Tracheostomy

Goals. We want to get these patients on self-care and out of the hospital as rapidly as possible. Three factors influence hospital discharge: 1) ability of patient (and spouse or friend) to care for trach, 2) ability to do without mist while still keeping secretions moists, 3) infection. Orders are written with these in mind: antibiotic ointment to the trach stoma tid; decrease mist use as rapidly as possible (this varies from patient to patient) by substituting saline drops; insist that patient and family participate in daily care by the fourth day.

Time	Routine
1) First 2 hours postoperative	Tracheostomy suctioning every 15 minutes
Next 4 hours	Tracheostomy suctioning every 30 minutes
First 24 hours	Continuous mist to tracheostomy; apply antibiotic to tracheostomy stoma
2) Second 24 hours	During waking hours — 20 minutes off mist 10 minutes on mist
	Apply antibiotic ointment to tracheostomy stoma
3) Third 24 hours	During waking hours — 40 minutes off mist 20 minutes on mist 5 ml normal saline down tracheostomy in middle of off-mist period
	Apply antibiotic ointment
4) Fourth 24 hours	During waking hours — off mist continually 5 ml normal saline down tracheostomy every two hours
	Apply antibiotic ointment
5) Fifth 24 hours	Home mist may be supplied at home by several commercial agencies for nighttime use

6) Train patient to clean own tracheostomy tube and to suction himself; train how to use both suction and mist machines.

7) Suggested criteria for ability of patient to return home:
   a) ability to care for tracheostomy, including cleaning the inner cannula, self-suctioning, wound care;
   b) patient must feel at ease with tracheostomy;
   c) no evidence of respiratory rate increase from that of admission;
   d) patient ambulating vigorously about ward;
   e) amount and character of secretions from tracheostomy not suggestive of pulmonary infection;
   f) have patient's sleeping habits improved since surgery?

8) Have Social Service arrange for suction and mist machines for patient to take home or have available when he returns home.

Upon anticipated discharge from the hospital some decisions need to be made about individual patients, specifically with regard to mist use. If there is no one at home besides the patient, he will need home mist for nighttime sleeping for about three weeks. If there is someone at home who can put 3 ml of saline into the trach tube every two to four hours for the first week or so, a mist machine will not be needed. A suction machine is needed, and we recommend purchase, not rental, since there will be an intermittent need for suction indefinitely. Purchase is less expensive than renting.

Appendix 1.
General Discussion

Is Sleep Apnea a Familial Disorder?

Dr Coccagna reported that there are families of Pickwickians, but as the Pickwickian syndrome does not automatically imply sleep apnea, the question of familial obesity must also be raised in any consideration of Pickwickians. Dr Guilleminault reported familial histories of heavy snoring, but no systematic studies have been done, and the epidemiology of the sleep apnea syndrome is nonexistent at this time. Similarly, few data have been collected on the incidence of sudden death in this population. At Stanford, from 150 sleep apneic patients of all types, five sudden, unexpected deaths during sleep have been reported. The Johns Hopkins study (McGregor et al) reported a statistical difference between the ages of death in the general population and the Pickwickian population, but a large-scale data collection has not yet been done.

Once the Diagnosis of Obstructive Apnea During Sleep Has Been Made, How and When Is the Decision To Perform a Tracheostomy Made?

No general guideline was obtained from this panel. As many patients were first seen or first correctly diagnosed by a sleep center, most of them were extremely sleepy. Daytime sleepiness was a documented life-threatening risk with multiple reports of automobile and work-related accidents. Not only extreme sleepiness but the occurrence of automatic behavior as well had markedly impaired their professional and social activities. It was agreed that marked social and professional disability due to sleepiness is one criterion for the decision for tracheostomy.

For the Stanford and Montefiore teams, the degree of cardiac abnormalities during sleep is a second factor. Dr Tilkian stressed, however, that to this time no tracheostomy has been recommended solely on the basis of arrhythmia. Each time major arrhythmia has been seen, disability also existed. Dr Weitzman mentioned being impressed by the fact that 50% of his obstructive sleep apneic patients had experienced myocardial infarction. He stressed that the cardiovascular risk in these patients must be weighed in the consideration of any therapeutic trial.

Sleep Apnea Syndromes, pages 353–355
© 1978 Alan R. Liss, Inc., 150 Fifth Avenue, New York, NY 10011

The degree of nocturnal oxygen desaturation and systemic and pulmonary arterial pressure increases may also be assessed in difficult borderline cases in the evaluation of possible cardiovascular risk. There was a consensus that obesity in itself was not an issue, but several investigators (Stanford, Montefiore, and Bologna teams) emphasized that patients had found it virtually impossible to lose weight before tracheostomy but had been successful in this endeavor, sometimes without a specific diet, following surgery.

While there were cases for whom all participants could agree on the course of clinical care, there was a grey zone of patients with intermittent apneas, mild to moderate clinical complaints (sometimes the complaint was raised only by the spouse), with some arrhythmias, and intermittent desaturation. For these patients therapeutic trials for varying numbers of months appeared acceptable to the majority of the panel.

On the problem of obesity, the question of whether it preceded or followed apnea was raised. Dr Guilleminault reported that heavy snoring is commonly acknowledged as the primary event, and Dr Lugaresi and Dr Coccagna agreed that there was a secondary progressive increase of weight. Apparently the increasing weight triggers a feedback loop which exacerbates the existing problem.

Referring to the problem of repetitive hypoxia, Dr Severinghaus questioned how long the body can stand being that hypoxic during sleep and if this repetitive nocturnal hypoxia can cause cerebral deterioration. Dr Weitzman reported two patients referred to the Montefiore Neurology Department not for sleepiness but because of progressive "dementia." Investigation revealed that the patients did not have significant degrees of organic dementia, but exhibited abnormal behavior related to severe sleepiness. This was reversed by tracheostomy.

Dr Guilleminault noted the confusion and changes of personality observed in several patients. Dr Severinghaus expressed puzzlement by the absence of long-term sequelae in view of the long histories of cerebral hypoxia. No objective information on the intellectual levels of these patients in earlier years is available. The Stanford group reported that approximately half of the children seen for a sleep apnea syndrome had some learning disability or slight mental retardation, and no great improvement was seen after treatment of the disorder.

Dr Weitzman addressed the issue of respiratory function in the aged and the possible relationship between snoring, possible apneic periods, and progressive intellectual deterioration in these older people. Most of the reported studies have been done on patients with a peak age of 42–45 years; it is possible that the two age extremes (children and the aged) are at higher risk for intellectual deterioration from hypoxia.

Should Chemoreceptor Testing During Sleep Be Done in These Patients?

Dr Severinghaus noted that the obstructive sleep apneic patients clearly have chemoreceptor responses which return them to a state wherein the airway opens

nd breathing resumes. The failure appears to be of the airway rather than of the
hemoreceptors. Some patients with very low oxygen saturation and marked
ypoventilation may have fringed chemoreceptor drives but, in the typical ob-
tructive patient group, this approach may not add much information. Dr Weil
uggested, however, that chemoreceptor testing may be of importance as some
sleep apneic patients have a notably abnormal tolerance to hypoxemia and/or
hypercapnia. The question was raised as to whether this slow response could be
related to cerebral hypoxia or to continuous sleep deprivation. The crux of these
investigations is whether there is a pharmacological approach to the diminution
or augmentation of these drives. Would acetazolamide, for example, stimulate
these patients?

The Workshop ended with the unanimous opinion that we should reconvene
in two years and again exchange our findings on the puzzling and intriguing
sleep apnea syndromes.

Appendix 2.
Polygraphic Aspects of Sleep Apnea

Wayne H Flagg and Stephen C Coburn

Polygraphic monitoring of respiratory status during sleep provides a definitive test for the presence of the sleep apnea syndrome. Subcategories of the syndrome, severity of nocturnal respiratory impairment, and disruption of normal sleep structure may all be appreciated from analysis of the polygraphic recording. Such monitoring of nocturnal respiration and related variables presents unique difficulties, requiring specialized equipment and techniques. Because correlations between covariants contribute significantly to the complete evaluation of patient status the successful simultaneous recording of all relevant parameters is necessary.

It is convenient to distinguish between polygraphic respiratory monitoring performed as an initial screening procedure, and the more intensive evaluations that may follow when the diagnosis of sleep apnea has been confirmed. For screening, diaphragmatic excursion and intercostal activity may be monitored indirectly by means of mercury capillary strain gauges attached to the patient's abdomen and thorax [1]. We have found it convenient to employ strain gauges of 7–10 cm in length, secured to the patient with surgical tape. The electrical interface between strain gauge and polygraph is simple (Fig 1A), and may be directly connected to the input of an AC preamplifier. (Model 7P5B AC preamplifier, Grass Instrument Company, Quincy, Massachusetts.) A qualitative measurement of airflow is provided by glass bead thermistors secured below the patient's nostrils and before the mouth; a simple interface to the polygraph is again employed (Fig 1B). Finally, the patient's arterial oxygen saturation is monitored by an ear oximeter (Waters Instruments, Inc, Rochester, Minnesota). The oximeter is coupled directly to the input of a polygraph DC preamplifier. It may, with care, be used for continuous monitoring during an all-night sleep recording.

Information obtained from the above measures is sufficient to indicate the presence or absence of sleep apnea, and also to distinguish in most cases among central, mixed, and upper airway (obstructive) sleep apnea. Desaturation, con-

Sleep Apnea Syndromes, pages 357–363
© 1978 Alan R. Liss, Inc., 150 Fifth Avenue, New York, NY 10011

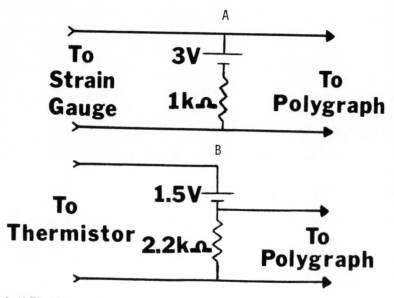

Fig 1. A) Electrical interface between strain gauge and polygraph. B) Electrical interface between thermistor and polygraph.

current with the apparent absence of respiratory effort as indicated by thoracic and abdominal strain gauges, is indicative of central sleep apnea. Cessation of airflow, accompanied by normal or increased respiratory effort, constitutes an upper airway (obstructive) apnea. Mixed apneic episodes may occur, and are so classified if the central component is of greater than ten-seconds duration. Establishment of both type and severity are often difficult and may indicate the need for further polygraphic monitoring.

A satisfactory estimation of the PaO_2 may be obtained from arterial blood oxygen saturation measurements. An instrument capable of adapting to baseline changes resulting from patient movement is essential in this context (Model 47201A ear oximeter, Hewlett-Packard, Waltham, Massachusetts). An appreciation of type may be obtained from measurement of endoesophageal pressure. This pressure may be determined by insertion of either an endoesophageal balloon or catheter-tip pressure transducer (Bio-Tec Instruments, Pasadena, California). Negative endoesophageal pressures occurring on inspiration possibly increasing in magnitude, with apparent absence of airflow, are definitive in establishing the presence of airway obstruction. Inspiration may be distinguished from expiration by monitoring percentage of CO_2 beneath the nose or below the mouth (Beckman Instruments, gas analyzer, Schiller Park, Illinois.) Polygraphically, a series of increasingly negative inspiratory esophageal pressures, following from and terminated by an interval during which the pressure variation with respiratory effort is consistent with waking values, constitutes the upper airway (obstructive) apneic cycle. In addition to the above respiratory parameters, the patient's arousal status must be monitored. Evaluation of the resulting record is difficult when significant pathology is present, particularly in the case of upper airway or mixed apnea. The EEG often indicates an arousal at termination of each apneic episode, and the cycle length of the episodes may be as short as 20 seconds, in which case no sleep may be scored by the Rechtschaffen-Kales (1968) sleep stage scoring criteria [2]. Moreover, much of the arousal time in a sleep apnea record is unscorable artifact, during which arousal status is unknown.

Problems arise in the definition of sleep stage transitions. The following modified rules are suggested to clarify the situation. An epoch following a clear stage 0 epoch, as judged by the standard rules, shall be scored stage 1, if it contains an interval scorable as stage 1 (by criteria other than duration), of greater duration than cumulative stage 0 contained on the same page (epoch). In other words, 50% of the scorable portion of an epoch (the nonartifact part) must meet the conventional criteria for stage 1. Stage 1 is continued through any arousal artifact that is not followed by clear stage 0, until the first sleep spindle, K complex, or rapid eye movement. If the sleep spindle or K complex occurs before 50% of the scorable portion of the epoch on which it occurs, that epoch is scored stage 2. Otherwise, it is scored the same as the preceding epoch, and the succeeding epoch is scored stage 2 unless there is an intervening arousal resulting in transition stage 0. Stage 2 is continued through any arousals not followed by transition stage 0. At the discretion of the scorer, stage 3—4 may not be scored, any epochs satisfying the conventional stage 3—4 criteria being regarded as continuations of stage 2. In a central apnea record containing minimal movement artifact, stage 3—4 may be scored according to the standard criteria. Stage REM following stage 2 is scored from the last sleep spindle or K complex preceding an interval containing a rapid eye movement not associated with an arousal or body movement, irrespective of intervening movement artifact. It continues until an interval of transitional stage 0 or stage 2 (defined the same as when following stage 1). Electromyogram (EMG) elevations from snoring or movement artifacts are ignored. A non-stage 2 epoch occurring between stage 0 (unambiguous or transitional) and an epoch containing an unambiguous rapid eye movement, when there is no intervening transitional stage 0, is scored stage 1 if the tonic EMG level (excluding snoring and movement associated increases) is greater than the tonic EMG level of the epoch on which the rapid eye movement occurs, or is scored stage REM if the tonic EMG level is less than or equal to that of the eye movement epoch. Transitional stage 0 is an interval of scorable record (ie, not obscured by artifact) that follows movement artifact or arousal that meets the conventional stage 0 criteria other than duration. Movement time is scored by conventional criteria. Body movements are not scored, and movement arousals are only considered when they satisfy the definition of transitional stage 0.

An appreciation of many of the cardiac abnormalities associated with the sleep apnea syndrome may be gained from continuous monitoring of the electrocardiogram (ECG) during sleep and wakefulness. A 24-hour continuous ECG recording is made, using a Holter monitor (Avionics, Irvine, California), and the data are computer-processed for comparison with the polygraphic record.

Further evaluation of hemodynamic status is obtained by simultaneous all-night monitoring of aortic and pulmonary arterial pressures, PaO_2, and the screening parameters. Any of the standard pressure transducers (eg, Model MP-15, Micron Instruments, Los Angeles, California) may be employed, coupled to optically isolated polygraph preamplifiers (Model 8805C pressure amplifier, Hewlett-Packard, Waltham, Massachusetts). For continuous all-night monitoring, a chart speed of 1–2.5 mm/sec is convenient. The pulmonary arterial pressure tracing is a significant aid in the evaluation of both severity and type of respiratory abnormality. A pressure tracing similar to that produced by an apneic episode of central type may be produced by voluntary cessation of respiration while awake. Baseline pressure data may be obtained by inclusion of an interval of wakefulness at the start of the polygraphic recording. Inclusion of a suitable monitoring electrode in the aortic arterial catheter permits continuous monitoring of arterial PaO_2 (multipurpose differential oxygen analyzer, Model 625-001, International Biophysics Corporation, Irvine, California). Simultaneous measurement of arterial pressures and PaO_2 permits an episode by episode evaluation of the sleep apnea syndrome.

Finally, the difficulties that arise in polygraphic monitoring should be mentioned. Both patient and equipment artifact may be expected to confuse and obscure the polygraphic record. Sway artifact in EEG and electrooculogram may be decreased by changing the polygraph amplifier band-pass characteristics. In many cases, especially where the patient is obese, it will prove difficult or impossible to eliminate ECG artifact from the EEG. Artifactual readings may be expected from the thermistor before the mouth due to head and/or mouth movement during a struggle for breath. Lastly, in some extremely obese patients, the presence of nearly continuous large body movements during sleep makes polygraphic monitoring and interpretation of any resulting records extremely challenging.

The placement of strain gauges is problematical, and position and orientation on the patient's thorax and abdomen must be chosen to optimize the recording. Care must also be taken that these devices remain securely attached. Both thermistors and a catheter for percentage CO_2 determination are easily dislodged by patient movements, resulting in erratic measurements.

Extreme care should be exercised that the arterial line associated with the PaO_2 measurement is flushed frequently. Clotting at the lumen of the arterial catheter results in erroneous pressure registration and misleading PaO_2 determinations. Flushing also helps to avoid lodging of the catheter against the arterial wall, with resulting erroneous measurements. The pulmonary arterial line is also subject to lodging against a vascular wall, falsifying pressure readings, and should be flushed frequently. The PaO_2 electrode is easily damaged by crimping, which will tend to result in fluid leakage. Finally, arterial pressure transducers should be located at the patient's chest height to avoid erroneous readings.

Figures 2–6 show examples of polygraphic recordings.

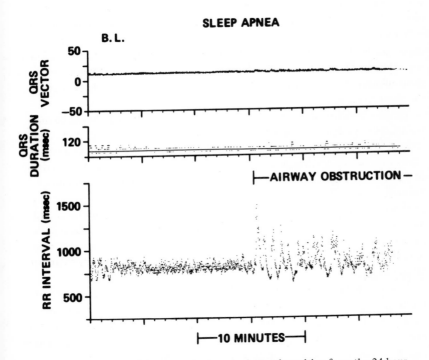

Fig 2. A typical segment of the computer-processed record resulting from the 24-hour Holter monitoring. Note cyclic sinus arrhythmia in the RR interval record, corresponding to an interval of upper airway sleep apnea.

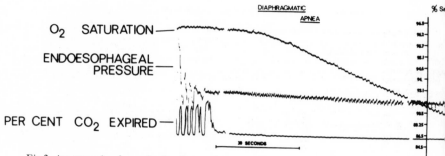

Fig 3. An example of an episode of central sleep apnea as represented by respiratory parameter monitoring in a noninvasive study. Oxygen saturation of arterial hemoglobin was determined by a Waters ear oximeter, the endoesophageal pressure from a Bio-Tec catheter-tip pressure transducer, and percentage CO_2 expired by a Beckman LB-1 gas analyzer.

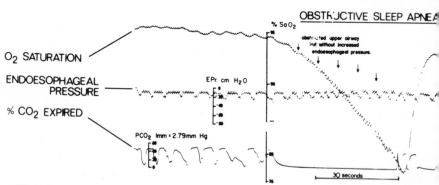

Fig 4. An example of an episode of upper airway sleep apnea as represented by respiratory parameter monitoring in a noninvasive study. The instrumentation was the same as in Figure 3.

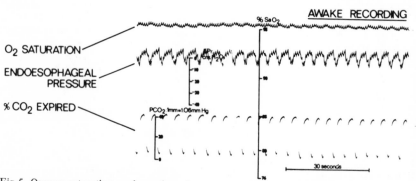

Fig 5. Oxygen saturation, endoesophageal pressure, and percentage CO_2 expired from a section of waking record obtained during a noninvasive screening recording. The instrumentation was the same as in Figures 3 and 4.

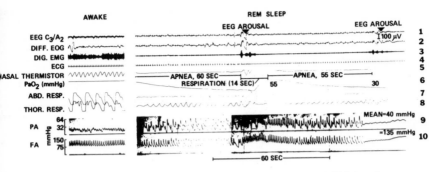

Fig 6. Examples of the polygraphic record obtained during waking and REM sleep in a complete hemodynamic monitoring, illustrating respiratory, arousal, and cardiac variables. Channels 9 and 10 were recorded on a separate polygraph and synchronized with channels 1 to 8 by means of a simultaneous time code (not shown). Channels 1 to 3 illustrate the electroencephalogram, electrooculogram, and electromyogram, respectively, from which the arousal state is determined. Channels 4, 9, and 10 represent the electrocardiogram, pulmonary, and femoral arterial pressures, respectively. Channels 5–8 illustrate airflow as determined by nasal thermistor, the arterial PaO_2, and the abdominal and thoracic strain gauge readings, respectively.

ACKNOWLEDGMENTS

This research was supported by National Institute of Neurological Diseases and Stroke grant NS 10727 and Public Health Service Research Grant RR-70 from the General Clinical Research Centers, Division of Research Resources.

REFERENCES

1. Shapiro A, Cohen HD: The use of mercury capillary length gauges for the measurement of the volume of thoracic and diaphragmatic components of human respiration: A theoretical analysis and a practical method. Trans NY Acad Sci 27:634–649, 1965.
2. Rechtschaffen A, Kales A: "A Manual of Standardized Terminology, Techniques, and Scoring for Sleep Stages of Human Subjects." Los Angeles: BIS/BRI, 1968.

Index

Abdominal muscle activity, 93, 95–
    97, 102, 104, 107, 112
Abnormal behavior during sleep, 3
Acetazolamide, 120, 122, 127, 355
Acidosis, blood, 138, 139, 321
Acidosis, respiratory, 7, 9, 179,
    182, 189, 312
Acromegaly, 10, 34, 37
Active sleep (*see also* Rapid eye
    movement sleep), 93, 96, 97,
    100, 101, 107, 108, 111, 113
Adductor activity, 80, 81
Afferent respiratory mechanism,
    47, 284
Airflow rates, 48, 301
Airway occlusion (*see also* Upper
    airway obstruction), 207, 211–
    217, 225, 226
Alkalosis, 56, 57, 59, 62, 120, 121,
    129, 132
Altered state of consciousness (*see
    also* Vigilance, level of), 24
Alveolar hypoventilation, 7, 13,
    44, 161, 262, 265, 289, 295,
    306, 333–345
Alveolar oxygen (partial) pressure,
    121
Aminophylline, 8
Amnesia (*see also* Memory deterior-
    ation), 25
Amphetamine, 267
Anatomic malformation, 15, 21,
    271
Anesthesia, 62, 73, 155, 219, 261,
    273, 348
Angiotensin, 319
Anxiety, 4, 37, 274, 345
Apnea (*see also* Obstructive,
    Central, Mixed sleep apnea),
    55, 56, 59, 60, 81, 112, 122,
    225, 235, 259, 264
Apnea Index, 2, 5, 6, 9, 10, 42,
    178, 299, 306, 311, 319, 323
Apneas, trains of, 153, 154

Apneusis, 62, 278, 282, 284, 286,
    287, 292
Arnold-Chiari syndrome, 280, 283,
    284
Arousal, 49, 51, 52, 60, 66, 100,
    106, 119, 124, 129, 141, 165,
    172, 188, 192, 216, 226, 244,
    359
Arrhythmias (*see also* Sinus arrhyth-
    mias), 188, 197–210, 235,
    242, 249
Arterial carbon dioxide (partial)
    pressure, 121, 127, 130,
    131, 136, 138, 267, 306, 310
Arterial pressure (*see also* Blood
    pressure), 178, 189, 263,
    266, 269, 318
Arterial Oxygen (partial) pressure,
    44, 121, 130, 186, 188,
    244, 267, 299, 305, 306, 310,
    319, 358
Artifact, 360
Asphyxia, vulnerability to, 93, 98,
    103, 111
Asystole, 202, 206, 349
Atelectasis, 132, 350
Atonia (*see also* Muscle tone), 230–
    232, 249, 252
Atrial fibrillation, 205
Atrioventricular block, 200, 205
Atropine, 182, 186, 197, 200, 202,
    205, 206, 319
Automatic behavior, 4, 24, 353
Automatic respiratory control sys-
    tem, 47, 58, 60
Automobile accidents, 4, 25
Autonomic insufficiency (*see also*
    Shy-Drager syndrome), 182
    317,
Autonomic nervous system, 199, 319
Autopsy, 7, 110, 199

Babies (*see also* Infants; Newborn),
    93, 101–113